Thematic Collections
in Biomedical Research

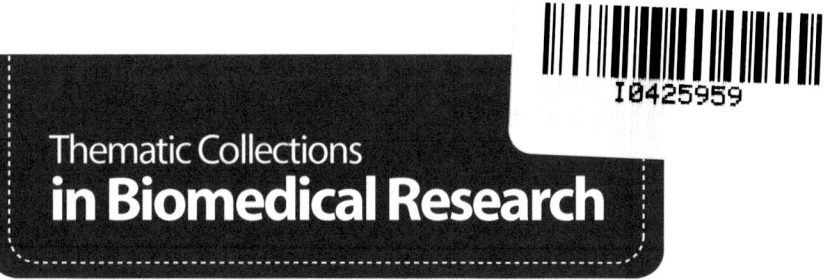
Biochemical biomarkers *in* Alzheimer's disease.

Dr. Samuel Barrack

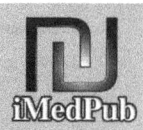

Title: *Biochemical biomarkers
in Alzheimer's disease*

Autor: Samuel Barrack

ISBN-13: 978-1-49227-446-9
ISBN-10: 1492274461

Cover design and Layout: design@imedpub.com

Maquetación: David Márquez
david.maquetacion@gmail.com

Publisher: Internet Medical Publishing
info@imedpub.com
http://imedpub.com/

First edition: 2013

Preface for Biomarkers for Alzheimer's disease

In view of the growing prevalence of AD worldwide, there is an urgent need for the development of better diagnostic tools and more effective therapeutic interventions. Indeed, much work in this field has been done during last decades. As such, a major goal of current clinical research in AD is to improve early detection of disease and presymptomatic detection of neuronal dysfunction, concurrently with the development of better tools to assess disease progression in this group of disorders. All these putative correlates are commonly referred to as AD-related biomarkers. The ideal biomarker should be easy to quantify and measure, reproducible, not subject to wide variation in the general population and unaffected by co-morbid factors. For evaluation of therapies, a biomarker needs to change linearly with disease progression and closely correlate with established clinico-pathological parameters of the disease.

There is growing evidence that the use of biomarkers will increase our ability to better indentify the underlying biology of AD, especially in its early stages. These biomarkers will improve the detection of the patients suitable for research studies and drug trials, and they will contribute to a better management of the disease in the clinical practice. Indeed, much work in this field has been done during last decades. The vast number of important applications, combined with the untamed diversity of already identified biomarkers, show that there is a pressing need to structure the research made on AD biomarkers into a solid, comprehensive and easy to use tool to de deployed in clinical settings.

To date there are few publications compiling results on this topic. That is why when I was asked to address this task I accepted inmediately. I am happy to present you a bundle of the best articles published about biomarkers for Alzheimer's disease in recent times.

Signed
Dr Samuel Barrack

Contents

1

Cerebrospinal Fluid PKR Level Predicts Cognitive Decline in Alzheimer's Disease

Julien Dumurgier[1,2,9], Francois Mouton-Liger[2,9], Pauline Lapalus[1], Magali Prevot[1], Jean-Louis Laplanche[3], Jacques Hugon[1,2*,9], Claire Paquet[1,2,9], for the Groupe d'Investigation du Liquide Cephalorachidien (GIL) Study Network

1 Clinical and Research Memory Center, Paris Nord Ile de France Saint Louis Lariboisière Fernand Hospital, AP-HP, University of Paris Diderot, Paris, France, 2 Institut du Fer à Moulin, Inserm UMR-S 839, Paris, France, 3 Department of Biochemistry Saint Louis Lariboisière Fernand Hospital, AP-HP, University of Paris Diderot, Paris, France

Abstract

The cerebrospinal fluid (CSF) levels of the proapoptotic kinase R (PKR) and its phosphorylated PKR (pPKR) are increased in Alzheimer's disease (AD), but whether CSF PKR concentrations are associated with cognitive decline in AD patients remain unknown. In this study, 41 consecutive patients with AD and 11 patients with amnestic mild cognitive impairment (aMCI) from our Memory Clinic were included. A lumbar puncture was performed during the following month of the clinical diagnosis and Mini-Mental State Examination (MMSE) evaluations were repeated every 6 months during a mean follow-up of 2 years. In AD patients, linear mixed models adjusted for age and sex were used to assess the cross-sectional and longitudinal associations between MMSE scores and baseline CSF levels of Aβ peptide (Aβ 1-42), Tau, phosphorylated Tau (p-Tau 181), PKR and pPKR. The mean (SD) MMSE at baseline was 20.5 (6.1) and MMSE scores declined over the follow-up (-0.12 point/month, standard error [SE] = 0.03). A lower MMSE at baseline was associated with lower levels of CSF Aβ 1–42 and p-Tau 181/Tau ratio. pPKR level was associated with longitudinal MMSE changes over the follow-up, higher pPKR levels being related with an exacerbated cognitive deterioration. Other CSF biomarkers were not associated with MMSE changes over time. In aMCI patients, mean CSF biomarker levels were not different in patients who converted to AD from those who did not convert. These results suggest that at the time of AD diagnosis, a higher level of CSF pPKR can predict a faster rate of cognitive decline.

Citation: Dumurgier J, Mouton-Liger F, Lapalus P, Prevot M, Laplanche J-L, et al. (2013) Cerebrospinal Fluid PKR Level Predicts Cognitive Decline in Alzheimer's Disease. PLoS ONE 8(1): e53587. doi:10.1371/journal.pone.0053587

Editor: Kewei Chen, Banner Alzheimer's Institute, United States of America

Received July 23, 2012; **Accepted** December 3, 2012; **Published** January 8, 2013

Funding: This study was supported by Assistance publique hopitaux de Paris and Inserm. The funders had no role in study design, data collection and analysis, decision to publish, or preparation of the manuscript.

Competing Interests: The authors have declared that no competing interests exist.

* E-mail: jacques.hugon@lrb.aphp.fr

⑨ These authors equally contributed to the work.

Introduction

Alzheimer's disease (AD) is classically marked by the progressive occurrence of memory disturbances followed by aphasia, apraxia and agnosia associated with behavioral symptoms [1]. It is difficult to predict clinically the rate of cognitive decline in affected patients [2]. The brain lesions in AD are characterized by senile plaques made of extracellular accumulated Aβ peptides, neurofibrillary tangles formed by hyperphorylated tau protein and synaptic and neuronal losses [3]. Over the past several years, the analysis of cerebrospinal fluid (CSF) biomarkers such as Aβ 1-42, Tau and phosphorylated Tau (p-Tau 181) has improved the accuracy of the clinical diagnosis, even at the early phase of the disease [4]. These CSF biomarkers reflect the magnitude of neuropathological lesions detected in AD brains [5,6]. Several cofounding factors, such as vascular lesions [7] or the cognitive reserve [8] can influence the evolution of cognitive signs in AD and may delay or precipitate the early symptoms. So far, it has been very difficult to find out a reliable biological marker in the blood or in the CSF that could predict the slope of cognitive deterioration in affected patients. The double-stranded RNA dependent protein kinase (PKR) is a ubiquitous cellular kinase that controls protein synthesis by phosphorylating the eukaryotic initiation factor 2α. PKR also controls viral infection, inflammation and when activated by autophosphorylation is a major factor of cell death [9]. Activated PKR is increased in AD brains [10] and PKR activation via Aβ 1-42, can also lead to the phosphorylation of Tau protein and during oxidative stress can modify β –secretase 1 (BACE1) protein levels, one of the main enzyme implicated in the formation of Aβ peptides [10–12]. We have recently shown that the levels of phosphorylated PKR (pPKR) were increased in the CSF of patients with AD and amnestic mild cognitive impairment (aMCI) compared to neurological disease controls, and that pPKR levels correlate with p-Tau 181 levels in AD patients [13]. All these results can argue in favor of a possible role of PKR in AD pathophysiology.

The goal of the present study was to determine in a longitudinal cohort of AD and aMCI patients the possible links between the rate of cognitive decline and the initial levels of CSF biomarkers including PKR and pPKR. Our results show that CSF pPKR concentration can predict the future cognitive decline in AD patients.

Materials and Methods

Patients

41 consecutive patients with a diagnosis of AD have been recruited from our outpatient Memory Clinic between January 2010 and January 2011, as previously described [13]. AD diagnosis was made according to NINCDS-ADRDA criteria [14] and was performed by a team of neurologists and neuropsychologists specialized in cognitive disorders. All patients were treated by cholinesterase inhibitors and/or by memantin when appropriate. Every 6 months, patients underwent neurological exams and neuropsychological assessments including a Mini-Mental State Examination (MMSE) evaluation. In addition, we also included 11 aMCI patients from our initial discovery cohort and we established the number of MCI patients who converted to AD at the end of the follow-up survey (June 2012), according to the NINCDS-ADRDA criteria [14].

This work has been approved by the Ethics Committee of Paris University Hospital (Bichat Hospital) and all patients or caregivers gave their written informed consent for this study. Next of kin, care takers or guardians consented on the behalf of participants whose capacity to consent was compromised. Usually, patients with mild AD forms signed the consent, for moderate AD forms patients and care givers signed the consent and in severe AD forms care takers signed the consent.

CSF Procedures

Lumbar punctures were performed in fasting patients in the following month after the clinical diagnosis. CSF was collected in 12 mL polypropylene tubes. Within 2 hours, CSF samples were centrifuged at 1800 g for 10 minutes at 4°C. An appropriate part of CSF was used for routine analysis, including total cell count, bacteriologic exam, and total protein and glucose levels. CSF was aliquoted in polypropylene tubes of 500 μL and stored at −80°C until further analysis. CSF Aβ 1-42, Tau, and p-Tau 181 were measured with Innotest sandwich enzyme-linked immunosorbent assay (ELISA) according to manufacturer's procedures (Innogenetics, Ghent, Belgium). Positivity criteria for biomarkers were defined by anomalies of Aß and T-tau or p181tau levels, according to the cutoffs of our center (Aß<500 pg/mL; T-tau>300 pg/mL; p181tau>65 pg/mL). PKR and pPKR CSF levels were analyzed by western blots procedures as previously reported (13). Results of PKR and pPKR are expressed in optical density units (ODU). All biological analyses were done in a single hospital laboratory. The biological team involved in the CSF analysis was unaware of the clinical diagnosis. The quality of CSF evaluations was validated by a European Consortium (Alzheimer's Association Quality Control [QC] Program for CSF Biomarkers).

Statistical Analysis

Linear mixed models were used to study the relationship between baseline levels of CSF biomarkers and repeated measurements of MMSE scores. The intercept and the slope (time) of the models were treated as random effects, allowing them to vary between individuals, with an unstructured covariance matrix. Time in months since baseline was included as a continuous linear term after verification that a quadratic term did not provide a better fit. We used z-scores to estimate standardized regression coefficients β that allow comparing the strength of the relations between MMSE and the different biomarkers. Models included one of the CSF biomarkers, age, sex, time and the interaction between time and the different parameters. Results were also shown using tertiles of patients according to CSF pPKR at baseline. In a complementary analysis, 11 patients with amnestic MCI, coming from our previously reported cohort [13], were assessed for conversion. These patients were categorized into two groups; those who have converted to AD (converters) or those who have not converted (non-converters) at the end of the follow-up period. Mean levels of the various CSF biomarkers between these 2 groups were compared using Kruskal-Wallis non parametric analysis.

P-values were two-tailed and values ≤0.05 considered as statistically significant. Analyses were performed using SAS 9.2 (SAS Institute, Cary, North Carolina, USA).

Results

Baseline characteristics of the study cohort are depicted in Table 1. Forty one AD patients were followed during a mean (SD) period of 25.7 (4.5) months. During this period, the mean (SD) number of MMSE evaluations was 4.5 (2.9) per patient. Their mean (SD) age was 69.9 (7.4) years, 61% of them were women, and their mean (SD) MMSE score was 20.5 (6.1).

Table 2 shows the results of age and sex adjusted linear mixed model estimates concerning the relationships between baseline CSF biomarkers and MMSE scores at baseline and during the follow-up survey. Lower levels of CSF Aβ 1-42 and p-Tau 181/Tau ratio were associated with lower baseline MMSE score, with standardized estimates β (SE) respectively equal to 2.5 (0.87) (p = 0.007) and 2.0 (0.97) (p = 0.048). In the longitudinal analysis, the mean (SE) decline of MMSE was −0.12 (0.03) point per month (p<0.001). Higher baseline level of CSF pPKR was associated with a more marked decline of MMSE over follow-up (β[SE] = −0.065 (0.032), p = 0.043). Other CSF biomarkers were not associated with MMSE change.

The Figure 1 illustrates the evolution of MMSE scores according to tertiles of CSF pPKR at baseline. Patients in the higher tertile (pPKR>100 optical density units) tended to have an exacerbated decline of MMSE compared to those in the lower tertile (pPKR<65 ODU) (p = 0.09).

Table 3 presents the results of mean biomarker levels in the 2 groups of aMCI patients. Their mean (SD) age was 76.9 (10.5) years, 7 were women, their mean (SD) MMSE was 24.1. Seven of them converted to AD, 4 were non-converters. None of these CSF biomarker reached statistical significance, however, CSF total

Table 1. Baseline characteristics of the study sample.

Characteristics	AD patients, n = 41
Age, years, mean (SD)	69.9 (7.4)
Women, n (%)	25 (61)
MMSE, mean (SD)	20.5 (6.1)
CSF biomarkers, pg/mL, mean (SD)	
Aβ 1-42	423.4 (152.2)
Tau	597.7 (340.2)
p-Tau 181	108.1 (54.3)
p-Tau 181/Tau ratio	0.20 (0.04)
CSF PKR, ODU, mean (SD)	
T-PKR	62.8 (19.3)
pPKR	88.5 (36.0)
Follow-up, months, mean (SD)	25.7 (4.5)
Number of MMSE evaluations, mean (SD)	4.5 (2.9)

doi:10.1371/journal.pone.0053587.t001

3

Table 2. General linear mixed models estimates of the relationship between baseline CSF biomarkers and MMSE score at baseline and over follow-up.

CSF biomarkers	Estimate (SE)[a]	P[a]
MMSE score at baseline		
Intercept	20.9 (1.1)	<0.001
Aβ 1-42	2.5 (0.87)	0.007
Tau	0.067 (0.96)	0.95
p-Tau 181	0.55 (0.81)	0.50
p-Tau 181/Tau ratio	2.0 (0.97)	0.048
T-PKR	−0.73 (0.96)	0.45
pPKR	−0.83 (0.89)	0.35
Change in MMSE over the follow-up		
Time (in month)	−0.122 (0.032)	<0.001
Aβ 1-42×Time	0.002 (0.033)	0.94
Tau×Time	−0.037 (0.037)	0.32
p-Tau 181×Time	−0.042 (0.041)	0.30
p-Tau 181/Tau ratio	0.007 (0.035)	0.84
T-PKR×Time	−0.009 (0.037)	0.81
pPKR×Time	−0.065 (0.032)	0.043

[a]Standardized estimates with their standard error (SE) computerized from mixed models adjusted for age, sex, CSF biomarker, and their interactions with time (one model per biomarker).
doi:10.1371/journal.pone.0053587.t002

PKR was the most discrimant biomarker between the 2 groups (converters, mean [SD] T-PKR = 94.8[37.6], non converters, mean [SD] T-PKR = 67.7[44.7], p = 0.09).

Discussion

Our results show that the level of CSF pPKR is associated with a more pronounced cognitive decline, as measured with the MMSE, in a cohort of patients newly diagnosed with AD. While CSF Aβ 1-42 levels and p-Tau 181/Tau ratio were cross-sectionally associated with MMSE score at the time of the diagnosis, pPKR was the only biomarker to be linked to the cognitive decline over the follow-up survey.

Several previous studies have reported an association between CSF biomarkers and cognitive change in AD, and results remain debated. In a previous study, one cluster of AD patients with extreme levels of CSF biomarkers were characterized by a faster progression of their cognitive deficit, no response to cholinesterase inhibitor treatment, and a higher mortality [15]. Another study using quintiles of patients found that CSF p-Tau 181/Tau ratio and Aβ 1-42 levels were associated with cognitive decline assessed by repeated MMSE, not with baseline MMSE [16]. CSF biomarkers have also been associated with longitudinal brain atrophy assessed by volumetric MRI [17–19]. Other potential CSF biomarkers of neuronal damage, such as Visinin-like protein-1, have also been linked to the rate of cognitive decline using terciles of patients [20,21].

In a previous study we have shown that CSF PKR and pPKR levels were increased in AD patients as compared to neurological disease controls [13]. The first question that can be addressed is why pPKR can predict the global cognitive decline in AD patients. As mentioned earlier, PKR, once activated, is a pro-apoptotic kinase that accumulates in degenerating neurons [22] and patients

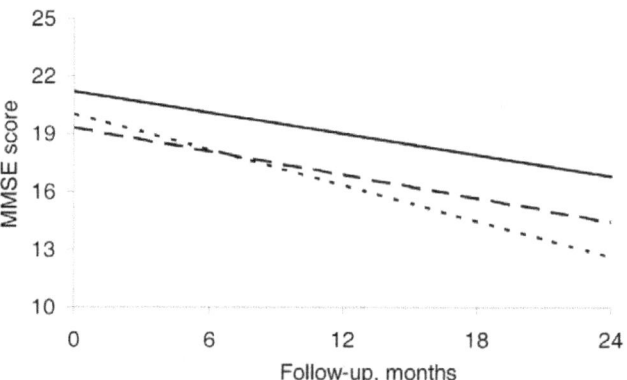

Figure 1. Predicted trajectories of MMSE score according to tertiles of CSF phosphorylated PKR. Mixed model is adjusted for age, sex, tertiles of CSF pPKR and their interactions with time in months. Solid line: lower tertile of pPKR (0–65 ODU), long-dashed sline: middle tertile of pPKR (65–100 ODU), short-dashed line : upper tertile of pPKR (>100 ODU). Cognitive decline is more pronounced in patients with high levels of CSF pPKR (short-dashed line).
doi:10.1371/journal.pone.0053587.g001

with very high CSF levels of pPKR could simply be affected by a more widespread neuronal death. Another factor that could contribute to exacerbated degradation of cognition is neuroinflammation. High levels of inflammatory cytokines with microglial activation have been detected in AD brains [23] and PKR is known to play a role in the production of pro-inflammatory cytokines through the induction of the transcription factor NKκB. [24] It is possible to assume that PKR, which is activated by Aβ [22], could contribute to the chronic over production of cytokines by immune competent cells such as microglia leading to detrimental consequences in neurons. A final factor that could explain our results is the relation between Tau phosphorylation and activated PKR [11]. The phosphorylation of PKR can indirectly lead to the phosphorylation of Tau protein and in turn could accentuate the toxic consequences of neurofibrillary tangles in affected neurons.

The second question that can be posed is to know if analyzing CSF pPKR levels could be useful at the onset of the clinical disease. Although classical biomarkers are very useful to predict the clinical outcome in patients with MCI [4], it appears that in demented patients, their usefulness to predict the cognitive decline in longitudinal surveys, is not well established. In addition, to dispose of a possible surrogate biomarker in clinical trials, might be a way to objectively assess the efficacy of a pharmacological approach. Further studies in other cohorts of patients will be necessary to confirm our findings and to establish the exact usefulness of the evaluation of CSF pPKR. Similarly, the assessment of CSF Aβ 1-42 and pPKR in preclinical AD might help to understand the relations between these two biomarkers with imaging studies [25].

There are some limitations in our study. Firstly, the number of patients included in our study remains limited. The lack of association between CSF biomarkers levels and conversion from MCI to AD we observed may be probably linked to the small number of MCI patients in our sample. A larger multicentric study including other types of dementia as well as MCI patients is needed to confirm the link between pPKR and the cognitive decline. Secondly, other indicators such as volumetric MRI or PET scan DFG glucose could also be compared with pPKR in future studies. Thirdly, the patients have been followed up during a mean period of time of 26 months. This is obviously limited and longer surveys are needed in order to detect exacerbated cognitive

Table 3. CSF biomarker levels in converters and non-converters MCI patients.

| CSF biomarkers | Patients with MCI | | | Statistic[a] | P-value[a] |
| | All | Converters | Non converters | | |
	(N = 11)	(N = 7)	(N = 4)		
Aβ 1-42, pg/mL, mean (SD)	608.7 (276.4)	657.7 (281.6)	523.0 (283.9)	1.76	0.18
Tau, pg/mL, mean (SD)	316.1 (124.2)	329.6 (45.0)	292.5 (214.9)	1.75	0.19
p-Tau 181 pg/mL mean (SD)	63.1 (18.8)	67.2 (14.3)	56.0 (25.8)	0.57	0.45
p-Tau 181/Tau ratio, mean (SD)	1.10 (0.37)	1.16 (0.36)	1.00 (0.43)	0.89	0.34
T-PKR, ODU, mean (SD)	75.3 (21.6)	82.2 (20.3)	63.3 (20.6)	2.89	0.09
pPKR, ODU, mean (SD)	84.9 (40.4)	94.8 (37.6)	67.7 (44.7)	1.75	0.19

[a]Kruskal-Wallis Test.
doi:10.1371/journal.pone.0053587.t003

decline. We did not include the neurological controls of our initial discovery cohort of patients because those patients were suffering from an heterogenous group of diseases with various clinical evolutions. In addition, apolipoprotein E genotyping should be performed in future studies to determine a possible influence of ApoE4 genotype on pPKR and other biomarker CSF levels [26].

In conclusion, we report that pPKR is a biological indicator of the cognitive decline in AD patients that 1- could be utilized to complement the current CSF biomarkers, 2- could be used in future clinical trials, 3 - could represent a possible pharmacological target for future therapeutic approaches [27].

Acknowledgments

List of the Groupe d'Investigation du LCR (GIL) Network Members: Catherine Belin, M.D., Department of Neurology Centre Hospitalo-Universitaire (CHU) Avicenne Assistance Publique –Hôpitaux de Paris (APHP) Bobigny France; Lucie Cabrejo, M.D., Department of Neurology CHU Bichat APHP, Paris France; Hugues Chabriat, M.D., Department of Neurology CHU Lariboisière APHP Paris; Sarah Benisty, M.D., Memory Center CHU Lariboisière APHP Paris; Olivier Drunat, M.D., Department of Psycho Geriatrics CHU Bretonneau APHP Paris; Katell Peoch, Department of Biochemistry Lariboisière Hospital Paris; Sarah Gourmaud MS Inserm U 839 Paris.

Author Contributions

Conceived and designed the experiments: FML JLL JH CP. Performed the experiments: FML CP. Analyzed the data: JD JH. Contributed reagents/materials/analysis tools: PL MP JLL. Wrote the paper: JD FML JH CP.

References

1. Burns A, Iliffe S (2009) Alzheimer's disease. Bmj 338: b158.
2. Ito K, Ahadieh S, Corrigan B, French J, Fullerton T, et al. (2010) Disease progression meta-analysis model in Alzheimer's disease. Alzheimers Dement 6: 39–53.
3. Duyckaerts C, Delatour B, Potier MC (2009) Classification and basic pathology of Alzheimer disease. Acta Neuropathol 118: 5–36.
4. Blennow K, Hampel H, Weiner M, Zetterberg H (2010) Cerebrospinal fluid and plasma biomarkers in Alzheimer disease. Nat Rev Neurol 6: 131–144.
5. Tapiola T, Pirtila T, Mehta PD, Alafuzofff I, Lehtovirta M, et al. (2000) Relationship between apoE genotype and CSF beta-amyloid (1–42) and tau in patients with probable and definite Alzheimer's disease. Neurobiol Aging 21: 735–740.
6. Seppala TT, Nerg O, Koivisto AM, Rummukainen J, Puli L, et al. (2012) CSF biomarkers for Alzheimer disease correlate with cortical brain biopsy findings. Neurology 78: 1568–1575.
7. Chui HC, Zarow C, Mack WJ, Ellis WG, Zheng L, et al. (2006) Cognitive impact of subcortical vascular and Alzheimer's disease pathology. Ann Neurol 60: 677–687.
8. Dumurgier J, Paquet C, Benisty S, Kiffel C, Lidy C, et al. (2010) Inverse association between CSF Abeta 42 levels and years of education in mild form of Alzheimer's disease: the cognitive reserve theory. Neurobiol Dis 40: 456–459.
9. Garcia MA, Meurs EF, Esteban M (2007) The dsRNA protein kinase PKR: virus and cell control. Biochimie 89: 799–811.
10. Mouton-Liger F, Paquet C, Dumurgier J, Bouras C, Pradier L, et al. (2012) Oxidative stress increases BACE1 protein levels through activation of the PKR-eIF2alpha pathway. Biochim Biophys Acta 1822: 885–896.
11. Bose A, Mouton-Liger F, Paquet C, Mazot P, Vigny M, et al. (2011) Modulation of tau phosphorylation by the kinase PKR: implications in Alzheimer's disease. Brain Pathol 21: 189–200.
12. Ill-Raga G, Palomer E, Wozniak MA, Ramos-Fernandez E, Bosch-Morato M, et al. (2011) Activation of PKR causes amyloid ss-peptide accumulation via de-repression of BACE1 expression. PLoS One 6: e21456.
13. Mouton-Liger F, Paquet C, Dumurgier J, Lapalus P, Gray F, et al. (2012) Increased Cerebrospinal Fluid Levels of Double-Stranded RNA-Dependant Protein Kinase in Alzheimer's Disease. Biol Psychiatry 71: 829–835.
14. McKhann GM, Knopman DS, Chertkow H, Hyman BT, Jack CR Jr, et al. (2011) The diagnosis of dementia due to Alzheimer's disease: recommendations from the National Institute on Aging-Alzheimer's Association workgroups on diagnostic guidelines for Alzheimer's disease. Alzheimers Dement 7: 263–269.
15. Wallin AK, Blennow K, Zetterberg H, Londos E, Minthon L, et al. (2010) CSF biomarkers predict a more malignant outcome in Alzheimer disease. Neurology 74: 1531–1537.
16. Kester MI, van der Vlies AE, Blankenstein MA, Pijnenburg YA, van Elk EJ, et al. (2009) CSF biomarkers predict rate of cognitive decline in Alzheimer disease. Neurology 73: 1353–1358.
17. Fjell AM, Walhovd KB, Fennema-Notestine C, McEvoy LK, Hagler DJ, et al. (2010) CSF biomarkers in prediction of cerebral and clinical change in mild cognitive impairment and Alzheimer's disease. J Neurosci 30: 2088–2101.
18. Wang L, Fagan AM, Shah AR, Beg MF, Csernansky JG, et al. (2011) Cerebrospinal Fluid Proteins Predict Longitudinal Hippocampal Degeneration in Early-stage Dementia of the Alzheimer Type. Alzheimer Dis Assoc Disord.
19. Henneman WJ, Vrenken H, Barnes J, Sluimer IC, Verwey NA, et al. (2009) Baseline CSF p-tau levels independently predict progression of hippocampal atrophy in Alzheimer disease. Neurology 73: 935–940.
20. Tarawneh R, D'Angelo G, Macy E, Xiong C, Carter D, et al. (2011) Visinin-like protein-1: diagnostic and prognostic biomarker in Alzheimer disease. Ann Neurol 70: 274–285.
21. Tarawneh R, Lee JM, Ladenson JH, Morris JC, Holtzman DM (2012) CSF VILIP-1 predicts rates of cognitive decline in early Alzheimer disease. Neurology 78: 709–719.
22. Chang RC, Suen KC, Ma CH, Elyaman W, Ng HK, et al. (2002) Involvement of double-stranded RNA-dependent protein kinase and phosphorylation of eukaryotic initiation factor-2alpha in neuronal degeneration. J Neurochem 83: 1215–1225.
23. Perry VH, Nicoll JA, Holmes C (2010) Microglia in neurodegenerative disease. Nat Rev Neurol 6: 193–201.
24. Zamanian-Daryoush M, Mogensen TH, DiDonato JA, Williams BR (2000) NF-kappaB activation by double-stranded-RNA-activated protein kinase (PKR) is mediated through NF-kappaB-inducing kinase and IkappaB kinase. Mol Cell Biol 20: 1278–1290.

25. Jack CR Jr, Knopman DS, Weigand SD, Wiste HJ, Vemuri P, et al. (2012) An operational approach to National Institute on Aging-Alzheimer's Association criteria for preclinical Alzheimer disease. Ann Neurol 71: 765–775.

26. Vemuri P, Wiste HJ, Weigand SD, Knopman DS, Shaw LM, et al. (2010) Effect of apolipoprotein E on biomarkers of amyloid load and neuronal pathology in Alzheimer disease. Ann Neurol 67: 308–316.

27. Hugon J, Paquet C, Chang RC (2009) Could PKR inhibition modulate human neurodegeneration? Expert Rev Neurother 9: 1455–1457.

Longitudinal Study of CSF Biomarkers in Patients with Alzheimer's Disease

Peder Buchhave[1,2], Kaj Blennow[3,4], Henrik Zetterberg[3,4], Erik Stomrud[1,2], Elisabet Londos[1,2], Niels Andreasen[5], Lennart Minthon[1,2], Oskar Hansson[1,2]*

1 Clinical Memory Research Unit, Department of Clinical Sciences Malmö, Lund University, Lund, Sweden, 2 Neuropsychiatric Clinic, Malmö University Hospital, Malmö, Sweden, 3 Institute of Neuroscience and Physiology, Department of Neurochemistry and Psychiatry, Sahlgrenska University Hospital, Göteborg University, Göteborg, Sweden, 4 Institute of Biomedicine, Department of Clinical Chemistry and Transfusion Medicine, Sahlgrenska University Hospital, Göteborg University, Göteborg, Sweden, 5 Karolinska Institutet, Department of Neurobiology, Caring Sciences and Society, Stockholm, Sweden

Abstract

Background: The CSF biomarkers tau and Aβ42 can identify patients with AD, even during the preclinical stages. However, previous studies on longitudinal changes of tau and Aβ42 in individual patients with AD and elderly controls report somewhat inconsistent results.

Methodology/Principal Findings: We investigated the levels of tau and Aβ42 at baseline and after 1 year in 100 patients with AD. In a second cohort of 45 AD patients we measured the CSF biomarkers at baseline and after 2 years. Moreover, in 34 healthy elderly controls the CSF biomarkers were followed for 4 years. The baseline levels of tau were increased with >60% in AD patients compared to controls ($p < 0.001$), while baseline Aβ42 levels were decreased with >50% ($p < 0.001$). In the AD group followed for 2 years, tau increased with 16% compared to the baseline levels ($p < 0.05$). However, the levels of tau were stable over 4 years in the controls. The levels of Aβ42 did not change significantly over time in any of the groups. In the patients with AD, tau was moderately associated with worse cognitive performance already at baseline ($p < 0.05$).

Conclusions/Significance: Tau and Aβ42 in CSF seem to reflect the underlying disease state in both early and late stages of AD. The slight increase in tau over time observed in the patients with AD is modest when compared to the relatively large difference in absolute tau levels between AD patients and controls. Therefore, these markers maintain their usefulness as state markers over time and might serve as surrogate markers for treatment efficacy in clinical trials.

Citation: Buchhave P, Blennow K, Zetterberg H, Stomrud E, Londos E, et al. (2009) Longitudinal Study of CSF Biomarkers in Patients with Alzheimer's Disease. PLoS ONE 4(7): e6294. doi:10.1371/journal.pone.0006294

Editor: Peter Heutink, VU University Medical Center and Center for Neurogenomics and Cognitive Research – VU University, the Netherlands

Received April 15, 2009; **Accepted** June 16, 2009; **Published** July 17, 2009

Funding: This work was supported by the Swedish Alzheimer foundation, Lund, Sweden; the Segerfalk Foundation; Stiftelsen Gamla Tjänarinnor; the Swedish Research Council (http://www.vr.se/2.69f66a93108e85f68d480000.html); Skane county council's research and development foundation; The Swedish Foundations of the National Board of Health and Welfare (http://www.socialstyrelsen.se/en/) and the Åke Wiberg Foundation. The funders had no role in study design, data collection and analysis, decision to publish, or preparation of the manuscript.

Competing Interests: The authors have declared that no competing interests exist.

* E-mail: oskar.hansson@med.lu.se

Introduction

Dementia is a growing health-economic issue worldwide. Alzheimer's disease (AD) accounts for most cases of dementia. The onset of AD is insidious. The molecular pathology probably starts 10–20 years before that patients with AD develop any symptoms. The major pathological features in the brains of AD patients are senile plaques, containing β-amyloid (Aβ), and neurofibrillary tangles with tau protein[1].

As novel therapies with possible disease-modifying effects are under development, there is an urgent need for surrogate markers to measure the potential biochemical effects of such therapies. Cerebrospinal fluid (CSF) tau and Aβ42 reflect the underlying disease state and might serve as such surrogate markers[2]. However, for this purpose, the intra-individual variation of the biomarker levels over time needs to be relatively small in order to identify treatment effects.

CSF biomarkers might also be used in the diagnostic work up of symptomatic AD patients, since the levels of tau are typically increased, while the levels of Aβ42 are decreased[2]. These biomarkers can also predict progression to AD in subjects suffering from mild cognitive impairment (MCI) with relatively high accuracy[3,4,5]. There is evidence of changes of CSF tau and Aβ42 in the even earlier, pre-symptomatic phase of the AD[6,7]. In conclusion, the CSF levels of tau and Aβ42 seem to be substantially altered very early in the disease process of AD. Numerous studies show that in groups of AD patients there is no strong correlation between the severity of the disease stage and the levels of tau and Aβ42, indicating that the levels of the CSF biomarkers do not change substantially over time in symptomatic AD patients[2]. However, previous longitudinal studies of the levels of tau in patients with AD show somewhat conflicting results[8,9,10,11,12,13,14,15]. Some studies have shown that the levels of CSF tau are stable over time[9,10,12], while others have shown that tau levels are increased at follow-up[8,13]. The results of studies on the stability of Aβ42 in AD have also been inconsistent - some studies have found no change over time[10,11], while others have found longitudinal increments[8] or decrements[14]. Because of the previous inconsistent results we conducted a longitudinal study in two rather large cohorts of patients with AD. Lumbar puncture was performed at baseline and after 1 year in 100 AD patients, while lumbar puncture was performed at baseline and after 2 year in 45 AD patients. Moreover, 34 healthy elderly controls underwent lumbar puncture at baseline and after 4 years.

Methods

Subjects

The study sample was recruited at the memory disorder clinic, Malmö University Hospital, Sweden. At baseline, physicians specialized in cognitive disorders performed a thorough physical, neurological and psychiatric examination, as well as a clinical interview, of each patient. Computed tomography (CT) or magnetic resonance imaging (MRI) of the brain was done, as well as routine blood analyses and analysis of *APOE* genotype. The patients were also evaluated with cognitive tests, including Mini-mental State Examination (MMSE).

The patients with AD fulfilled the DSM-IIIR criteria of dementia[16] and the criteria of probable AD defined by NINCDS-ADRDA[17]. Their cognitive symptoms could not be explained by other pathology.

The recruited 119 AD patients had undergone lumbar puncture two times with an interval of 6–30 months. In 100 of these patients, the time from baseline to the second lumbar puncture was approximately one year (6–18 months) and they are subsequently called the one-year AD cohort. In 45 AD patients the interval between baseline and follow-up lumbar puncture was two years (18–30 months) and they are subsequently called the two-year AD cohort 2. In 26 of the AD patients there were follow-up lumbar punctures performed at both one and two years and they are included in both of the cohorts. All patients were during the follow-up period continuously tested with cognitive tests including MMSE.

For the age-matched control population the inclusion criteria were: (i) absence of memory complaints or any other cognitive symptoms, (ii) preservation of general cognitive functioning, and (iii) no active neurological or psychiatric disease. At baseline, 36 controls with MMSE scores over 27 were included. The controls were followed clinically and evaluated with MMSE after 4 years, in order to rule out development of cognitive decline. At follow-up, two patients exhibited significant cognitive dysfunction and were therefore excluded. The remaining 34 controls had MMSE scores ≥27 at follow-up. Lumbar puncture was performed at baseline and after 4 years (range 3.7–4.2).

Ethics Statement

All patients gave written informed consent to participate in the study. The study was conducted according to the provisions of the Helsinki Declaration and approved by the ethics committee of Lund University, Sweden.

Analyses of levels of tau and Aβ42

The CSF samples were collected by lumbar puncture. The first 12 mL of CSF was collected in a polypropylene tube, directly transported to the local laboratory for centrifugation at $2000 \times g$ at $+4°C$ for 10 min. The supernatant was pipetted off, gently mixed to avoid potential gradient effects, and aliquoted in 1 mL portions in polypropylene tubes that were stored at $-80°C$ pending biochemical analyses, without being thawed and re-frozen.

In the AD patients, CSF total tau (T-tau) concentration was determined using a sandwich ELISA (Innotest hTAU-Ag, Innogenetics, Gent, Belgium) specifically constructed to measure all tau isoforms irrespectively of phosphorylation status, as previously described[18]. CSF Aβ1-42 levels were determined using a sandwich ELISA (Innotest® ß- amyloid (1–42), Innogenetics, Gent, Belgium), specifically constructed to measure Aβ containing both the first and 42nd amino acid, as previously described[11]. In the 1-year AD cohort repeated measurement of CSF tau and CSF Aβ42 were done in 100 and 97 subjects, respectively. In the 2-year AD cohort repeated measurement of CSF tau and Aβ42 were done in 45 and 42 subjects, respectively.

In the cognitively normal controls, the concentrations of tau and Aβ42 in CSF was determined with xMAP technology using the INNO-BIA AlzBio3 kit (Innogenetics, Ghent, Belgium)[4]. Results from the Luminex xMAP system were converted to ELISA levels based on previously published conversion factors[19].

Statistical analyses

To compare continuous baseline data between the cohorts, non-parametric Kruskal-Wallis ANOVA was performed, followed by Mann-Whitney U-test. Pearson's x^2 test was used for dichotomous variables. Wilcoxon signed-rank test was used to compare baseline and follow-up data in the cohorts. Spearman's correlation coefficient was used for correlation analyses. The statistical analyses were accomplished with SPSS for Windows, version 16.0.

Results

Baseline CSF levels of tau and Aβ42

The baseline demographic variables of the two AD cohorts and the age-matched controls are given in table 1. Both the baseline CSF levels of tau in the 1-year AD cohort (693 ± 301 ng/l) and in the 2-year AD cohort (663 ± 308 ng/l) were significantly elevated with 61–68%, when compared to the baseline levels in the control group (412 ± 232 ng/l; $P < 0.001$) (table 2). In contrast, the baseline CSF levels of Aβ42 in the 1-year AD cohort (275 ± 103 ng/l) and in the 2-year AD cohort (288 ± 103 ng/l) were significantly reduced with 56–58%, when compared to the baseline levels in the control group (659 ± 179 ng/l; $P < 0.001$) (table 2). Furthermore, the above described alterations of tau and Aβ42 were highly significant both in AD patients with low and high scores on MMSE at baseline, when compared to the healthy controls (data not shown).

Longitudinal changes of the CSF levels of tau and Aβ42 in the AD patients

The levels of CSF tau were non-significantly higher at follow-up compared to the baseline levels in the 1-year AD cohort ($P > 0.05$; table 2, figure 1). Also the levels of CSF Aβ42 were non-significantly higher at follow-up in this group ($P > 0.05$; table 2, figure 1). In the 2-year AD cohort, the levels of CSF tau were significantly increased with 15.8% at follow-up, when compared to the baseline levels ($p = 0.03$; table 2, figure 1). Furthermore, the CSF levels of Aβ42 were non-significantly increased at follow-up compared to baseline in this group ($P > 0.05$; table 2, figure 1).

Longitudinal changes of the CSF levels of tau and Aβ42 in the controls

At follow-up, the CSF levels of tau were slightly and non-significantly lower compared to the baseline levels (table 2, figure 1). A modest and non-significant decrease of Aβ42 was also observed during follow-up (table 2, figure 1).

Table 1. Demographic characteristics of the AD patients and the age-matched controls at baseline and follow-up.

	Controls, n = 34	1-year AD cohort, n = 100	2-year AD cohort, n = 45
Age, years	72±8.3	74±7.2	73±7.1
Sex, M/F	10/24	36/64	22/23
APOE ε4 carrier, %	26.5	67.7[a]	75.6[a]
Follow-up time, y	3.8±0.1	1.2±0.2	2.1±0.2
MMSE, baseline (0–30 p)	29.3±1.0	21.8±4.8[a]	23.4±4.4[a]
MMSE, follow-up (0–30 p)	28.7±1.2	20.4±5.6	20.2±6.9

Values are means±SD, except as noted otherwise.
[a]p<0.001 vs Controls.
Abbreviations: 1-year AD cohort, AD patients with approximately one year between baseline and follow-up lumbar puncture; 2-year AD cohort, AD patients with approximately two years between baseline and follow-up lumbar puncture; Controls, healthy controls followed for 4 years; APOE ε4 carrier, at least one apolipoprotein E ε4 allele; MMSE, Mini-Mental State Examination.
doi:10.1371/journal.pone.0006294.t001

Associations between the levels of tau and Aβ42 in CSF and cognitive performance

In the 1-year AD cohort, high levels of CSF tau at baseline, but not Aβ42, correlated moderately to poor baseline performance on the cognitive test MMSE ($r_s = -0.22$, p<0.05). In the 2-year AD cohort, similar correlations between the baseline levels of tau, but not Aβ42, and MMSE performance ($r_s = -0.40$, p<0.01) were found. However, baseline levels of tau or Aβ42 did not correlate with cognitive deterioration over time as measured with repeated MMSE during the clinical follow-up (p>0.05). Moreover, changes in tau or Aβ42 levels over time did not correlate with the rate of cognitive deterioration (p>0.05).

Discussion

We found that the baseline levels of CSF tau were increased with around 60% in AD patients compared to controls, while baseline CSF Aβ42 levels were decreased with more than 50%. In AD patients, tau increased with 16% over two years and CSF tau was moderately associated with worse cognitive performance already at baseline. However, the levels of tau were stable over 4 years in the controls. The levels of Aβ42 did not change significantly over time in any of the groups and did not correlate with baseline cognitive performance.

Biomarkers for neurodegenerative disorders can be divided into markers of disease state and markers of disease stage or rate[20].

Markers of disease state, usually called diagnostic biomarkers, facilitate detection of a certain biological disease in populations of individuals with similar symptoms (e.g. memory impairment) caused by different conditions. A disease state marker should ideally exhibit a high diagnostic accuracy over the entire course of the disease process. Both CSF tau and Aβ42 fulfill the requirements for disease state markers of AD, because these biomarkers exhibit reasonably high specificity and sensitivity for both early and late stages of AD[2]. The results of the present study suggest that CSF Aβ42 is not a marker of disease stage or rate, since the levels are stable over time in individual patients with AD and do not correlate with cognitive function. Similarly, previous studies show that the amyloid load in the brain of AD patients, as assessed with repeated positron emission tomography (PIB-PET) measurements, keeps stable over time despite cognitive decline[21]. It might be that Aβ42 levels in both the CSF and the brain are altered during the very early preclinical stages of AD and are thereafter relatively stable during the symptomatic course of the disease.

The present study suggests that tau levels in CSF increase slightly over time. In agreement, Stefani and collaborators have found that CSF tau levels are associated with the disease stage of AD[22], a finding supported by the moderate correlation between cognitive performance and CSF tau found in the present study. Therefore, it might be that CSF tau, in addition to being a robust disease state marker, to some degree reflects the disease stage.

Table 2. Baseline and follow-up levels of CSF tau and Aβ42 in the AD patients and age-matched controls.

	Controls, n = 34	1-year AD cohort, n = 100	2-year AD cohort, n = 45
Baseline Tau, ng/L	412±232	693±301[a]	663±308[a]
Follow-up Tau, ng/L	399±194	731±402	768±528[b]
Longitudinal difference, Tau, %	−3.2	+5.5	+15.8
Baseline Aβ42, ng/L	659±179	275±103[a]	288±103[a]
Follow-up Aβ42, ng/L	651±168	296±132	321±137
Longitudinal difference, Aβ42, %	−1.2	+7.6	+11.5

Values are means±SD except if noted otherwise.
[a]p<0.001 vs Controls.
[b]p<0.05 vs baseline.
Abbreviations: CSF, cerebrospinal fluid; 1-year AD cohort, subjects with Alzheimer's disease with an interval between baseline and follow-up lumbar puncture of approximately one year; 2-year AD cohort, subjects with Alzheimer's disease with an interval between baseline and follow-up lumbar puncture of approximately two years. Controls, healthy controls followed for 4 years.
doi:10.1371/journal.pone.0006294.t002

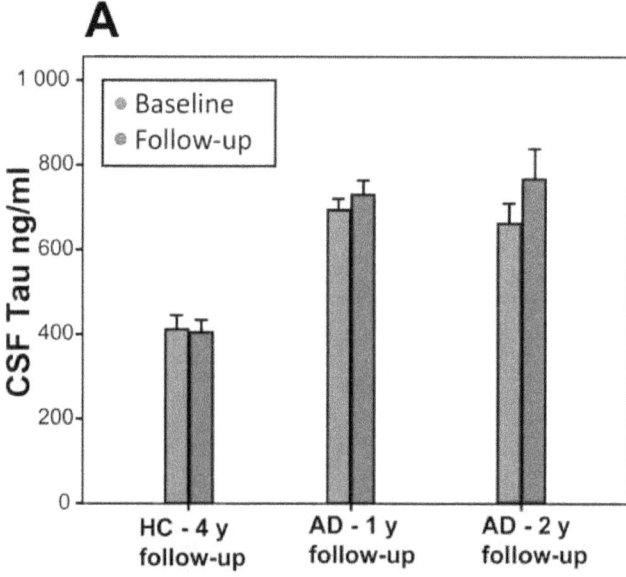

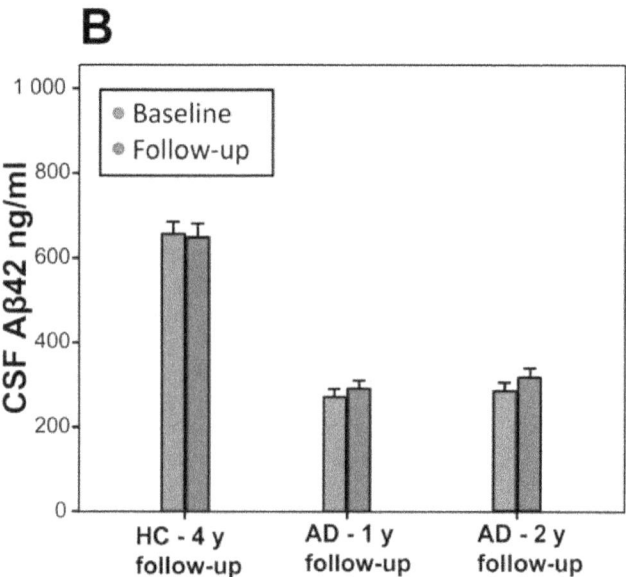

Figure 1. Longitudinal change of CSF tau and Aβ42. The figure shows the mean baseline and follow-up levels of CSF tau (panel A) and CSF Aβ42 (panel B) in healthy controls (HC), that were followed for 4 years (y), and in two cohorts of patients with Alzheimer's disease (AD) that were followed for one or two years, respectively. Error bars represent standard errors of the mean. The figure illustrates that differences between controls and AD patients by far surpass the within-group differences over time.
doi:10.1371/journal.pone.0006294.g001

These observations are supported by neuropathological studies showing that tau-containing neurofibrillary tangles, but not amyloid plaques, are associated with the cognitive function of AD patients[23]. However, other methods such as cognitive tests or measures of brain atrophy or cerebral blood flow are likely to prove to be more valuable as disease stage markers of AD[24,25,26], and CSF biomarkers should primarily be used as diagnostic markers detecting the underlying disease state[2]. Therefore, different methods should be combined when defining the disease state and stage of individual patients with cognitive dysfunction.

CSF biomarkers, such as tau and Aβ42, could possibly also be used as *surrogate markers* in clinical therapeutic AD trials. Surrogate biomarkers should be involved in the early pathophysiologic cascade and they ought to inform on biological interactions with the molecular target of the drug in humans [20]. Future disease-modifying therapies against AD may halt the degenerative process, but are not expected to have direct symptomatic effects. As a result no short-term cognitive improvements are expected in such trials. Therefore, large patient populations and extensive treatment periods will be required to identify treatment effects on clinical parameters. Data from smaller pilot investigations, using biomarkers as endpoint to determine whether a certain drug is reaching and acting on its biological target in patients with AD, would be very valuable when making a go/no-go decision for an expensive clinical trial with clinical improvement as the endpoint[2]. However, the markers used as surrogate markers in such trials must have a low intra-individual variation over time. The present study confirms previous investigations that the changes of CSF tau and Aβ42 is very modest over time in individual patients with AD[8,9,10,11,12,13,14], which might indicate that these CSF biomarkers may serve as sensitive tools to identify and monitor even minor biochemical changes induced by treatments that are directed against these targets, such as Aβ immunotherapy. For example, recently Lannfelt and colleagues found that PBT2 (a metal-protein attenuating compound) reduced the levels of Aβ42 in CSF, but not plasma, of patients with AD, indicating that the drug had a central effect on Aβ metabolism[27].

In conclusion, CSF tau and Aβ42 seem to reflect the underlying disease state in both early and late stages of AD. The slight increase in tau over time observed in patients with AD is modest when compared to the relatively large difference in absolute tau levels observed between AD patients and controls, indicating that tau and Aβ42 do not primarily reflect the progression of the disease over time. Therefore, these markers might serve as surrogate markers for treatment efficacy in clinical trials.

Author Contributions

Conceived and designed the experiments: PB KB HZ EL NA LM OH. Performed the experiments: KB HZ. Analyzed the data: PB OH. Contributed reagents/materials/analysis tools: KB HZ ES EL LM. Wrote the paper: PB.

References

1. Blennow K, de Leon MJ, Zetterberg H (2006) Alzheimer's disease. Lancet 368: 387–403.
2. Zetterberg H, Blennow K (2008) Biological CSF Markers of Alzheimer's Disease. Handb Clin Neurol 89: 261–268.
3. Hansson O, Zetterberg H, Buchhave P, Andreasson U, Londos E, et al. (2007) Prediction of Alzheimer's disease using the CSF Abeta42/Abeta40 ratio in patients with mild cognitive impairment. Dement Geriatr Cogn Disord 23: 316–320.
4. Hansson O, Zetterberg H, Buchhave P, Londos E, Blennow K, et al. (2006) Association between CSF biomarkers and incipient Alzheimer's disease in patients with mild cognitive impairment: a follow-up study. Lancet Neurol 5: 228–234.
5. Hampel H, Teipel SJ, Fuchsberger T, Andreasen N, Wiltfang J, et al. (2004) Value of CSF beta-amyloid1-42 and tau as predictors of Alzheimer's disease in patients with mild cognitive impairment. Mol Psychiatry 9: 705–710.

6. Fagan AM, Roe CM, Xiong C, Mintun MA, Morris JC, et al. (2007) Cerebrospinal fluid tau/beta-amyloid(42) ratio as a prediction of cognitive decline in nondemented older adults. Arch Neurol 64: 343–349.

7. Stomrud E, Hansson O, Blennow K, Minthon L, Londos E (2007) Cerebrospinal fluid biomarkers predict decline in subjective cognitive function over 3 years in healthy elderly. Dement Geriatr Cogn Disord 24: 118–124.

8. Bouwman FH, van der Flier WM, Schoonenboom NS, van Elk EJ, Kok A, et al. (2007) Longitudinal changes of CSF biomarkers in memory clinic patients. Neurology 69: 1006–1011.

9. Sunderland T, Wolozin B, Galasko D, Levy J, Dukoff R, et al. (1999) Longitudinal stability of CSF tau levels in Alzheimer patients. Biol Psychiatry 46: 750–755.

10. Blennow K, Zetterberg H, Minthon L, Lannfelt L, Strid S, et al. (2007) Longitudinal stability of CSF biomarkers in Alzheimer's disease. Neurosci Lett 419: 18–22.

11. Andreasen N, Hesse C, Davidsson P, Minthon L, Wallin A, et al. (1999) Cerebrospinal fluid beta-amyloid(1–42) in Alzheimer disease: differences between early- and late-onset Alzheimer disease and stability during the course of disease. Arch Neurol 56: 673–680.

12. Andreasen N, Minthon L, Clarberg A, Davidsson P, Gottfries J, et al. (1999) Sensitivity, specificity, and stability of CSF-tau in AD in a community-based patient sample. Neurology 53: 1488–1494.

13. Kanai M, Matsubara E, Isoe K, Urakami K, Nakashima K, et al. (1998) Longitudinal study of cerebrospinal fluid levels of tau, A beta1–40, and A beta1–42(43) in Alzheimer's disease: a study in Japan. Ann Neurol 44: 17–26.

14. Huey ED, Mirza N, Putnam KT, Soares H, Csako G, et al. (2006) Stability of CSF beta-amyloid(1–42) and APOE genotype in Alzheimer patients. Dement Geriatr Cogn Disord 22: 48–53.

15. Zetterberg H, Pedersen M, Lind K, Svensson M, Rolstad S, et al. (2007) Intra-individual stability of CSF biomarkers for Alzheimer's disease over two years. J Alzheimers Dis 12: 255–260.

16. association AP (1987) Diagnostic and Statistical Manual of Mental Disorders. Arlington, VA, USA: American Psychiatric Association.

17. McKhann G, Drachman D, Folstein M, Katzman R, Price D, et al. (1984) Clinical diagnosis of Alzheimer's disease: report of the NINCDS-ADRDA Work Group under the auspices of Department of Health and Human Services Task Force on Alzheimer's Disease. Neurology 34: 939–944.

18. Blennow K, Wallin A, Agren H, Spenger C, Siegfried J, et al. (1995) Tau protein in cerebrospinal fluid: a biochemical marker for axonal degeneration in Alzheimer disease? Mol Chem Neuropathol 26: 231–245.

19. Olsson A, Vanderstichele H, Andreasen N, De Meyer G, Wallin A, et al. (2005) Simultaneous measurement of beta-amyloid(1–42), total tau, and phosphorylated tau (Thr181) in cerebrospinal fluid by the xMAP technology. Clin Chem 51: 336–345.

20. Fox N, Growdon JH (2004) Biomarkers and surrogates. Neurorx 1: 181.

21. Engler H, Forsberg A, Almkvist O, Blomquist G, Larsson E, et al. (2006) Two-year follow-up of amyloid deposition in patients with Alzheimer's disease. Brain 129: 2856–2866.

22. Stefani A, Martorana A, Bernardini S, Panella M, Mercati F, et al. (2006) CSF markers in Alzheimer disease patients are not related to the different degree of cognitive impairment. J Neurol Sci 251: 124–128.

23. Giannakopoulos P, Herrmann FR, Bussiere T, Bouras C, Kovari E, et al. (2003) Tangle and neuron numbers, but not amyloid load, predict cognitive status in Alzheimer's disease. Neurology 60: 1495–1500.

24. Fleisher AS, Sowell BB, Taylor C, Gamst AC, Petersen RC, et al. (2007) Clinical predictors of progression to Alzheimer disease in amnestic mild cognitive impairment. Neurology 68: 1588–1595.

25. Jack CR Jr, Shiung MM, Gunter JL, O'Brien PC, Weigand SD, et al. (2004) Comparison of different MRI brain atrophy rate measures with clinical disease progression in AD. Neurology 62: 591–600.

26. Hansson O, Buchhave P, Zetterberg H, Blennow K, Minthon L, et al. (2007) Combined rCBF and CSF biomarkers predict progression from mild cognitive impairment to Alzheimer's disease. Neurobiol Aging 30: 165–170.

27. Lannfelt L, Blennow K, Zetterberg H, Batsman S, Ames D, et al. (2008) Safety, efficacy, and biomarker findings of PBT2 in targeting Abeta as a modifying therapy for Alzheimer's disease: a phase IIa, double-blind, randomised, placebo-controlled trial. Lancet Neurol 7: 779–786.

Increased Levels of Antigen-Bound β-Amyloid Autoantibodies in Serum and Cerebrospinal Fluid of Alzheimer's Disease Patients

Madalina Maftei[1,2,9], Franka Thurm[3,4,5,9], Cathrin Schnack[6], Hayrettin Tumani[6], Markus Otto[6], Thomas Elbert[3], Iris-Tatjana Kolassa[4,7]*, Michael Przybylski[1]*, Marilena Manea[1,7]*, Christine A. F. von Arnim[6]*

1 Laboratory of Analytical Chemistry and Biopolymer Structure Analysis, Department of Chemistry, University of Konstanz, Konstanz, Germany, 2 Steinbeis Research Center for Biopolymer Analysis, University of Konstanz, Konstanz, Germany, 3 Department of Psychology, University of Konstanz, Konstanz, Germany, 4 Clinical and Biological Psychology, Institute of Psychology and Education, University of Ulm, Ulm, Germany, 5 Department of Psychology, TU Dresden, Dresden, Germany, 6 Department of Neurology, University of Ulm, Ulm, Germany, 7 Zukunftskolleg, University of Konstanz, Konstanz, Germany

Abstract

Recent studies have suggested a protective role of physiological β-amyloid autoantibodies (Aβ-autoantibodies) in Alzheimer's disease (AD). However, the determination of both free and dissociated Aβ-autoantibodies in serum hitherto has yielded inconsistent results regarding their function and possible biomarker value. Here we report the application of a new sandwich enzyme-linked immunosorbent assay (ELISA) for the determination of antigen-bound Aβ-autoantibodies (intact Aβ-IgG immune complexes) in serum and cerebrospinal fluid (CSF) of a total number of 112 AD patients and age- and gender-matched control subjects. Both serum and CSF levels of Aβ-IgG immune complexes were found to be significantly higher in AD patients compared to control subjects. Moreover, the levels of Aβ-IgG complexes were negatively correlated with the cognitive status across the groups, increasing with declining cognitive test performance of the subjects. Our results suggest a contribution of IgG-type autoantibodies to Aβ clearance in vivo and an increased immune response in AD, which may be associated with deficient Aβ-IgG removal. These findings may contribute to elucidating the role of Aβ-autoantibodies in AD pathophysiology and their potential application in AD diagnosis.

Citation: Maftei M, Thurm F, Schnack C, Tumani H, Otto M, et al. (2013) Increased Levels of Antigen-Bound β-Amyloid Autoantibodies in Serum and Cerebrospinal Fluid of Alzheimer's Disease Patients. PLoS ONE 8(7): e68996. doi:10.1371/journal.pone.0068996

Editor: Christoph Kleinschnitz, Julius-Maximilians-Universität Würzburg, Germany

Received March 17, 2013; Accepted June 4, 2013; Published July 18, 2013

Funding: This research was funded as an interdisciplinary project within the WIN-Kolleg (Junior Academy for Young Scholars and Scientists) of the Heidelberg Academy of Sciences, Heidelberg, Germany, awarded to I.-T. Kolassa, M. Manea and C.A.F. von Arnim, by the Zukunftskolleg (I.-T. Kolassa, now alumna, and M. Manea) and Research Center Proteostasis (M. Przybylski), University of Konstanz. I.-T. Kolassa is now at the University of Ulm, F. Thurm is now at the TU Dresden. The funders had no role in study design, data collection and analysis, decision to publish, or preparation of the manuscript.

Competing Interests: The authors have declared that no competing interests exist.

* E-mail: marilena.manea@uni-konstanz.de (MM); iris.kolassa@uni-ulm.de (I-TK); christine.arnim@uni-ulm.de (CAFVA); michael.przybylski@uni-konstanz.de (MP)

⑨ These authors contributed equally to this work.

Introduction

Alzheimer's disease (AD) is the most prevalent form of dementia among the aging population. Its long preclinical phase and the lack of biomarkers that would allow an early diagnosis pose great challenges for the development of effective therapeutic approaches. The neuropathology of AD is characterized by the accumulation of intracellular neurofibrillary tangles and extracellular beta-amyloid (Aβ) plaques, associated with axonal, dendritic and synaptic degeneration [1–4]. Several species of aggregated Aβ, such as small oligomers, annular oligomers and fibrils, precede the formation of amyloid plaques in the AD brain. The small Aβ oligomers, consisting of 3–50 monomer units, appear to be the most neurotoxic species [5].

In transgenic mouse models of AD, both active immunization with full-length Aβ peptides or Aβ fragments [6–9] and passive immunization with monoclonal anti-Aβ-antibodies [10–12] were effective in preventing Aβ-aggregation, clearing amyloid plaques and improving cognitive performance. Based on the promising preclinical results, immunotherapy has been proposed as a possible therapeutic approach for AD [13,14]. A phase II multicenter clinical trial of active immunization with preaggregated Aβ42 (AN1792(QS-21) vaccine) showed a reduction of amyloid plaque burden and slower cognitive decline in AD patients. However, the trial was interrupted due to the occurrence of meningoencephalitis in some of the immunized participants [14,15]. A follow-up study of the AN1792 clinical trial with yearly assessments and post-mortem neuropathological examinations indicated progression of AD-related neurodegeneration and cognitive decline, despite vaccination [16]. Another study reporting the clinical effects of a phase IIa immunotherapeutic trial of AN1792 showed similar results, but also revealed a significantly higher score in one of the neuropsychological test batteries in antibody responders compared to the placebo group, suggesting that Aβ-immunotherapy may be useful for the treatment of AD [17]. Several clinical trials are carried out to further evaluate the therapeutic potential of Aβ-based active immunization and to assess the effect of passive immunization with anti-Aβ-antibodies in AD patients [18]. Two phase 3 clinical trials designed to evaluate the efficacy and safety of a humanized N-terminal anti-Aβ monoclonal antibody, Bapineuzumab, in patients with mild to moderate AD have recently been completed (http://clinicaltrials.gov). Results presented at the 16th EFNS congress in Stockholm showed that the treatment with Bapineuzumab did not reach clinical endpoints (no significant benefit on cognitive or functional performance); however, reduced CSF levels of phospho-tau were observed in the Bapineuzumab-treated group (http://www.stevenderoover.be/EFNS/Presentations/EFNS2012/WC220/; http://www.stevenderoover.be/EFNS/Presentations/EFNS2012/WC219/). Considering the difficulty to find an efficient treatment that would improve the cognitive functions of AD patients, a promising approach would be the administration of potential drugs (e.g., antibodies) at the earliest possible stage, before or just after the onset of AD symptoms, in order to prevent the disease progression [19].

Recently, physiological antibodies binding Aβ (Aβ-autoantibodies) have been detected in serum and CSF of AD patients and healthy individuals [20–24], as well as in intravenous immunoglobulin preparations (IVIg), which are fractionated blood products used for the treatment of immune deficiencies and other disorders [25]. Dodel et al. [26] reported that administration of Aβ-autoantibodies led to reduced plaque formation and improvement of behavior in a mouse model of AD. Moreover, in AD patients, promising effects on cognition were observed in small pilot trials involving passive immunization with IVIg [20,23,27]. These findings suggest that Aβ-autoantibodies might exert a protective function against AD and could play an important role in AD treatment.

In addition to their potential therapeutic applications for AD, the biomarker value of Aβ-autoantibodies was also investigated. Currently available data on the serum/plasma levels of Aβ-autoantibodies in AD patients compared to healthy individuals are controversial. Several groups found that the serum levels of free, non-antigen-bound Aβ-autoantibodies were lower in AD patients than in controls [28–30], while others reported either higher values [31] or no difference [32,33]. So far, there is only one reported study on the CSF levels of free Aβ-autoantibodies, showing decreased values in AD patients compared to control subjects [34]. Gustaw et al. [35] suggested that the presence of Aβ-autoantibodies not only in free, non-antigen-bound state, but also as preformed immune complexes with Aβ-peptides, may be a possible reason for these controversial results. Subsequent serum determinations of Aβ-autoantibodies after acidic dissociation of the Aβ-immune complexes indicated higher levels of Aβ-autoantibodies in AD patients compared to controls [35,36]. However, using a similar procedure, Klaver et al. [37] found no difference between the groups.

Based on the finding that Aβ-autoantibodies recognize the Aβ (21–37) epitope [38,39], unlike the antibodies produced by active immunization that bind the Aβ (4–10) epitope [40], we have recently developed a sandwich ELISA for the determination of intact Aβ-IgG immune complexes and applied it for the analysis of serum samples from healthy individuals aged 18 to 89 years. The serum levels of Aβ-IgG immune complexes were not correlated with age or cognitive performance of healthy adults [41]. To date, there are no other reports on the determination of Aβ-IgG immune complexes in serum or CSF by ELISA.

In the present study, we have employed the sandwich ELISA to determine the levels of Aβ-IgG immune complexes in both serum and CSF of AD patients and age- and gender-matched control subjects and evaluated their correlations with the neuropsychological performance and age of the study participants, as well as their diagnostic power.

Materials and Methods

Ethics Statement

This study was approved by the ethics committee of the University of Ulm, Germany, and conducted according to the guidelines outlined in the Declaration of Helsinki. Prior to participation, written informed consent was obtained.

Participants

Demographic data are depicted in Table 1. Altogether, 58 AD patients were recruited at the Memory Clinic of the Hospital for Neurology of the University of Ulm, Germany. Patients underwent a comprehensive clinical neurological examination, a routine blood analysis, structural imaging (MRI or CT), apolipoprotein E (APOE) genotyping and a detailed neuropsychological assessment, including the Mini Mental State Examination test (MMSE, range 0–30 points; [42]) and the Alzheimer's Disease Assessment Scale - Cognitive subscale (ADAS-Cog, range 0–70 errors; e.g., [43]). Probable AD was diagnosed according to NINCDS-ADRDA [44] and DSM-IV-TR criteria [45]. Furthermore, 54 unrelated age- and gender-matched control subjects were recruited at the same site and did not display any cognitive or neurological deficits following thorough clinical and neuropsychological examination.

Determination of Aβ42 and Total tau (T-tau) Levels in CSF

The collection of CSF samples by lumbar puncture and the pre-analytical processing were performed using a standardized protocol [46]. In brief, CSF samples were collected into polypropylene tubes, centrifuged immediately and stored at

Table 1. Demographic and clinical characteristics of Alzheimer's disease patients (AD) and controls (C).

	Serum donors database		CSF donors database	
	AD (n = 45)	C (n = 42)	AD (n = 37)	C (n = 29)
Age (years)	70.0±7.5	68.7±7.4	69.3±7.4	71.1±5.8
Gender (% male)	33.3	33.3	40.5	51.7
APOE (% ε4)	58.5	15.2	52.9	16.7
	(n = 41)	(n = 33)	(n = 34)	(n = 12)
MMSE	19.7±4.4	29.2±0.8	19.6±5.2	28.8±1.4
	(n = 44)	(n = 37)	(n = 37)	(n = 24)
ADAS-Cog	27.0±8.3	8.8±2.9	24.7±10.8	8.5±3.6
	(n = 30)	(n = 25)	(n = 20)	(n = 11)
CSF Aβ42 (pg/mL)	499±177	999±322	520±193	951±327
	(n = 44)	(n = 36)	(n = 36)	(n = 23)
CSF T-tau (pg/mL)	786±381	288±132	744±377	300±109
	(n = 44)	(n = 36)	(n = 36)	(n = 23)
Serum Aβ-IgG (OD)[a]	0.569±0.2	0.463±0.2		
	(n = 45)	(n = 42)		
CSF Aβ-IgG (OD)[b]			0.449±0.2	0.348±0.2
			(n = 37)	(n = 29)

Values are mean ± standard deviation. For gender and APOE status, percentages per group are given. ADAS-Cog - Alzheimer Disease Assessment Scale-Cognitive Subscale (range 0–70 errors); MMSE - Mini Mental Status Examination (range 0–30 points); OD - optical density.
[a]Diluted 1:100.
[b]Diluted 1:1.
doi:10.1371/journal.pone.0068996.t001

−80°C. The CSF levels of total tau (T-tau) were determined using a sandwich ELISA (INNOTEST® hTau Ag, Innogenetics, Belgium), by which both normally phosphorylated and non-phosphorylated tau were detected. The assay was performed according to the manufacturers' instructions and the laboratory reference ranges were as follows: <200 ng/L and <300 ng/L for control individuals below 65 and older than 65 years, respectively. The concentrations of total tau in the analyzed CSF samples were estimated from standard curves obtained for each assay. Tau levels >350 ng/L were regarded as indicative of a neurodegenerative process. The analytical sensitivity of the assay was 75 pg/mL, and the intra-assay and inter-assay variations were <8%. The CSF levels of Aβ (1–42) (Aβ42) were determined using a commercially available sandwich ELISA kit (INNOTEST® β-amyloid(1–42), Innogenetics, Belgium), according to the protocol supplied with the kit. CSF Aβ42 concentrations of the samples were estimated from standard curves obtained for each assay. Aβ42 levels below 550 ng/L were regarded as abnormal.

ELISA Determination of Aβ-IgG Immune Complexes in Serum and CSF

Serum levels of Aβ-IgG immune complexes were determined by sandwich ELISA, as previously reported [41]. The method is based on the different epitope specificities of the Aβ-autoantibodies, that recognize Aβ (21–37) and of a mouse monoclonal 6E10 antibody (mAb 6E10), that binds to Aβ (3–8) (Figure 1). Briefly, 96-well ELISA plates were coated overnight with the mAb 6E10 (Covance, Emeryville, CA, USA) followed by blocking the unspecific binding sites with 5% bovine serum albumin (BSA, w/v), 0.1% Tween-20 (v/v) in phosphate buffered saline (PBS, pH 7.4). Subsequently, human serum samples, diluted 1:100 with blocking buffer, were applied in triplicates. For detection, a horseradish peroxidase (HRP)-conjugated goat anti-human IgG (H+L) antibody (Pierce, Rockford, IL, USA) showing no cross-reactivity with mouse IgG and o-phenylenediamine (OPD, Merck, Darmstadt, Germany) as enzymatic substrate were used. The optical density (OD) was measured at 450 nm on a Wallac 1420 Victor^2 ELISA Plate Counter (Perkin Elmer, Rodgau, Germany). The described sandwich ELISA was also optimized for the analysis of CSF samples. Two washing buffers, PBS-Tween (0.05% Tween-20 in PBS, v/v) and PBS-Triton (0.1% Triton X-100 in PBS, v/v) and various CSF dilutions (1:300, 1:100, 1:30, 1:10, 1:3 and 1:1) were tested. The highest OD response was obtained using PBS-Tween for washing and 1:1 CSF dilution.

For both serum and CSF determinations, triplicate 3-fold dilutions from a stock solution (7 μg/μL in blocking buffer) of human serum γ-globulin (immunoglobulin preparation, Calbiochem, Merck, Darmstadt, Germany) were used as reference, to allow data to be normalized between plates and different experiments. The non-specific binding (NSB) of the IgG preparation and analyte samples was assessed from triplicate wells containing all components except the mAb 6E10. The average OD values, NSB subtraction, standard deviation (SD) and intra−/inter-assay coefficients of variation (CV) were calculated with the

WorkOut2.0 software (Perkin Elmer, Rodgau, Germany). Both serum and CSF determinations of Aβ-IgG immune complexes showed intra-assay CVs<10% and inter-assay CVs<15%. For the newly developed CSF ELISA, the cut-off values of the assay, defined as the linearity limits of the reference curve (R^2>0.97), were as follows: 0.065 min. and 1.129 max. Since there is no unique method for expressing ELISA responses and arbitrary units are derived from absorbance readings, we considered it adequate to present the results of Aβ-IgG determinations in serum and CSF as OD values.

Data Analysis

Statistical analysis was performed using the R statistical software package of The R Foundation of Statistical Computing (www.r-project.org; version 2.11.1 for Mac OS X, GUI 1.34 Leopard).

Welch's two-sample t-tests (two-tailed with modified degrees of freedom) were applied to examine differences in demographic and cognitive data between AD patients and controls. Analysis of variance with group as factor and age as covariate were computed in order to investigate differences in the levels of Aβ-IgG immune complexes between both groups. Models' residuals were tested for normality using the Shapiro-Wilk normality test. For categorical variables, Pearsons's Chi-squared (χ^2) test was computed. Pearson's r product moment correlation coefficient was calculated in order to investigate possible associations of serum and CSF levels of Aβ-IgG immune complexes with age and neuropsychological performance (MMSE, ADAS-Cog). The diagnostic power of the Aβ-IgG immune complexes in serum and CSF was calculated using receiver-operating characteristic (ROC) curve analysis (package Daim and pROC for R; [47,48]). All tests for statistical significance referred to a significance level with α ≤0.05.

Results

Demographic and Clinical Characteristics of Alzheimer's Disease Patients and Controls

Demographic and clinical characteristics of Alzheimer's disease patients and controls are shown in Table 1 and Table S1 in the Supporting Information. The statistical evaluation indicated a similar distribution of age ($t_{(85)} = 0.79$, $p = 0.43$ for serum donors; $t_{(64)} = -1.12$, $p = 0.27$ for CSF donors) and gender ($\chi^2_{(1)} = 0.05$, $p = 0.82$ for serum donors; $\chi^2_{(1)} = 0.43$, $p = 0.51$ for CSF donors) in the AD and the control group. As expected, AD patients scored lower in the MMSE ($t_{(47)} = -14.00$, $p<0.0001$ for serum donors; $t_{(44)} = -10.16$, $p<0.0001$ for CSF donors) and committed more errors in the ADAS-Cog neuropsychological test battery ($t_{(37)} = 11.30$, $p<0.0001$ for serum donors; $t_{(26)} = 6.12$, $p<0.0001$ for CSF donors) than the control subjects. They also presented significantly lower levels of Aβ42 ($t_{(69)} = -9.39$, $p<0.0001$) and higher levels of T-tau ($t_{(69)} = 8.88$, $p<0.0001$) in CSF. Furthermore, an increased incidence of APOE ε4 allele was observed in the AD cases ($\chi^2_{(1)} = 15.26$, $p<0.0001$).

In the following paragraphs we compare the levels of Aβ-IgG immune complexes in serum and CSF samples from AD patients and age- and gender-matched control subjects. Since old age and APOE ε4 status are considered to be associated with an increased risk of AD pathology [49], we also included age as covariate into the group comparison and further investigated potential differences between the levels of Aβ-IgG immune complexes in serum and CSF with respect to APOE genotype.

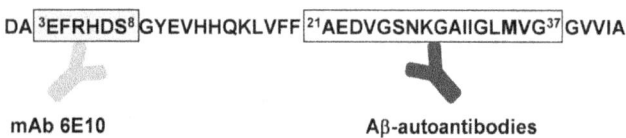

DA ³EFRHDS⁸ GYEVHHQKLVFF ²¹AEDVGSNKGAIIGLMVG³⁷ GVVIA

mAb 6E10   Aβ-autoantibodies

Figure 1. Epitope specificities of the coating antibody (mAb 6E10) and the Aβ-autoantibodies.
doi:10.1371/journal.pone.0068996.g001

Aβ-IgG Immune Complexes in Serum of AD Patients and Control Subjects

Two samples (from one AD patient and one control subject) were excluded from the statistical analysis, since the Aβ-IgG levels exceeded the ELISA cut-off values.

Higher levels of Aβ-IgG immune complexes were determined in serum of AD patients compared to the controls ($F_{(1,84)} = 4.94$, $p = 0.03$; Table 1, Figure 2A). According to ROC curve analyses, the serum Aβ-IgG levels discriminate the AD patients from the control subjects with 81% specificity and 44% sensitivity ($AUC = 0.63$, 95% CI: 0.75–0.51; Figure 2B). When the assay sensitivity was set to 80%, specificity reached a maximum of 33%.

A

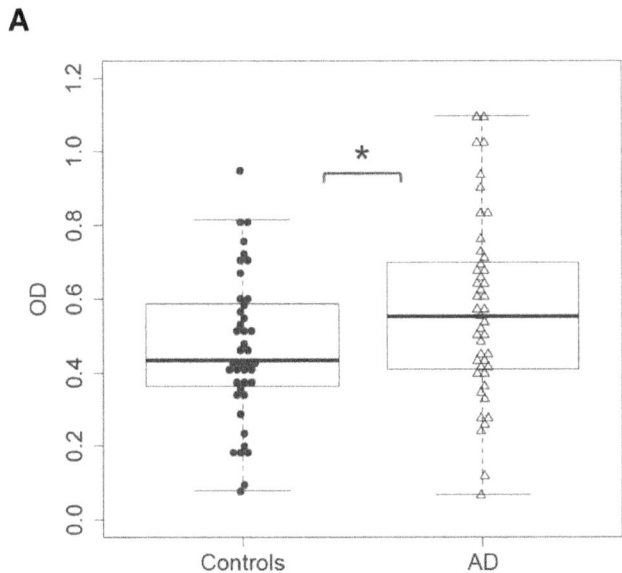

B

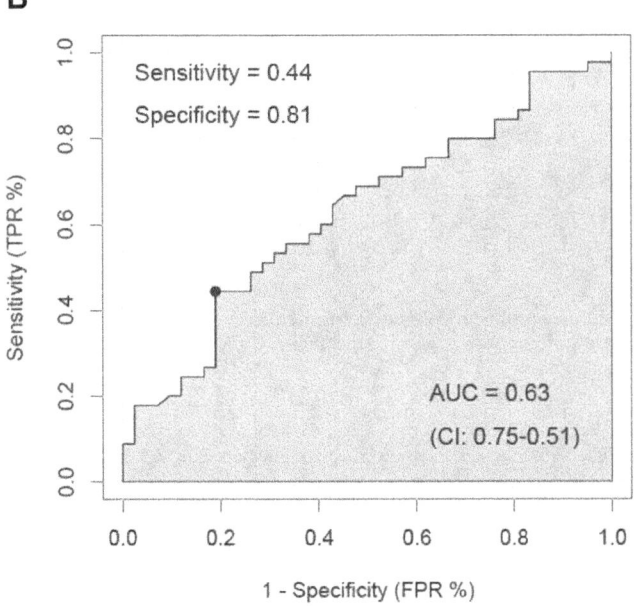

Figure 2. Aβ-IgG immune complexes in serum. (**A**) Comparison between the levels of Aβ-IgG immune complexes (OD at 450 nm) in serum of AD patients and control subjects; (**B**) ROC curve analysis; x-axis: 1-specificity (FPR: false positive rate), y-axis: sensitivity (TPR: true positive rate), AUC - area under the curve; * $p \leq 0.05$.
doi:10.1371/journal.pone.0068996.g002

The serum levels of Aβ-IgG immune complexes increased with advancing age in the AD patients ($r = 0.37$, $p = 0.01$) but not in the controls ($r = -0.14$, $p = 0.38$; Figure 3A). Furthermore, they were negatively correlated with the MMSE scores ($r = -0.23$, $p = 0.04$; Figure 3B) and positively with the ADAS-Cog scores across groups ($r = 0.32$, $p = 0.02$; Figure 3C), i.e., reaching higher values with decreasing cognitive test performance. There was no difference between the serum levels of Aβ-IgG immune complexes in the case of APOE ε4 (homo- and heterozygotes) and non-APOE ε4 carriers, either in the AD or the control group.

Aβ-IgG Immune Complexes in CSF from AD Patients and Control Subjects

The levels of Aβ-IgG immune complexes were higher in AD patients compared to the controls ($F_{(1,63)} = 4.98$, $p = 0.03$; Table 1, Figure 4A). ROC curve analyses indicated 59% specificity and 70% sensitivity ($AUC = 0.65$, 95% CI: 0.79–0.52; Figure 4B) for the diagnostic discrimination of the assay between AD cases and controls. When specificity of the Aβ-IgG determinations was set to 80%, sensitivity reached a maximum of 33%. When sensitivity was set to 80%, specificity reached a maximum of 31%. The ratio of the CSF to serum levels of the Aβ-IgG immune complexes showed 82% specificity and 50% sensitivity in ROC curve analysis ($AUC = 0.67$, 95% CI: 0.83–0.50). When sensitivity was set to 80%, specificity was only 35%. The ROC curve analysis of the CSF T-tau/Aβ42 concentration ratio showed 91% specificity and 93% sensitivity ($AUC = 0.97$, 95% CI: 0.10–0.94).

The CSF levels of Aβ-IgG immune complexes across all subjects were negatively correlated with the MMSE scores ($r = -0.30$, $p = 0.02$) and positively correlated with the ADAS-Cog test scores ($r = 0.48$, $p = 0.006$), increasing with the decline of cognitive performance (Figure 5A, B). Furthermore, they were positively correlated with the Aβ42 concentration in CSF of AD patients ($r = 0.35$, $p = 0.04$; Figure S1 in the Supporting Information), but not of control subjects. A highly significant positive correlation was observed across groups between the levels of Aβ-IgG immune complexes in CSF and serum ($r = 0.54$, $p = 0.0002$; Figure S2 in the Supporting Information). There was no effect of age or APOE ε4 (homo- and heterozygote) genotype on the Aβ-IgG levels in the CSF of either AD patients or control subjects.

Discussion

AD-related pathological processes start well before the onset of clinical manifestations [2,4,50,51]. Hence, the identification and evaluation of biochemical markers that enable an early diagnosis should be of substantial value. CSF levels of Aβ42 and tau protein are currently the only reliable biomarkers for the diagnosis of AD, with sufficient sensitivity and specificity [52], while efforts to establish less invasive blood-derived biomarkers have been hitherto unsuccessful. Reports on potential serum-biomarkers for AD diagnosis have provided contradictory results and it is unclear whether changes in the periphery reflect pathologies within the brain [53–55]. Thus, studies of Aβ42 levels in serum of AD patients showed both reduced [56,57] and increased values [58,59] compared to control subjects, while other reports indicated no differences between groups [60,61]. Also, no correlation was found between the serum Aβ42 levels and the Aβ42 levels in CSF of AD patients and healthy individuals [62,63], the accumulation of Aβ peptides in AD brain [64] or the progression of cognitive deterioration in AD [65,66]. Furthermore, research focused on blood protein signatures recently revealed that epidermal growth factor (EGF), platelet-derived growth factor (PDG-BB) and macrophage inflammatory protein 1δ (MIP-1δ) differentiated

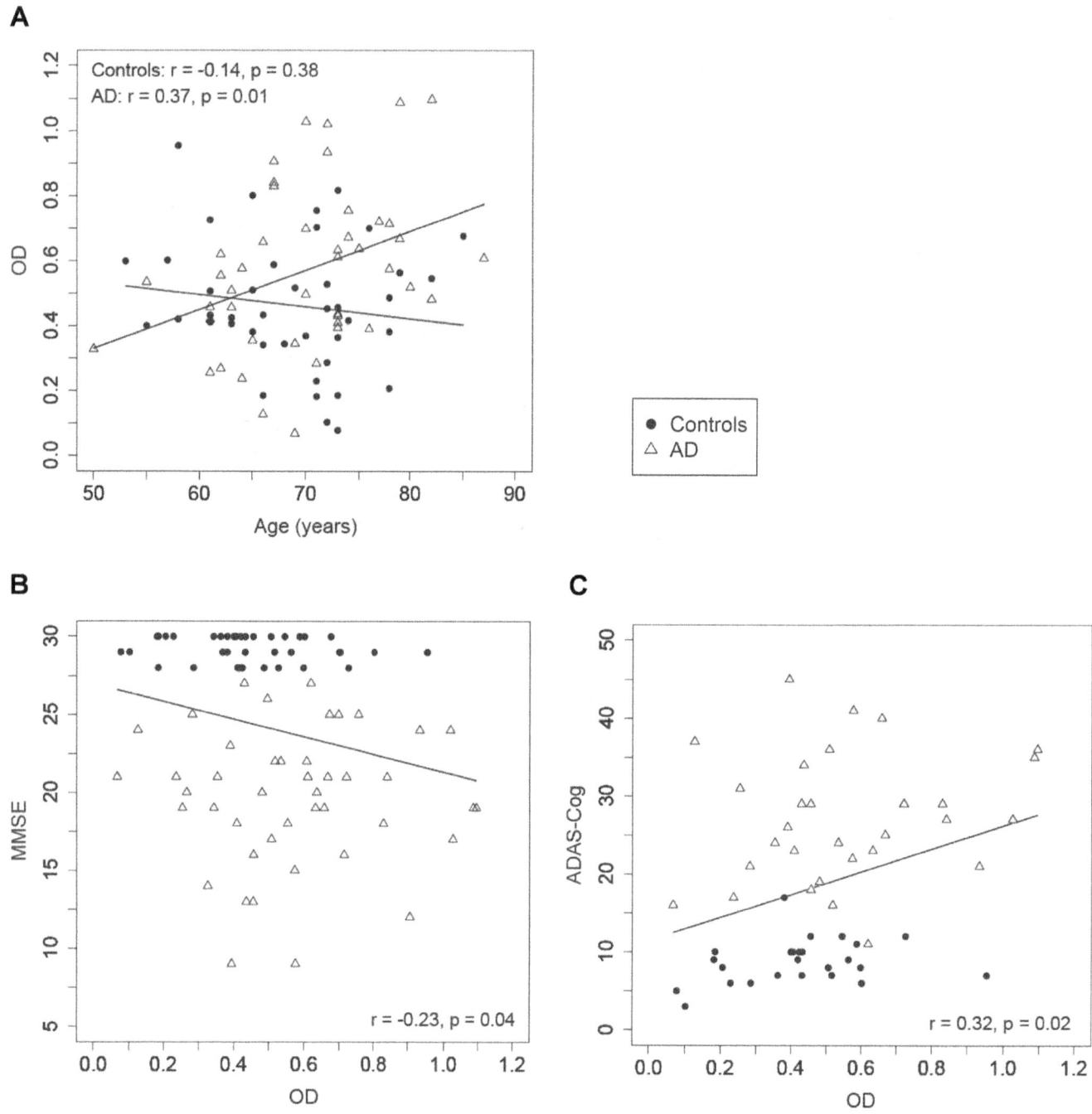

Figure 3. Correlations of serum levels of Aβ-IgG immune complexes with age and cognitive performance. Correlation analysis of serum levels of Aβ-IgG immune complexes (OD at 450 nm) with (**A**) age of AD patients and control subjects, respectively; (**B**) MMSE score (range 0–30 points) across all subjects and (**C**) ADAS-Cog score (range 0–70 errors) across all subjects.
doi:10.1371/journal.pone.0068996.g003

AD from control subjects, but not from patients with other types of dementia [67].

Physiological Aβ-autoantibodies have been detected in serum and CSF [20–24,27] and generated a high interest as a potential biomarker for AD, however with hitherto inconsistent results. In AD patients compared to controls, the serum levels of free, non-antigen-bound Aβ-autoantibodies were found to be reduced [28–30,34], enhanced [31] or unchanged [32,33]. Other studies reported increased levels of Aβ-autoantibodies after acidic dissociation of preformed Aβ-immune complexes in serum of AD patients [35,36]. Nevertheless, these results could not be reproduced by Klaver et al. [37], who found no difference in the levels of dissociated Aβ-autoantibodies between AD and control subjects.

Due to the postulated imbalance between Aβ production and removal in AD [11], we have evaluated the contribution of Aβ-autoantibodies to Aβ-clearance and the diagnostic potential of Aβ-IgG immune complexes. Our method could be applied as an alternative or complementary approach to the previously reported direct ELISAs for the determination of total Aβ-autoantibodies levels. It does not require additional sample preparation steps such as acidic dissociation and may provide valuable information on possible problems related to antibody avidity and clearance of the immune complexes. Another important aspect is the subtraction of

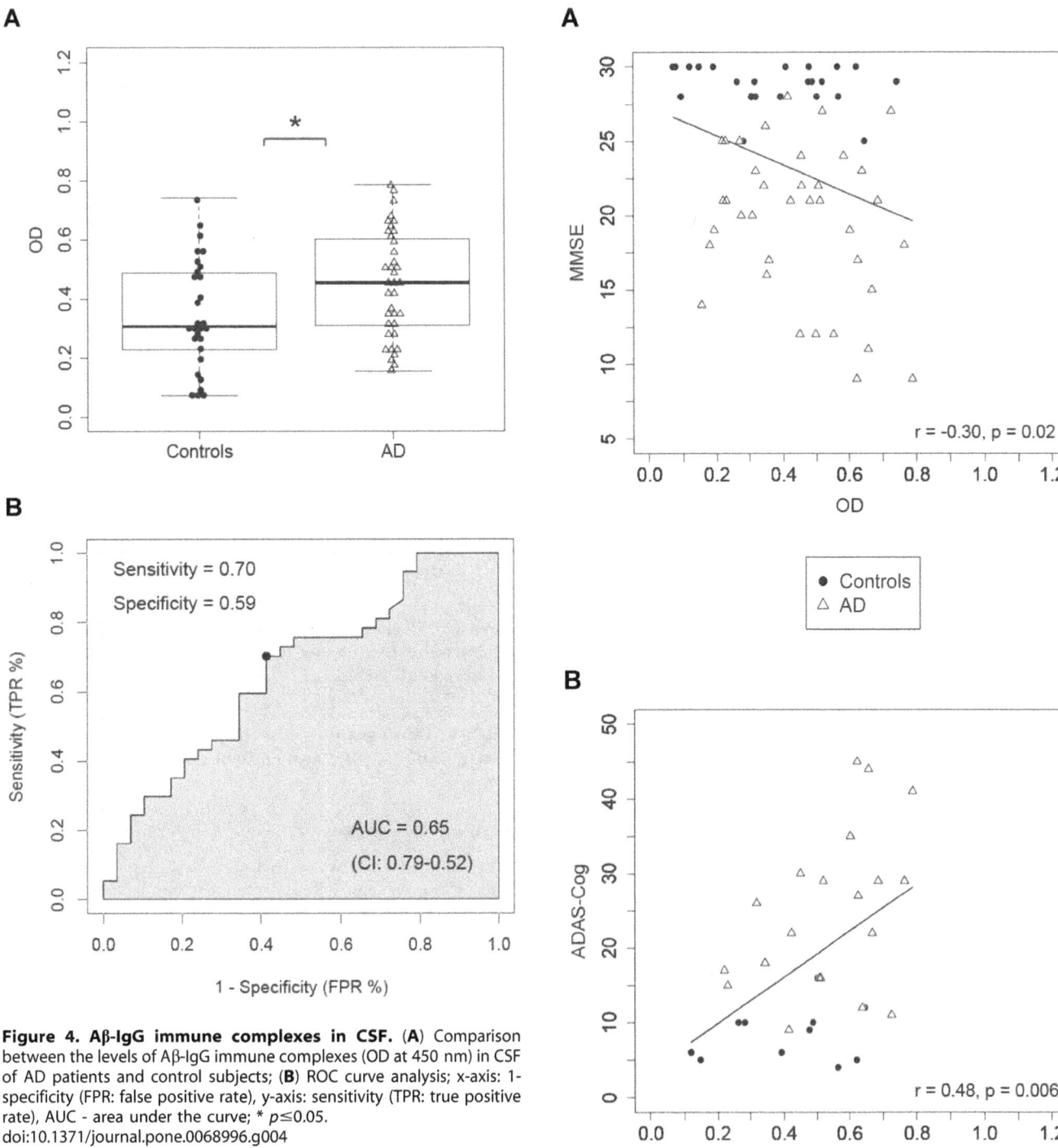

Figure 4. Aβ-IgG immune complexes in CSF. (A) Comparison between the levels of Aβ-IgG immune complexes (OD at 450 nm) in CSF of AD patients and control subjects; **(B)** ROC curve analysis; x-axis: 1-specificity (FPR: false positive rate), y-axis: sensitivity (TPR: true positive rate), AUC - area under the curve; * $p \leq 0.05$.
doi:10.1371/journal.pone.0068996.g004

Figure 5. Correlations of CSF levels of Aβ-IgG immune complexes with the cognitive performance. Correlation analysis of CSF levels of Aβ-IgG immune complexes (OD at 450 nm) with **(A)** MMSE score (range 0–30 points) across all subjects and **(B)** ADAS-Cog score (range 0–70 errors) across all subjects.
doi:10.1371/journal.pone.0068996.g005

the NSB from the OD response of each sample, a procedure previously reported only in a few ELISA studies of Aβ-autoantibodies [37]. We initially optimized and employed the sandwich ELISA protocol for the analysis of serum samples from healthy adults aged 18–89 years [41]. In the present study, the experimental procedure was also optimized for CSF analysis and applied to determine the levels of Aβ-IgG immune complexes in serum and CSF samples from a total number of 112 AD patients and age- and gender-matched control subjects. Aβ-IgG immune complexes were detected in all serum and CSF samples, suggesting a contribution of IgG-type Aβ-autoantibodies to Aβ clearance *in vivo*. Higher Aβ-IgG levels were found in both serum and CSF of AD patients compared to controls, in agreement with two previous studies [35,36] that revealed increased total levels of Aβ-

autoantibodies in AD patients. An elevated antibody production would be expected in response to Aβ accumulation, which is either due to deficient clearance mechanisms [68,69] or to an increased formation of Aβ peptides. The latter is mainly the case in familial AD, owing to genetic mutations of amyloid precursor protein (APP) and presenilin 1 and 2, but it can also occur in sporadic AD, where it was suggested to be partially caused by the enhanced expression and activity of APP cleaving enzyme 1 (BACE 1) [70]. The progression of the disease, despite increased Aβ-IgG levels in serum and CSF of AD patients, could indicate defective clearance mechanisms, leading to the accumulation of Aβ-IgG immune complexes in AD. In healthy individuals, antigen-bound antibodies are captured by macrophages through Fc receptor-mediated recognition and transferred to mastocytes in liver or spleen for degradation during the process of "immune adhesion", which is regulated by antibody avidity [10,71]. A possible explanation for the apparent clearance deficiency of Aβ-IgG immune complexes is provided by the observations of Jianping et al. [72] who found the avidity of Aβ-autoantibodies to be lower in AD patients than in healthy controls and suggested that this could impair the removal of Aβ-IgG immune complexes by macrophages.

Our results further revealed that serum and CSF levels of Aβ-IgG immune complexes were negatively correlated with the cognitive performance of the study participants. Thus, subjects with higher Aβ-IgG levels had weaker performances during MMSE screening and ADAS-Cog neuropsychological testing. The increased levels of Aβ-IgG immune complexes and their inverse correlation with the cognitive status would point to a pathological process, potentially associated with defective clearance mechanisms, as discussed above. Thereby, the reported cognitive improvements of AD patients treated with IVIg [20,23,27] might be partially attributed to the replacement of deficient Aβ-autoantibodies by passive immunization.

In agreement with our previous work [41], serum Aβ-IgG levels were not correlated with the age of control subjects. In the AD group, however, increased age was associated with higher levels of Aβ-IgG immune complexes in serum and might therefore represent a factor for reduced Aβ clearance in AD. A positive correlation with age was also reported by Gustaw-Rothenberg et al. [36] for the difference values between the Aβ-autoantibody levels before and after acidic dissociation of the Aβ-IgG immune complexes, which might be comparable with the levels of intact Aβ-IgG immune complexes.

As shown in Figure S1 in the Supporting Information, our results also indicated a positive correlation between the CSF levels of Aβ-IgG immune complexes and Aβ42 peptide. Furthermore, we found a strong correlation across groups between the serum and CSF levels of Aβ-IgG immune complexes. Considering the dilution factors applied in ELISA, the Aβ-IgG levels were approximately 100 fold lower in CSF than in serum, suggesting that the Aβ-autoantibodies are produced and bind to Aβ mainly in the periphery.

In summary, we report here for the first time the determination of intact Aβ-IgG immune complexes in serum and CSF of AD patients and age- and gender-matched control subjects, employing a sandwich ELISA approach. Our results showed higher serum and CSF levels of Aβ-IgG immune complexes in AD patients relative to controls; however, due to the variability within groups leading to overlapping values, the Aβ-IgG levels displayed only moderate discrimination powers in ROC analyses. A possible application of serum Aβ-IgG immune complexes for AD diagnosis in a panel of blood-derived biomarkers remains to be further tested. Nevertheless, the correlation of both serum and CSF Aβ-IgG levels with the cognitive status across groups represents a valuable characteristic and it would be interesting to assess their potential use for predicting conversion to AD or evaluating the efficacy of therapeutic interventions in AD (e.g., passive immunization with intravenous immunoglobulin preparations containing Aβ-autoantibodies).

Our findings additionally suggest an increased immune response in AD, presumably associated with deficiencies in the clearance of Aβ-IgG immune complexes. A better understanding of the mechanisms causing the apparent accumulation of Aβ-IgG immune complexes could reveal in future studies new approaches for diagnosis or targeted treatment of AD.

Supporting Information

Figure S1   Correlation analysis between the levels of Aβ-IgG immune complexes (OD at 450 nm) and Aβ42 in CSF of AD patients.
(TIF)

Figure S2   Correlation analysis between the levels of Aβ-IgG immune complexes (OD at 450 nm) in serum and CSF across all subjects.
(TIF)

Table S1   Demographic and clinical data of Alzheimer's disease patients (AD) and control subjects (C).
(XLS)

Acknowledgments

We thank all participants for their willingness to take part in this study. We also thank Dagmar Vogel, Refika Aksamija, Christa Ondratschek, Rehane Mojib and Alice Pabst for their support in pre-analytical processing and in Aβ42 and T-tau determinations in CSF samples.

Author Contributions

Conceived and designed the experiments: CAFVA M. Manea I-TK MP TE M. Maftei. Performed the experiments: M. Maftei M. Manea. Analyzed the data: FT M. Maftei CS M. Manea MP CAFVA I-TK HT MO. Wrote the paper: FT M. Maftei M. Manea CAFVA MP I-TK. Critically revised the manuscript: FT M. Maftei CS M. Manea MP CAFVA I-TK TE HT MO. Approved the final version of the manuscript: FT M. Maftei CS M. Manea MP CAFVA I-TK TE HT MO.

References

1. Selkoe DJ (2000) Toward a comprehensive theory for Alzheimer's disease. Hypothesis: Alzheimer's disease is caused by the cerebral accumulation and cytotoxicity of amyloid beta-protein. Ann N Y Acad Sci 924: 17–25.
2. Thal DR, Rüb U, Orantes M, Braak H (2002) Phases of A beta-deposition in the human brain and its relevance for the development of AD. Neurology 58: 1791–1800.
3. Braak E, Griffing K, Arai K, Bohl J, Bratzke H, et al. (1999) Neuropathology of Alzheimer's disease: what is new since A. Alzheimer? Eur Arch Psychiatry Clin Neurosci Suppl. 249: 14–22.
4. Villemagne VL, Burnham S, Bourgeat P, Brown B, Ellis KA, et al. (2013) Amyloid β deposition, neurodegeneration, and cognitive decline in sporadic Alzheimer's disease: a prospective cohort study. Lancet Neurol 12: 357–367.
5. Finder VH, Glockshuber R (2007) Amyloid-beta aggregation. Neurodegener Dis 4: 13–27.
6. Janus C, Pearson J, McLaurin J, Mathews PM, Jiang Y, et al. (2000) A beta peptide immunization reduces behavioural impairment and plaques in a model of Alzheimer's disease. Nature 408: 979–982.
7. Morgan D, Diamond DM, Gottschall PE, Ugen KE, Dickey C, et al. (2000) A beta peptide vaccination prevents memory loss in an animal model of Alzheimer's disease. Nature 408: 982–985.
8. Sigurdsson EM, Scholtzova H, Mehta PD, Frangione B, Wisniewski T (2001) Immunization with a nontoxic/nonfibrillar amyloid-beta homologous peptide reduces Alzheimer's disease-associated pathology in transgenic mice. Am J Pathol 159: 439–447.
9. Schenk D, Barbour R, Dunn W, Gordon G, Grajeda H, et al. (1999) Immunization with amyloid-beta attenuates Alzheimer-disease-like pathology in the PDAPP mouse. Nature 400: 173–177.
10. Bard F, Cannon C, Barbour R, Burke RL, Games D, et al. (2000) Peripherally administered antibodies against amyloid beta-peptide enter the central nervous

system and reduce pathology in a mouse model of Alzheimer disease. Nat Med 6: 916–919.

11. DeMattos RB, Bales KR, Cummins DJ, Dodart JC, Paul SM, et al. (2001) Peripheral anti-A beta antibody alters CNS and plasma A beta clearance and decreases brain A beta burden in a mouse model of Alzheimer's disease. PNAS 98: 8850–8855.

12. Dodart J-C, Bales KR, Gannon KS, Greene SJ, DeMattos RB, et al. (2002) Immunization reverses memory deficits without reducing brain Abeta burden in Alzheimer's disease model. Nat Neurosci 5: 452–457.

13. Morgan D (2011) Immunotherapy for Alzheimer's disease. J Intern Med 269: 54–63.

14. Schenk D (2002) Amyloid-beta immunotherapy for Alzheimer's disease: the end of the beginning. Nat Rev Neurosci 3: 824–828.

15. Hock C, Konietzko U, Streffer JR, Tracy J, Signorell A, et al. (2003) Antibodies against beta-amyloid slow cognitive decline in Alzheimer's disease. Neuron 38: 547–554.

16. Holmes C, Boche D, Wilkinson D, Yadegarfar G, Hopkins V, et al. (2008) Long-term effects of Abeta42 immunisation in Alzheimer's disease: follow-up of a randomised, placebo-controlled phase I trial. Lancet 372: 216–223.

17. Gilman S, Koller M, Black RS, Jenkins L, Griffith SG, et al. (2005) Clinical effects of Abeta immunization (AN1792) in patients with AD in an interrupted trial. Neurology 64: 1553–1562.

18. Mangialasche F, Solomon A, Winblad B, Mecocci P, Kivipelto M (2010) Alzheimer's disease: clinical trials and drug development. Lancet Neurol 9: 702–716.

19. Garber K (2012) Genentech's Alzheimer's antibody trial to study disease prevention. Nat Biotechnol 30: 731–732.

20. Relkin NR, Szabo P, Adamiak B, Burgut T, Monthe C, et al. (2009) 18-Month study of intravenous immunoglobulin for treatment of mild Alzheimer disease. Neurobiol Aging 30: 1728–1736.

21. Taguchi H, Planque S, Nishiyama Y, Symersky J, Boivin S, et al. (2008) Autoantibody-catalyzed hydrolysis of amyloid beta peptide. J Biol Chem 283: 4714–4722.

22. Du Y, Wei X, Dodel R, Sommer N, Hampel H, et al. (2003) Human anti-beta-amyloid antibodies block beta-amyloid fibril formation and prevent beta-amyloid-induced neurotoxicity. Brain 126: 1935–1939.

23. Dodel RC, Du Y, Depboylu C, Hampel H, Frölich L, et al. (2004) Intravenous immunoglobulins containing antibodies against beta-amyloid for the treatment of Alzheimer's disease. J Neurol Neurosurg Psychiatry 75: 1472–1474.

24. Bacher M, Depboylu C, Du Y, Noelker C, Oertel WH, et al. (2009) Peripheral and central biodistribution of (111)In-labeled anti-beta-amyloid autoantibodies in a transgenic mouse model of Alzheimer's disease. Neurosci Lett 449: 240–245.

25. Jolles S, Sewell WAC, Misbah SA (2005) Clinical uses of intravenous immunoglobulin. Clin Exp Immunol 142: 1–11.

26. Dodel R, Balakrishnan K, Keyvani K, Deuster O, Neff F, et al. (2011) Naturally occurring autoantibodies against beta-amyloid: investigating their role in transgenic animal and in vitro models of Alzheimer's disease. J Neurosci 31: 5847–5854.

27. Dodel R, Neff F, Noelker C, Pul R, Du Y, et al. (2010) Intravenous immunoglobulins as a treatment for Alzheimer's disease: rationale and current evidence. Drugs 70: 513–528.

28. Song M, Mook-Jung I, Lee H, Min J, Park M (2007) Serum anti-amyloid-beta antibodies and Alzheimer 's disease in elderly Korean patients. J Int Med Res 35: 301–306.

29. Weksler ME, Relkin N, Turkenich R, Larusse S, Ling Z, et al. (2002) Patients with Alzheimer disease have lower levels of serum anti-amyloid peptide antibodies than healthy elderly individuals. Exp Gerontol 37: 943–948.

30. Brettschneider S, Morgenthaler NG, Teipel SJ, Fischer-Schulz C, Bürger K, et al. (2005) Decreased serum amyloid beta(1–42) autoantibody levels in Alzheimer's disease, determined by a newly developed immuno-precipitation assay with radiolabeled amyloid beta(1–42) peptide. Biol Psychiatry 57: 813–816.

31. Mruthinti S, Buccafusco JJ, Hill WD, Waller JL, Jackson TW, et al. (2004) Autoimmunity in Alzheimer's disease: increased levels of circulating IgGs binding Abeta and RAGE peptides. Neurobiol Aging 25: 1023–1032.

32. Hyman BT, Smith C, Buldyrev I, Whelan C, Brown H, et al. (2001) Autoantibodies to amyloid-beta and Alzheimer's disease. Ann Neurol 49: 808–810.

33. Baril L, Nicolas L, Croisile B, Crozier P, Hessler C, et al. (2004) Immune response to Abeta-peptides in peripheral blood from patients with Alzheimer's disease and control subjects. Neurosci Lett 355: 226–230.

34. Du Y, Dodel R, Hampel H, Buerger K, Lin S, et al. (2001) Reduced levels of amyloid beta-peptide antibody in Alzheimer disease. Neurology 57: 801–805.

35. Gustaw KA, Garrett MR, Lee H-G, Castellani RJ, Zagorski MG, et al. (2008) Antigen-antibody dissociation in Alzheimer disease: a novel approach to diagnosis. J Neurochem 106: 1350–1356.

36. Gustaw-Rothenberg K, Siedlak S, Bonda D (2010) Dissociated amyloid-beta antibody levels as a serum biomarker for the progression of Alzheimer's disease: A population-based study. Exp Gerontol 45: 47–52.

37. Klaver AC, Coffey MP, Smith LM, Bennett DA, Finke JM, et al. (2011) ELISA measurement of specific non-antigen-bound antibodies to Abeta1–42 monomer and soluble oligomers in sera from Alzheimer's disease, mild cognitively impaired, and noncognitively impaired subjects. J Neuroinflammation 8: 93.

38. Przybylski M, Stefanescu R, Manea M, Perdivara I, Cozma C, et al. (2007) New molecular approaches for immunotherapy and diagnosis of Alzheimer's disease based on epitope-specific serum beta-amyloid antibodies. 7th Austral. Pept. Symposium, Cairns, abstr. p. 32.

39. Dodel R, Bacher M, Przybylski M, Stefanescu R, Manea M (2008) Diagnosis of Alzheimer's disease and other neurodementing disorders. Patent International Application No.: PCT/IB2008/000456, Pub. No.: WO/2008/084402, European Patent Office. Available: http://ip.com/patapp/EP1944314A1. Accessed 13 November 2011.

40. McLaurin J, Cecal R, Kierstead ME, Tian X, Phinney AL, et al. (2002) Therapeutically effective antibodies against amyloid-beta peptide target amyloid-beta residues 4–10 and inhibit cytotoxicity and fibrillogenesis. Nat Med 8: 1263–1269.

41. Maftei M, Thurm F, Leirer VM, Von Arnim C a F, Elbert T, et al. (2012) Antigen-bound and free β-amyloid autoantibodies in serum of healthy adults. PloS One 7: e44516.

42. Folstein MF, Folstein SE, McHugh PR (1975) "Mini-mental state". A practical method for grading the cognitive state of patients for the clinician. J Psychiatr Res 12: 189–198.

43. Ihl R, Weyer G (1993) Die Alzheimer Disease Assessment Scale (ADAS). [The Alzheimer Disease Assessment Scale (ADAS).]. Beltz Test: Weinheim.

44. McKhann G, Drachman D, Folstein M, Katzman R, Price D, et al. (1984) Clinical diagnosis of Alzheimer's disease: report of the NINCDS-ADRDA Work Group under the auspices of Department of Health and Human Services Task Force on Alzheimer's Disease. Neurology 34: 939–944.

45. American Psychiatric Association (2000) Diagnostic and statistical manual of mental disorders. 4th ed. te. Washington, DC: Author.

46. Brettschneider J, Petzold A, Schottle D, Claus A, Riepe M, et al. (2006) The neurofilament heavy chain (NfH) in the cerebrospinal fluid diagnosis of Alzheimer's disease. Dement Geriatr Cogn Disord 21: 291–295.

47. Potapov S, Adler W, Lausen B (2009) Daim: Diagnostic accuracy of classification models. R package version 1.0.0. Available:http://cran.r-project.org/package = Daim. Accessed 8 August 2011.

48. Robin X, Turck N, Hainard A, Tiberti N, Lisacek F, et al. (2011) pROC: an open-source package for R and S+ to analyze and compare ROC curves. BMC Bioinformatics 12: 77.

49. Lindsay J, Laurin D, Verreault R, Hébert R, Helliwell B, et al. (2002) Risk factors for Alzheimer's disease: a prospective analysis from the Canadian Study of Health and Aging. Am J Epidemiol 156: 445–453.

50. Braak H, Braak E (1991) Neuropathological stageing of Alzheimer-related changes. Acta Neuropathol 82: 239–259.

51. Jack CR, Knopman DS, Jagust WJ, Petersen RC, Weiner MW, et al. (2013) Tracking pathophysiological processes in Alzheimer's disease: an updated hypothetical model of dynamic biomarkers. Lancet Neurol 12: 207–216.

52. Tapiola T, Alafuzoff I, Herukka S-K, Parkkinen L, Hartikainen P, et al. (2009) Cerebrospinal fluid beta-amyloid 42 and tau proteins as biomarkers of Alzheimer-type pathologic changes in the brain. Arch Neurol 66: 382–389.

53. Zetterberg H, Blennow K, Hanse E (2010) Amyloid beta and APP as biomarkers for Alzheimer's disease. Exp Gerontol 45: 23–29.

54. Mehta PD (2007) Amyloid beta protein as a marker or risk factor of Alzheimer's disease. Curr Alzheimer Res 4: 359–363.

55. Irizarry MC (2004) Biomarkers of Alzheimer disease in plasma. NeuroRx 1: 226–234.

56. Seppälä TT, Herukka S-K, Hänninen T, Tervo S, Hallikainen M, et al. (2010) Plasma Abeta42 and Abeta40 as markers of cognitive change in follow-up: a prospective, longitudinal, population-based cohort study. J Neurol Neurosurg Psychiatry 81: 1123–1127.

57. Xu W, Kawarabayashi T, Matsubara E, Deguchi K, Murakami T, et al. (2008) Plasma antibodies to Abeta40 and Abeta42 in patients with Alzheimer's disease and normal controls. Brain Res 1219: 169–179.

58. Matsubara E, Ghiso J, Frangione B, Amari M, Tomidokoro Y, et al. (1999) Lipoprotein-free amyloidogenic peptides in plasma are elevated in patients with sporadic Alzheimer's disease and Down's syndrome. Ann Neurol 45: 537–541.

59. Mayeux R, Tang MX, Jacobs DM, Manly J, Bell K, et al. (1999) Plasma amyloid beta-peptide 1–42 and incipient Alzheimer's disease. Ann Neurol 46: 412–416.

60. Fukumoto H, Tennis M, Locascio JJ, Hyman BT, Growdon JH, et al. (2003) Age but not diagnosis is the main predictor of plasma amyloid beta-protein levels. Arch Neurol 60: 958–964.

61. Tamaoka A, Fukushima T, Sawamura N, Ishikawa K, Oguni E, et al. (1996) Amyloid beta protein in plasma from patients with sporadic Alzheimer's disease. J Neurol Sci 141: 65–68.

62. Mehta PD, Pirttila T, Patrick BA, Barshatzky M, Mehta SP (2001) Amyloid beta protein 1–40 and 1–42 levels in matched cerebrospinal fluid and plasma from patients with Alzheimer disease. Neurosci Lett 304: 102–106.

63. Mehta PD, Pirttila T (2005) Increased cerebrospinal fluid A beta38/A beta42 ratio in Alzheimer disease. Neurodegener Dis 2: 242–245.

64. Fagan AM, Mintun MA, Mach RH, Lee S-Y, Dence CS, et al. (2006) Inverse relation between in vivo amyloid imaging load and cerebrospinal fluid Abeta42 in humans. Ann Neurol 59: 512–519.

65. Mehta PD, Pirttila T, Mehta SP, Sersen EA, Aisen PS, et al. (2000) Plasma and cerebrospinal fluid levels of amyloid beta proteins 1–40 and 1–42 in Alzheimer disease. Arch Neurol 57: 100–105.

66. Sundelöf J, Giedraitis V, Irizarry MC, Sundström J, Ingelsson E, et al. (2008) Plasma beta amyloid and the risk of Alzheimer disease and dementia in elderly men: a prospective, population-based cohort study. Arch Neurol 65: 256–263.
67. Björkqvist M, Ohlsson M, Minthon L, Hansson O (2012) Evaluation of a previously suggested plasma biomarker panel to identify Alzheimer's disease. PLoS One 7: e29868.
68. Holtzman DM, Herz J, Bu G (2012) Apolipoprotein e and apolipoprotein e receptors: normal biology and roles in Alzheimer disease. Cold Spring Harb Perspect Med 2: a006312.
69. Wang Y-J, Zhou H-D, Zhou X-F (2006) Clearance of amyloid-beta in Alzheimer's disease: progress, problems and perspectives. Drug Discov Today 11: 931–938.
70. Li R, Lindholm K, Yang L-B, Yue X, Citron M, et al. (2004) Amyloid beta peptide load is correlated with increased beta-secretase activity in sporadic Alzheimer's disease patients. PNAS 101: 3632–3637.
71. Magga J, Puli L, Pihlaja R, Kanninen K, Neulamaa S, et al. (2010) Human intravenous immunoglobulin provides protection against Aβ toxicity by multiple mechanisms in a mouse model of Alzheimer's disease. J Neuroinflammation 7: 90.
72. Jianping L, Zhibing Y, Wei Q, Zhikai C, Jie X, et al. (2006) Low avidity and level of serum anti-Abeta antibodies in Alzheimer disease. Alzheimer Dis Assoc Disord 20: 127–132.

CSF T-Tau/Aβ₄₂ Predicts White Matter Microstructure in Healthy Adults at Risk for Alzheimer's Disease

Barbara B. Bendlin[1,2]*, Cynthia M. Carlsson[1,2], Sterling C. Johnson[1,2], Henrik Zetterberg[3], Kaj Blennow[3], Auriel A. Willette[1,2], Ozioma C. Okonkwo[1,2], Aparna Sodhi[1,2], Michele L. Ries[1,2], Alex C. Birdsill[1,2], Andrew L. Alexander[4,5,6], Howard A. Rowley[7], Luigi Puglielli[1,2], Sanjay Asthana[1,2], Mark A. Sager[1,2]

1 Geriatric Research, Education and Clinical Center (GRECC), William S. Middleton Memorial Veteran's Hospital, Madison, Wisconsin, United States of America, 2 Wisconsin Alzheimer's Disease Research Center, Department of Medicine, University of Wisconsin, Madison, Wisconsin, United States of America, 3 Institute of Neuroscience and Physiology, Department of Psychiatry and Neurochemistry, The Sahlgrenska Academy at University of Gothenburg, Sweden, 4 University of Wisconsin School of Medicine and Public Health, Department of Medical Physics, Madison, Wisconsin, United States of America, 5 University of Wisconsin School of Medicine and Public Health, Department of Psychiatry, Madison, Wisconsin, United States of America, 6 Waisman Laboratory for Brain Imaging and Behavior, Madison, Wisconsin, United States of America, 7 University of Wisconsin School of Medicine and Public Health, Department of Radiology, Madison, Wisconsin, United States of America

Abstract

Cerebrospinal fluid (CSF) biomarkers T-Tau and Aβ₄₂ are linked with Alzheimer's disease (AD), yet little is known about the relationship between CSF biomarkers and structural brain alteration in healthy adults. In this study we examined the extent to which AD biomarkers measured in CSF predict brain microstructure indexed by diffusion tensor imaging (DTI) and volume indexed by T1-weighted imaging. Forty-three middle-aged adults with parental family history of AD received baseline lumbar puncture and MRI approximately 3.5 years later. Voxel-wise image analysis methods were used to test whether baseline CSF Aβ₄₂, total tau (T-Tau), phosphorylated tau (P-Tau) and neurofilament light protein predicted brain microstructure as indexed by DTI and gray matter volume indexed by T1-weighted imaging. T-Tau and T-Tau/Aβ₄₂ were widely correlated with indices of brain microstructure (mean, axial, and radial diffusivity), notably in white matter regions adjacent to gray matter structures affected in the earliest stages of AD. None of the CSF biomarkers were related to gray matter volume. Elevated P-Tau and P-Tau/Aβ₄₂ levels were associated with lower recognition performance on the Rey Auditory Verbal Learning Test. Overall, the results suggest that CSF biomarkers are related to brain microstructure in healthy adults with elevated risk of developing AD. Furthermore, the results clearly suggest that early pathological changes in AD can be detected with DTI and occur not only in cortex, but also in white matter.

Citation: Bendlin BB, Carlsson CM, Johnson SC, Zetterberg H, Blennow K, et al. (2012) CSF T-Tau/Aβ₄₂ Predicts White Matter Microstructure in Healthy Adults at Risk for Alzheimer's Disease. PLoS ONE 7(6): e37720. doi:10.1371/journal.pone.0037720

Editor: Yong He, Beijing Normal University, Beijing, China

Received December 15, 2011; **Accepted** April 23, 2012; **Published** June 6, 2012

Funding: This project was supported in part by the National Institute on Aging (R01 AG027161 [MAS], K23 AG026752 [CMC]; ADRC P50 AG033514 [SA]), the University of Wisconsin Institute for Clinical and Translational Research, funded through a National Center for Research Resources/National Institutes of Health Clinical and Translational Science Award, 1UL1RR025011, a program of the National Center for Research Resources, United States National Institutes of Health, and the Swedish Research Council. The project was also facilitated by the facilities and resources at the Geriatric Research, Education, and Clinical Center (GRECC) of the William S. Middleton Memorial Veterans Hospital, Madison, WI. GRECC MS # 2011-19. The funders had no role in study design, data collection and analysis, decision to publish, or preparation of the manuscript.

Competing Interests: Dr. Blennow has served on scientific advisory boards for Adlyfe Inc., Bayer Schering Pharma, Bristol-Myers Squibb, and Merz Pharmaceuticals GmbH; received a speaker honorarium from Pfizer Inc.; serves as a consultant for Wyeth, AstraZeneca, Bristol-Myers Squibb, and Eli Lilly and Company; and has received research support from Pfizer Inc., Innogenetics, the Swedish Research Council, Västra Götalandsregionen, Sweden, the Swedish Brain Power Project, the Swedish Council for Working Life and Social Research, the Swedish Alzheimer Foundation, Stiftelsen för Gamla Tjänarinnor, and the King Gustaf V and Queen Victoria Foundation. Dr. Zetterberg has served on a scientific advisory board for GlaxoSmithKline; serves as an Associate Editor for the Journal of Alzheimer's Disease; and receives research support from the Swedish Research Council, the Alzheimer's Association, and the Royal Swedish Academy of Sciences. This does not alter the authors' adherence to all the PLoS ONE policies on sharing data and materials.

* E-mail: bbb@medicine.wisc.edu

Introduction

Distinguishing pathologically aging elders from those who will age normally is a key challenge in preventing Alzheimer's disease (AD). Several cerebrospinal fluid (CSF) markers that are presumably related to the core pathology in AD show promise for early detection of the disease. Lower levels of CSF Aβ₄₂, higher CSF total tau (T-Tau), and higher tau phosphorylated at threonine 181 (P-Tau₁₈₁), as well as biomarker ratios (T-Tau/Aβ₄₂ or P-Tau/Aβ₄₂) distinguish patients from controls [1,2,3,4,5] and predict conversion from mild cognitive impairment (MCI) to AD [1,2,6,7,8,9]. When evaluated in cognitively healthy individuals, these biomarkers also appear to be related to cognitive function

[10,11], and measures of brain health that include cortical thinning [12], ventricular expansion and atrophy [11,13,14,15,16].

While studies resulting from volumetric imaging have been very useful for revealing gross structural changes, it is possible that some of the earliest brain changes involved in AD are subtle and below the detection threshold for volumetric imaging. Sensitive to water molecule motion, maps derived from diffusion tensor imaging (DTI) [17] provide unique information on brain microstructure. Mean diffusivity (MD) provides an index of isotropic diffusion of water molecules, and fractional anisotropy (FA) provides a measure of the degree of diffusion anisotropy, both of which may be altered by tissue damage. Maps based on the principal diffusivities that compose the diffusion tensor may provide additional information on microstructural alterations. The principal diffusivity ($\lambda 1$), or axial diffusivity, represents water diffusion that is parallel to axons and may be altered by axonal injury; radial diffusivity (an average of $\lambda 2$ and $\lambda 3$), represents water diffusion that is perpendicular to axonal fibers and is thus linked to the microstructure of myelin [18,19,20,21,22,23,24,25,26]. DTI has been used to measure disease-related changes in patients with AD [27,28,29,30,31,32,33,34,35,36,37,38,39], as well as alterations in people with MCI [37,40,41,42,43,44,45,46]. Using DTI, microstructural differences have also been detected in presumed presymptomatic AD including participants with APOE4 genotype [47,48,49] family history of AD [50,51], or a combination of both risk factors [52].

In the present study, we examined the relationship between brain microstructure indexed by DTI and proteins associated with brain health in CSF collected in healthy middle-aged and older adults from the Wisconsin Registry for Alzheimer's Prevention [53]. Additionally, because T1-weighted imaging may inform upon atrophy, we assessed the extent to which biomarkers in CSF were related to volume as assessed via T1-weighted imaging. Based on their utility in distinguishing AD patients from controls [1,2,3,4,5], the CSF biomarkers considered in this study were T-Tau, P-Tau$_{181}$, and Aβ_{42}. In addition to these markers of AD pathology, we analyzed CSF for a structural protein of neurons that is predominantly localized in large-caliber axons (and thus likely sensitive to axonal degeneration in white matter): neurofilament light chain protein (NFL) [54]. We hypothesized that baseline CSF measures of these markers would be related to brain health as measured with DTI, especially in brain regions that are affected early in the AD process–principally temporal and cingulate gray and white matter. We expected higher T-Tau and P-Tau and lower Aβ_{42} in CSF would be related to lower FA, higher MD, and altered radial and axial diffusivity in AD-sensitive brain regions. Additionally, we expected that NFL, being sensitive to axonal alteration, would be especially related to axial diffusivity–reflecting altered axonal health. Although the brain regions affected in AD are well known, the relationship between CSF biomarkers and brain health is a relatively new area of study, accordingly we used voxel-wise analyses (corrected for multiple comparisons) [55] to assess relationships across the entire brain.

Materials and Methods

Study procedures were approved by the University of Wisconsin Health Sciences Institutional Review Board and were in accordance with U.S. federal regulations. All participants provided written informed consent.

Participants

We enrolled 47 participants, four of whom were excluded due to unexpected abnormalities found on their MRI scan by the reviewing radiologist (HAR). The remaining 43 middle- to older-aged participants were 37 years of age to 66 years of age at time of lumbar puncture and CSF collection (mean = 53.67, SD = 7.77); and 42 to 71 years of age at time of follow-up scan (mean = 57.61, SD = 8.03). There were 12 men and 31 women. As a group, participants were well educated (mean = 16.26 years, SD = 2.60). All participants were from the Wisconsin Registry for Alzheimer's Prevention (WRAP) [53] and had at least one parent with AD. WRAP is a registry of cognitively normal adults who are followed longitudinally and comprise individuals who have at least one

parent with late onset AD and a group of controls with no family history of AD [53]. To verify the diagnosis of AD in parents of WRAP participants, parental medical records (and autopsy reports where available) were reviewed by a multidisciplinary diagnostic consensus panel. A diagnosis of AD in parents was made using standard clinical criteria [56,57]. There were no families included with known autosomal dominant mutations. In the final sample, three participants had parents who were diagnosed with AD at autopsy, while the remaining clinical diagnoses were confirmed during a consensus meeting. Twelve participants (28%) were carriers of the $\varepsilon 4$ allele of the apolipoprotein E (APOE4) gene. Inclusion criteria for all subjects consisted of the following: prior visit for lumbar puncture, normal cognitive function determined by neuropsychological evaluation, no contraindications for MRI and a subsequent normal MRI scan, no current diagnosis of major psychiatric disease or other major medical conditions (e.g., diabetes, myocardial infarction, or recent history of cancer), and no history of head trauma.

Neuropsychological Testing

As part of their participation in WRAP, participants received at least one comprehensive neuropsychological assessment. Neuropsychological testing occurred an average of 1.80 years (SD = 1.28 years) out from the MR scan and 2.06 years (SD = 1.20 years) out from their lumbar puncture. In order to screen for changes in cognitive status, participants who were >3 months out from a neuropsychological testing visit also received the Mini Mental State Examination (MMSE) [58] upon the day of scan. We prospectively identified a subset of tests to examine memory, executive function, and speed of processing. These tests were *BVMT (Brief Visuospatial Memory Test, Revised)* total raw score, and delayed recall, which index visuospatial learning and memory [59]; *COWAT* (Controlled Oral Word Association Test; [60]) seconds to complete/raw score, to assess verbal fluency; *Trail Making Test A & B*, to assess motor speed, sequencing, and vigilance and in Trails B, the additional functions of rapid set shifting, serial retention and integration, verbal problem solving, and planning [61]; Wechsler Adult Intelligence Scale Working Memory Index–a composite of arithmetic, digit span, and letter number sequencing [62]–to assess the ability to hold information in working memory; *RAVLT (Rey Auditory Verbal Learning test)* total over the five learning trials, recognition, and 20 minute delayed recall raw scores [63] to assess immediate and delayed verbal memory.

CSF Collection

The CSF collection was performed via lumbar puncture at a baseline visit in a simvastatin trial [64] an average of 3.41 years prior to brain imaging (SD = 1.19 yrs). CSF samples were collected in the morning after a 12-hour overnight fast, aliquoted in sterile polypropylene collection tubes, and stored in a $-80°$C freezer. The samples were subsequently sent in one batch to the Sahlgrenska University Hospital at the University of Gothenburg in Sweden for analysis. CSF T-Tau, P-Tau$_{181}$, and Aβ_{42} analysis was accomplished via xMAP technology and utilizing the INNO-BIA AkzBio3 kit (Innogenetics) as previously described [65]. The xMAP technology is based on flow cytometric separation of antibody-coated microspheres that are labeled with a specific mixture of two fluorescent dyes. xMAP allows for simultaneous measurement of several analytes in the same tube, has low intra- and inter-assay variability, and high reproducibility even at low concentrations. NFL was analyzed using the sandwich ELISA method described in [66] with a limit of quantification of 125 ng/L. All analyses were performed on one occasion by certified laboratory technicians. Intra-assay coefficients of variation were below 10% for all analytes.

Magnetic Resonance Imaging

Participants were invited for brain imaging on the condition that baseline CSF samples were available for analysis. Participants were imaged on a General Electric 3.0 Tesla Discovery MR750 (Waukesha, WI) MRI system with an 8-channel head coil and parallel imaging (ASSET). DTI was acquired using a diffusion-weighted, spin-echo, single-shot, echo planar imaging pulse sequence in 40 encoding directions, B0 = 1300, with eight non-diffusion weighted reference images. The cerebrum was covered using contiguous 2.5 mm thick axial slices, FOV = 24 cm, TR = 8000, E = 67.8, matrix = 96×96, resulting in isotropic 2.5 mm voxels. High order shimming was performed prior to the DTI acquisition to optimize the homogeneity of the magnetic field across the brain and to minimize EPI distortions. A T1-weighted volume was acquired in the axial plane with a 3D fast spoiled gradient-echo (3D EFGRE) sequence using the following parameters: TI = 450 ms; TR = 8.1 ms; TE = 3.2 ms; flip angle = 12°; acquisition matrix = 256×256×156, FOV = 260 mm; slice thickness = 1.0 mm.

MRI Processing

Diffusion-weighted DICOM images were converted into NIFTI format using AFNI (http://afni.nimh.nih.gov/). FA, MD, and lambda maps ($\lambda1$, $\lambda2$ & $\lambda3$) were generated via the FMRIB Software Library (FSL) (http://www.fmrib.ox.ac.uk/fsl/fdt/index.html using the following procedures: (1) image distortions in the DTI data caused by eddy currents were corrected; (2) estimation of diffusion tensors was achieved using DTIFIT; (3) three-dimensional maps of FA, MD, and the 3 eigenvalues ($\lambda1$, $\lambda2$ & $\lambda3$) were computed from the tensors from step (2). Each participant's FA map was aligned to an FA template in Montreal Neurological Institute (MNI) space, comprised of an average of 121 FA maps acquired from healthy participants with similar demographics as the study cohort. Transformations were achieved via 12-parameter affine transformation and nonlinear deformation using Statistical Parametric Mapping software (SPM8 available at http://www.fil.ion.ucl.ac.uk/spm). Estimated transforms from each participant's FA map warping were applied to the participant's remaining DTI maps (MD, $\lambda1$, $\lambda2$ & $\lambda3$) resulting in a transformation of all the original images into MNI space. The normalized FA maps were used to visually inspect for accurate normalization using the "check registration" function in SPM and selecting specific fiber tracts for comparison (corpus callosum, cingulum, superior longitudinal fasciculus). $\lambda2$ & $\lambda3$ maps were averaged to create radial diffusivity maps, and $\lambda1$ was the axial diffusivity map.

Processing of the T1-weighted images was performed using a six class segmentation tool in SPM8. Processing involved bias correction and iterative normalization and segmentation of the original anatomic images [67] into distinct tissue classes (gray matter, white matter, cerebrospinal fluid, skull, fat tissue, and image background) using spatial prior information. Gray matter tissue segments were normalized to MNI template space via a 12-parameter affine transformation and nonlinear deformation (with a warp frequency cutoff of 25). The segmented and normalized gray matter maps were "modulated", which involves scaling the final gray matter maps by the amount of contraction or expansion required to warp the images to the template. The final result was a gray matter probability map for each participant in which the total amount of gray matter remained the same as in the original images. The spatially normalized gray matter maps were

smoothed using an 8-mm Gaussian kernel before being entered into the statistical analysis.

Statistical Analysis

In order to test the relationship between CSF proteins, age, and cognitive function, we performed linear correlation analysis using SPSS (Release 19.0.0, Chicago, SPSS Inc.). CSF biomarkers were log transformed to normalize distribution prior to inclusion in analysis. Differences in CSF protein levels based on APOE status and gender were tested using independent t-tests in SPSS. In order to test the extent to which CSF biomarkers were associated with brain health as indexed by the DTI maps and T1-weighted imaging, voxel-wise linear regression models were implemented via statistical modules available in SPM8. The independent variables were $A\beta_{42}$, total tau (T-Tau), phosphorylated tau (P-Tau$_{181}$), T-Tau/$A\beta_{42}$, and P-Tau$_{181}$/$A\beta_{42}$, while the dependent variables consisted of participants' DTI maps and gray matter probability maps. Due to relatively low levels of NFL in the majority of participants (NFL<125 ng/L; N = 33), NFL was treated as a categorical variable. The detection limit of the assay is NFL<125 ng/L, thus we used this as a cut-point to determine the groups. Differences in brain health based on NFL was tested using voxel-wise ANCOVA, where DTI maps or gray matter probability maps were the dependent variable and the groups were NFL>125 ng/L, and NFL<125 ng/L. Age (at time of MR scan) and gender were included as covariates in all models due to known effects on brain microstructure [68,69,70,71]. Because the imaging was performed in a group of participants that had been randomized in a simvastatin trial, only baseline (pre-simvastatin) CSF measures were used and a treatment vs. placebo covariate was included in the statistical models. All analyses were thresholded at p<.05 corrected for multiple comparisons using false discovery rate (FDR) correction [72]. In order to exclude small clusters and increase the anatomical plausibility of the results, a cluster size threshold of 50 contiguous voxels was used and analyses were restricted to gray and white matter using a binary brain mask. The binary brain mask was computed by thresholding the SPM brain mask in MNI space (which contains voxels that vary from 0 percent to 100 percent probability of brain) at a threshold of.5 or greater (50% probability or greater of being brain). Furthermore, analysis of the gray matter probability maps used an absolute threshold masking of 0.1 to exclude voxels with a low probability of being gray matter.

Results

Demographics, Neuropsychological Function, and CSF Biomarkers

There was a significant positive correlation (P<.05) between age at time of lumbar puncture and T-Tau, T-Tau/$A\beta_{42}$, and P-Tau$_{181}$/$A\beta_{42}$ (Pearson correlation coefficients for age and CSF markers are shown in **Table 1**). Men and women did not differ on CSF biomarker levels of T-Tau, P-Tau$_{181}$, $A\beta_{42}$, T-Tau/$A\beta_{42}$, or P-Tau$_{181}$/$A\beta_{42}$. There was a significant difference in T-Tau and $A\beta_{42}$ between APOE4 positive and APOE4 negative participants, where T-Tau was higher in the non-carriers (m = 4.25) compared to carriers (m = 3.90), t(41) = 2.038, p<.05, and $A\beta_{42}$ was lower in the carriers (m = 5.57) compared to non-carriers (m = 5.83), t(41) = 3.062, p<.05. APOE4 carriers and non-carriers did not differ on age (p = .78).

All participants were cognitively normal as determined by comprehensive neuropsychological testing and as assessed by MMSE (MMSE $\geq$27). Controlling for age and education, linear correlation analysis indicated that baseline CSF biomarker levels

Table 1. Linear correlation among CSF biomarkers and age.

		Age	T-Tau	P-Tau$_{181}$	Aβ$_{42}$	T-Tau/Aβ$_{42}$
Age	Pearson Correlation					
T-Tau	Pearson Correlation	0.367 *				
P-Tau$_{181}$	Pearson Correlation	0.253	0.585 Ŧ			
Aβ$_{42}$	Pearson Correlation	−0.147	0.256	0.228		
T-Tau/Aβ$_{42}$	Pearson Correlation	0.443 *	0.856 Ŧ	0.459 *	−0.281	
P-Tau$_{181}$/Aβ$_{42}$	Pearson Correlation	0.326 *	0.436 *	0.854 Ŧ	−0.310 *	0.599 Ŧ

Significant correlation at P<.05 *.
Significant at p<.001 Ŧ.
doi:10.1371/journal.pone.0037720.t001

were related to a subset of the neuropsychological test scores. WAIS Working Memory Index (scaled for age and education) was positively correlated with T-Tau (r = .307, p<.05) and with T-Tau/Aβ$_{42}$ (r = 0.303, p = .051). However, a scatter-plot revealed that the participant with the highest tau value (>2 SD higher than the mean) performed well on working memory–skewing the results. When this participant was removed from the analysis, the relationships were no longer significant. RAVLT recognition score was negatively correlated with both P-Tau$_{181}$ (r = −.379, p<.05) and P-Tau$_{181}$/Aβ$_{42}$ (r = −.362, p<.05) but was not related to T-Tau, Aβ$_{42}$, or their ratio. No other RAVLT sub-scores or other neuropsychological tests were significantly correlated with the CSF markers.

Imaging Results

Voxel-wise regression analysis indicated that both T-Tau and T-Tau/Aβ$_{42}$ showed robust and widespread positive relationships with several of the DTI measures, specifically MD, axial and radial diffusion. These relationships were extensive in white matter and were prevalent in temporal, parietal and frontal lobes. The locations of peak T-value for MD and FA clusters obtained in the voxel-wise analysis are tabulated in **Table 2** (axial and radial diffusivity results are tabulated in **Table S1**). The brain regions where CSF T-Tau/Aβ$_{42}$ predicted MD values in the voxel-wise regression analysis are shown in **Figure 1**; the positive relationship between T-Tau/Aβ$_{42}$ and MD is shown in **Figure 2** in scatter plots from a subset of the significant clusters found in the voxel-wise regression analysis. The regional overlap between T-Tau and T-Tau/Aβ$_{42}$ SPM result maps (MD, axial and radial diffusivity) was extensive, and is summarized in terms of percent overlap in **Table 3**.

At a statistical threshold of p<.05 (FDR corrected for multiple comparisons) there was no relationship between T-Tau or T-Tau/Aβ$_{42}$ and FA. Furthermore, neither P-Tau$_{181}$ nor P-Tau/Aβ$_{42}$ were related to any of the DTI measures (FA, MD, axial or radial diffusivity). Higher Aβ$_{42}$ in CSF was related to higher FA in medial frontal gyrus, but not related to MD, axial or radial diffusivity. Participants with NFL>125 ng/L showed a single region of higher FA in middle temporal gyrus white matter compared to control, with no differences in MD, axial or radial diffusivity. Complete results (cluster extent, T-value, and locations) for all CSF measures and FA and MD maps are in **Table 2** (axial and radial diffusivity results are tabulated in **Table S1**). None of the CSF biomarkers predicted gray matter volume as indexed by the modulated gray matter probability maps (FDR p<.05).

Discussion

General

AD-related CSF biomarkers are linked with global and regional brain volumes in healthy elderly [12,13,14]. In this study, we assessed the relationship between brain tissue microstructure measured with DTI and AD-related CSF biomarkers. Additionally, we assessed the relationship between CSF biomarkers and gray matter volume. Our group has previously found that cognitively healthy people with parental family history of AD show microstructural brain differences compared to those without risk for AD [50]. In this study, we found that CSF biomarkers previously associated with AD are related to brain tissue microstructure in similar regions as those previously found to be associated with parental family history.

While gray matter volume was not related to any of the CSF biomarkers in this study, CSF biomarkers were related to white matter health as indexed by DTI; interestingly, the regions of significant association were mostly *adjacent* to critical gray matter structures that are known to be affected in AD. This was especially true for T-Tau and T-Tau/Aβ$_{42}$, where higher CSF levels were related to higher axial, radial, and mean diffusivity in a large swath of temporal lobe white matter adjacent to hippocampus. Several studies now point toward early involvement of white matter in AD development, including human studies on AD risk [48,49,50,52,73], and studies on a triple transgenic mouse model of AD indicating white matter changes may precede other measurable pathology in AD [74,75]. In contrast, studies conducted in AD and memory impaired patients have found that CSF biomarker levels are related to gray matter structures including hippocampus, entorhinal cortex [76], and posterior cingulate cortex [77]. One possibility is that early AD pathology involves axonal or myelin degeneration and that cortical change is only measurable at later disease stages or in more elderly individuals.

White Matter Degeneration in AD: Myelin and Axons

White matter degeneration in diagnosed AD is confirmed by several human post mortem studies [78,79,80,81]. MRI enabled ante mortem studies substantiate post mortem findings, showing decreased regional white matter volumes in AD compared to controls [82,83,84,85,86,87,88,89,90,91,92] and differences in water diffusion properties in white matter [27,28,29,30,31,32,33,34,35,36,37,93]. White matter alterations in confirmed AD are a combination of axonal and myelin alteration, yet it is unknown whether white matter changes are secondary to damage of the neuronal soma, involve primary axonal

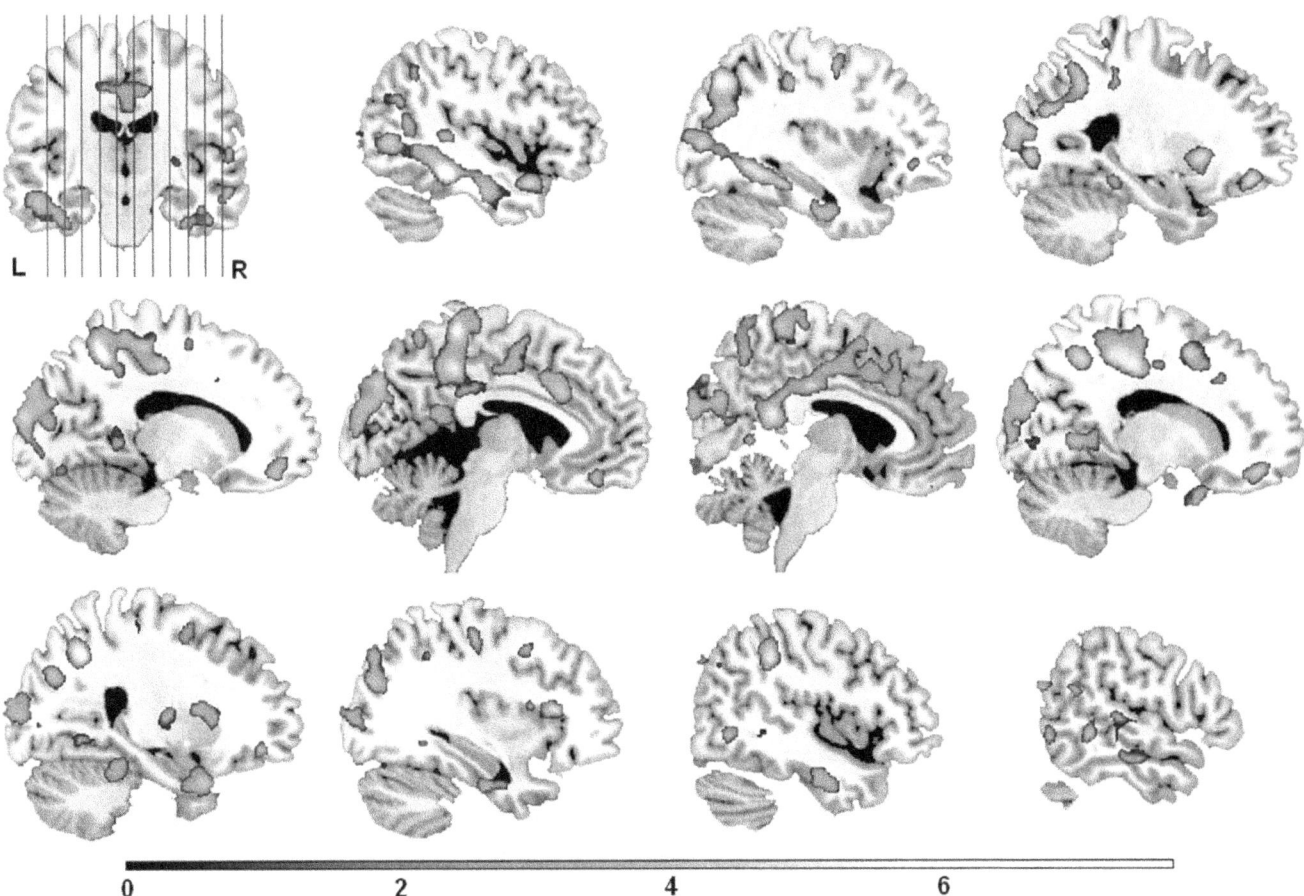

Figure 1. CSF T-Tau/Aβ42 and mean diffusivity. Higher T-Tau/Aβ42 at baseline was associated with increased mean diffusivity in follow-up scanning in several brain regions, encompassing both gray and white matter. As shown above, this relationship was especially prominent in temporal lobe white matter adjacent to hippocampus, but also encompassing gray and white matter in frontal and parietal lobes, portions of occipital white matter, and small clusters in cerebellum. Results are FDR corrected for multiple comparisons (p<.05) and displayed here with a cluster size threshold of 20 or more voxels. Sections are shown in sagittal view beginning from the left side of the brain to right. Variations in the color map reflect the size of the T-statistic (indexed by the color bar at bottom).
doi:10.1371/journal.pone.0037720.g001

degeneration [94,95], are linked with myelin degeneration [39,46,96,97,98], or represent some combination of these events.

In our study we measured the relationship between CSF biomarkers and DTI measures that are presumably related to axonal health (axial diffusivity) and myelin health (radial diffusivity). We found that both T-Tau and T-Tau/Aβ42 predicted axial and radial diffusivity, suggesting these CSF biomarkers are potentially related to both neuronal axon integrity and health of oligodendrocyte synthesized myelin. Furthermore, the analyses of axial, radial, and mean diffusivity produced statistical maps that were highly overlapping, suggesting that alterations in one cell component (e.g. neuronal axons) could very well be associated with related alterations in another cell component (myelin).

Although CSF measures of myelin were not available to us in this study, we assessed axonal degeneration via CSF measured neurofilament light protein. Neurofilament proteins are major constituents of the axonal cytoskeleton, consisting of three polypeptides; light (NFL), medium and heavy subunits. NFL proteins are most related to large-caliber axons [99] and when axons are damaged, NFL is released into CSF. NFL proteins measured in CSF are significantly higher in AD compared to controls [66,100,101,102,103,104]. In our study,a group comparison based on CSF NFL levels yielded a single region of difference in middle temporal gyrus white matter, where participants with

higher CSF NFL showed higher FA. Although we expected that the group with presumably greater axonal degeneration would show lower FA, it's possible that early stage axonal degeneration in the presence of intact myelin could lead to higher anisotropy. Another possibility is a loss of crossing fibers in this region–which could lead to higher FA. Although we did not find a relationship between CSF NFL and the mean, radial, and axial diffusivity maps at a relatively conservative statistical threshold, analyses performed at uncorrected (for multiple comparisons) thresholds did show differences between NFL groups. Interestingly, the group with higher CSF NFL showed higher axial diffusivity in cingulum and white matter adjacent to hippocampus. Because only ten participants in our study had NFL levels greater than the detection limit of 125 ng/L, we were likely underpowered to find these subtle differences at corrected thresholds and further work will be needed to expand upon these preliminary findings.

Classic Pathology: Abnormal Phosphorylation of Tau and Amyloid Deposition

In AD, abnormal phosphorylation of tau protein and deposition of amyloid are considered primary processes underlying neuronal degeneration. Hyperphosphorylation of tau and its subsequent release from the cell means markers of tau measured in CSF increase compared to controls [105]. In contrast, CSF markers of

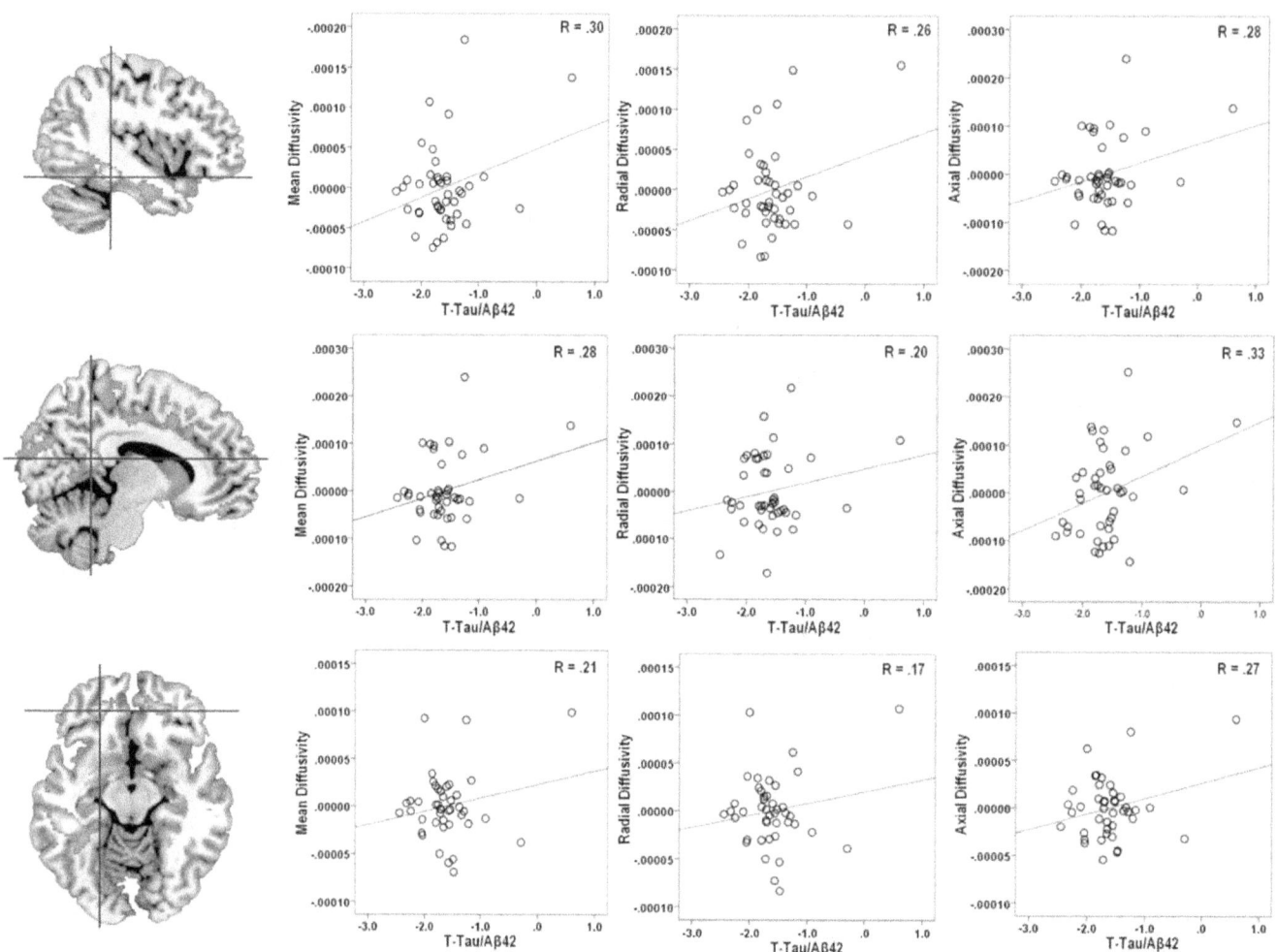

Figure 2. T-Tau/Aβ42 Plotted against mean, radial, and axial diffusivity. Shown here are the results of the voxel-wise analysis, where regions with color overlay are those where higher T-Tau/Aβ42 was associated with higher diffusivity (mean, radial, and axial). In order to illustrate the relationship between T-Tau/Aβ42 and the diffusivity maps, we extracted diffusion values from representative regions of significant correlation in the voxel-wise analysis and plotted them against T-Tau/Aβ42. Shown on the top row are diffusion values extracted from the left temporal lobe (x = −42, y = −34, z = −16) plotted against T-Tau/Aβ42. In the middle row are diffusion values extracted from right posterior cingulum bundle (x = 8, y = −46, z = 16) plotted against T-Tau/Aβ42. In the bottom row are diffusion values extracted from left inferior frontal white matter (x = −22, y = 43, z = −12) plotted against T-Tau/Aβ42. Blue crosshairs overlaid on the brain sections indicate the location of the extracted values. Each point in the scatter represents diffusion values from one participant (n = 43). T-Tau/Aβ42 values were log-transformed and mean, radial, and axial diffusivity values were adjusted for age at time of scan, sex, and treatment (CSF data were collected at baseline in a Simvastatin treatment trial, data from the prevention trial are not shown here).
doi:10.1371/journal.pone.0037720.g002

amyloid decrease as amyloid is deposited in the brain [3,4,106,107]. In our study, we found widespread relationships between elevated CSF T-Tau and altered measures of brain tissue microstructure indexed by mean, radial, and axial diffusivity, with somewhat similar but also distinctive patterns occurring for T-Tau/Aβ$_{42}$ (up to 70% overlap in the radial diffusivity maps). Although the localized source of tau protein measured in CSF is unknown, higher levels in our study were related to higher diffusion across temporal, parietal, and frontal lobes–particularly in white matter. We speculate CSF tau protein may have originated from axons in these brain regions, but we can not rule out that tau may have also originated from oligodendroglia [108]. Phosphorylation of tau is associated with the development of glial tangles in human patients with AD [109,110,111], as well as in animals expressing mutant tau [112,113,114]. Interestingly, CSF levels of tau phosphorylated at threonine 181 did not show a relationship with any of the DTI measures at the p<.05$_{FDR}$ threshold. Although some studies suggest that CSF P-Tau$_{181}$ does

not correlate with neuropathological burden in AD [115], in our study it is possible that the relationship between P-Tau$_{181}$ and tissue microstructure was too subtle to survive our statistical threshold. Indeed, when we performed exploratory analyses at uncorrected (for multiple comparisons) thresholds, higher P-Tau$_{181}$ was associated with altered tissue microstructure. Furthermore, P-Tau$_{181}$ and P-Tau$_{181}$/Aβ$_{42}$ were the only biomarkers related to memory function in this study. Nonetheless, considering alternative sites of tau phosphorylation will likely be important for understanding early AD and in AD biomarker development.

While T-Tau and T-Tau/Aβ$_{42}$ showed widespread relationships with the DTI measures, CSF Aβ$_{42}$ was associated with lower anisotropy of water (FA) only in medial frontal cortex and underlying white matter. Deposition of brain amyloid in AD likely involves frontal involvement at the earliest stages [116], which presumably could have resulted in altered tissue microstructure in this study. Studies using amyloid imaging in this cohort are

Table 2. Regions where CSF biomarkers were significantly correlated with FA and MD in the voxel-wise analyses.

	MNI coordinates x y z	Peak T value	k (mm^3)
T-Tau & Fractional Anisotropy	×	×	×
T-Tau & Mean Diffusivity			
R Parietal Lobe WM	26, −59, 42	7.89	13890
R Medial Frontal Gyrus	16, 7, 52	6.37	478
L Middle Frontal Gyrus	−24, 43, −14	5.83	259
R Middle Temporal Gyrus	58, −42, −1	5.33	159
L Frontal Lobe, WM	−18, −4, 59	5.25	154
R Corpus Callosum	12, −45, 12	5.23	414
R Medial Frontal WM	12, 46, −18	5.21	207
L Superior Temporal Gyrus WM	−60, −23, 7	4.73	112
R Lentiform Nucleus, Putamen	26, −9, 7	4.45	256
R Superior Temporal Gyrus WM	60, −24, −1	4.39	145
L Temporal Lobe WM	−52, −13, −21	4.37	143
L Inferior Frontal Gyrus	−40, 25, 3	4.25	56
R Fusiform WM	38, −71, −21	4.06	83
R Entorhinal WM	20, 11, −28	3.99	110
R Lingual Gyrus	28, −61, −4	3.96	74
R Middle Temporal Gyrus	46, −63, −6	3.91	52
L Inferior Parietal Lobule	−52, −41, 40	3.75	63
P-Tau & Fractional Anisotropy	×	×	×
P-Tau & Mean Diffusivity	×	×	×
Aβ$_{42}$ & Fractional Anisotropy			
L,R Medial Frontal Gyrus	0 11 −24	6.27	66
Aβ$_{42}$ & Mean Diffusivity	×	×	×
T-Tau/Aβ$_{42}$ & Fractional Anisotropy	×	×	×
T-Tau/Aβ$_{42}$ & Mean Diffusivity			
L Temporal Lobe WM	−44 −36 −13	7.71	11374
R Uncus	20 9 −27	6.11	286
L Middle Frontal Gyrus WM	−22 43 −12	5.69	257
R Insula WM	36 26 11	5.50	229
R Supramarginal Gyrus WM	44 −39 39	5.17	225
R Medial Frontal Gyrus WM	12 46 −16	5.09	204
R Middle Temporal Gyrus	58 −42 −1	5.07	126
L Superior Temporal Gyrus	−42 13 −22	5.05	157
L Putamen	−24 14 0	5.01	100
R Middle Temporal Gyrus	48 −63 −4	4.87	105
R Superior Temporal Gyrus WM	58 −24 5	4.68	154
L Superior Temporal Gyrus WM	−62 −21 7	4.54	109
R Temporal Lobe WM	42 −6 −31	4.48	209
L Superior Temporal Gyrus WM	−62 −43 14	4.41	99
R Superior Occipital Gyrus WM	34 −77 26	4.23	409
R Occipital Lobe WM	28 −59 −4	4.20	87
R Middle Temporal Gyrus WM	56 −14 −16	4.04	76
R Precentral Gyrus WM	34 −22 51	3.91	100
L Frontal Lobe WM	−30 −35 39	3.82	100
R Cerebellum, Anterior Lobe	24 −37 −21	3.78	118
R Putamen	28 −10 3	3.76	82
P-Tau/Aβ$_{42}$ & Fractional Anisotropy	×	×	×
P-Tau/Aβ$_{42}$ & Mean Diffusivity	×	×	×

Table 2. Cont.

	MNI coordinates x y z	Peak T value	k (mm³)
NFL & Fractional Anisotropy			
L Middle Temporal Gyrus WM	−42 −65 11	6.66	40
NFL & Mean Diffusivity	–	–	–

MNI: Montreal Neurological Institute; k: cluster size; T-Tau: Total Tau; P-Tau: Phosphorylated Tau; WM: White Matter; L: Left; R: Right.
× No relationship with any regions at FDR corrected threshold p<.05.
– No group differences in any region at FDR corrected threshold p<.05.
doi:10.1371/journal.pone.0037720.t002

expected to shed further light on regional amyloid deposition in the earliest stages of AD.

CSF Biomarkers in Cognitively Healthy Adults

In healthy older adults, levels of AD biomarkers measured in CSF are related to age, cognition, structural brain volume, and AD risk factors including APOE4 status [10,117,118] and family history [51]. In our sample of healthy adults with elevated risk for AD, we found significant positive correlations between age and T-Tau, T-Tau/$A\beta_{42}$, and P-Tau$_{181}$/$A\beta_{42}$. Alone, $A\beta_{42}$ was not related to age. We also found that both T-Tau and $A\beta_{42}$ differed between APOE4 carriers and non-carriers. Similar to previous studies, $A\beta_{42}$ was lower in the carriers compared to non-carriers–conceivably suggesting greater amyloid deposition in the group at greater risk for AD. Interesting, we found that the APOE4 carriers in this sample showed lower T-Tau compared to non-carriers. These T-Tau findings are consistent with our previous report on CSF biomarkers in middle-aged at-risk adults [119]. Although APOE4 has been linked with higher T-Tau in some studies [120,121], our sample differs in that all of the participants were positive for parental family history of AD–a group which in middle age shows higher T-Tau levels than the general population [51]. Further studies will be needed to dissociate the effects of APOE and family history of AD on CSF biomarkers in middle-age.

All of the participants in our study tested cognitively normal. Among the cognitive tests, only recognition memory was related to any of the CSF measures. Participants with higher P-Tau$_{181}$ and P-Tau$_{181}$/$A\beta_{42}$ levels had lower recognition on a list learning test (RAVLT). Glodzik et al. have also found a relationship between P-Tau (P-Tau$_{231}$) and memory function [11], and combined use of P-Tau$_{181}$ and $A\beta_{42}$ has also been shown to predict longitudinal subjective memory impairment in healthy elderly [122]. Because our study was cross-sectional and restricted to cognitively healthy participants, the limited range and variability of the cognitive scores may have impacted our power to detect relationships between the CSF biomarkers and other cognitive tests in our study.

Previous brain imaging studies in healthy adults have found that CSF biomarkers are related to volumetric measures. Healthy elderly individuals from ADNI with low CSF $A\beta_{42}$ levels have significantly higher whole brain loss over time, ventricular expansion, and greater rates of hippocampal atrophy [14]. Fjell et al. [13] also examined CSF biomarker and brain relationships in healthy elderly individuals from ADNI. Lower $A\beta_{42}$ correlated with 1-year change in several regions including putamen, thalamus, superior temporal cortex, cingulate, and frontal brain regions, whereas higher T-Tau/$A\beta_{42}$ was related to atrophy in amygdala, paracentral cortex, and ventricular regions. Higher P-Tau was related to 1-year change in amygdala, paracentral cortex, posterior cingulate, and pallidum. Fjell et al.'s study is also one of the few to show a relationship between P-Tau and cerebral white matter, with higher P-Tau predicting lower white matter volume. P-Tau reported in these studies was assayed for tau phosphorylated at threonine 181, although a similarly aged healthy cohort evaluated at baseline and 2 years later by Glodzik et al. [11] has shown that P-Tau$_{231}$ is also associated with longitudinal medial temporal lobe volume decline and memory function.

In our study of adults with parental family history of AD and a high frequency of APOE4, we found relationships between CSF measures and DTI in several brain regions shown in previous volumetric studies of healthy participants, including temporal, cingulate, and frontal cortices. We did not find a relationship between the CSF biomarkers and gray matter volume (indexed by T1-weighted imaging) in any brain regions, possibly due to the younger age of our cohort in whom tissue changes are likely to be more subtle and less easily detected with volumetric imaging. Using DTI, we had the additional advantage of being able to

Table 3. Percent of regional overlap between statistical parametric mapping result maps.

	T-Tau & MD	T-Tau & Rad.	T-Tau & Ax.	T-Tau/$A\beta_{42}$ & Ax.	T-Tau/$A\beta_{42}$ & Rad.
T-Tau/$A\beta_{42}$ & MD*	66%	74%	60%	85%	95%
T-Tau/$A\beta_{42}$ & Rad. Diff.	57%	70%	49%	68%	
T-Tau/$A\beta_{42}$ & Ax. Diff.	54%	58%	58%		
T-Tau & Ax. Diff.	84%	83%			
T-Tau & Rad. Diff.	70%				

All results maps were the product of a linear correlation analysis, where the CSF measures (T-Tau and T-Tau/Aβ42) were used to predict the diffusion measures (MD, axial and radial diffusivity). T-Tau: Total Tau; MD: Mean Diffusivity; Rad: Radial; Ax: Axial; Diff: Diffusivity.
*Result map shown in Figure 1.
doi:10.1371/journal.pone.0037720.t003

evaluate potentially subtle effects in white matter, and these relationships were robust and widespread.

Limitations

While the results of this study are promising, potential limitations should be noted. We adopted a voxel-wise approach in order to assess the extent to which CSF biomarkers were related to brain microstructure and volume across gray and white matter tissue. While we took great care to evaluate for potential errors during registration of the DTI maps to a common template, methods that employ registration to a template may be susceptible to subtle error and statistical effects may be influenced by the size of smoothing filters used in voxel-wise analyses. As a further comment on the DTI results, we would like to note that this study used a tensor model which resolves a single fiber direction within each voxel. We found very robust results when analyzing the MD, axial, and radial diffusivity maps, compared to the FA maps. Due to the complex architecture of white matter, employing FA derived from the tensor model may not have captured the full information available with alternative methods of DTI acquisition and higher order modeling [123]. We should also note that our population was composed solely of participants with parental family history of AD and the frequency of APOE4 was 28%. While this group is at increased risk for AD and thus provides a powerful cohort for examining AD biomarkers, the lack of family history negative participants and high frequency of APOE4 potentially limits the generalizability of our results to a healthy population in addition to limiting our ability to measure relationships between CSF biomarkers and brain measures that are independent of AD risk. Additionally, although our study was longitudinal in the sense that baseline CSF was collected followed by MRI acquisition approximately three and a half years later, simultaneous MRI and CSF collection over two or more time points would have yielded greater power to map out longitudinal change in these measures. Based on the results of this study, additional longitudinal work is warranted. Finally, while our results begin to address the

pattern of white matter changes that may occur in the earliest stages of AD, employing white matter biomarker assays in larger cohorts of older adults is expected to clarify the nature of white matter changes in the earliest disease stages.

Summary

CSF biomarkers previously associated with AD are related to brain tissue microstructure. This study supports an emerging theory that brain white matter alterations are an early event in AD pathogenesis. The mechanisms that underlie white matter alterations and the nature of these alterations deserve further study.

Supporting Information

Table S1   Regions where CSF biomarkers were significantly correlated with axial and radial diffusivity in the voxel-wise analyses.
(DOC)

Acknowledgments

The authors gratefully acknowledge Amy Hawley, Nancy Davenport, Erik Kastman, Hanna Blazel, and Jennifer Oh, as well as the support of researchers and staff at the Waisman Center, University of Wisconsin-Madison, for their assistance in recruitment, data collection, and data analysis. Above all, we wish to thank our dedicated volunteers for their participation in this research.

Author Contributions

Conceived and designed the experiments: BBB CMC LP. Performed the experiments: BBB CMC HZ KB AAW MLR ALA HAR SA MAS. Analyzed the data: BBB CMC HZ KB AAW ACB MLR AS ALA SCJ. Contributed reagents/materials/analysis tools: HZ KB ALA. Wrote the paper: BBB CMC SCJ HZ KB AAW OCO AS MLR ACB ALA HAR LP SA MAS.

References

1. De Meyer G, Shapiro F, Vanderstichele H, Vanmechelen E, Engelborghs S, et al. (2010) Diagnosis-independent Alzheimer disease biomarker signature in cognitively normal elderly people. Arch Neurol 67: 949–956.

2. Shaw LM, Vanderstichele H, Knapik-Czajka M, Clark CM, Aisen PS, et al. (2009) Cerebrospinal fluid biomarker signature in Alzheimer's disease neuroimaging initiative subjects. Ann Neurol 65: 403–413.

3. Galasko D, Chang L, Motter R, Clark CM, Kaye J, et al. (1998) High cerebrospinal fluid tau and low amyloid beta42 levels in the clinical diagnosis of Alzheimer disease and relation to apolipoprotein E genotype. Arch Neurol 55: 937–945.

4. Sunderland T, Linker G, Mirza N, Putnam KT, Friedman DL, et al. (2003) Decreased beta-amyloid1–42 and increased tau levels in cerebrospinal fluid of patients with Alzheimer disease. Jama 289: 2094–2103.

5. Smach MA, Charfeddine B, Ben Othman L, Lammouchi T, Dridi H, et al. (2009) Evaluation of cerebrospinal fluid tau/beta-amyloid(42) ratio as diagnostic markers for Alzheimer disease. Eur Neurol 62: 349–355.

6. Davatzikos C, Bhatt P, Shaw LM, Batmanghelich KN, Trojanowski JQ (2011) Prediction of MCI to AD conversion, via MRI, CSF biomarkers, and pattern classification. Neurobiol Aging.

7. Hampel H, Teipel SJ, Fuchsberger T, Andreasen N, Wiltfang J, et al. (2004) Value of CSF beta-amyloid1–42 and tau as predictors of Alzheimer's disease in patients with mild cognitive impairment. Mol Psychiatry 9: 705–710.

8. Hansson O, Zetterberg H, Buchhave P, Andreasson U, Londos E, et al. (2007) Prediction of Alzheimer's disease using the CSF Abeta42/Abeta40 ratio in patients with mild cognitive impairment. Dement Geriatr Cogn Disord 23: 316–320.

9. Mattsson N, Zetterberg H, Hansson O, Andreasen N, Parnetti L, et al. (2009) CSF biomarkers and incipient Alzheimer disease in patients with mild cognitive impairment. Jama 302: 385–393.

10. Fagan AM, Roe CM, Xiong C, Mintun MA, Morris JC, et al. (2007) Cerebrospinal fluid tau/beta-amyloid(42) ratio as a prediction of cognitive decline in nondemented older adults. Arch Neurol 64: 343–349.

11. Glodzik L, de Santi S, Tsui WH, Mosconi L, Zinkowski R, et al. (2011) Phosphorylated tau 231, memory decline and medial temporal atrophy in normal elders. Neurobiol Aging.

12. Desikan RS, Sabuncu MR, Schmansky NJ, Reuter M, Cabral HJ, et al. (2010) Selective disruption of the cerebral neocortex in Alzheimer's disease. PLoS One 5: e12853.

13. Fjell AM, Walhovd KB, Fennema-Notestine C, McEvoy LK, Hagler DJ, et al. (2010) Brain atrophy in healthy aging is related to CSF levels of Abeta1–42. Cereb Cortex 20: 2069–2079.

14. Schott JM, Bartlett JW, Fox NC, Barnes J (2010) Increased brain atrophy rates in cognitively normal older adults with low cerebrospinal fluid Abeta1–42. Ann Neurol 68: 825–834.

15. Ott BR, Cohen RA, Gongvatana A, Okonkwo OC, Johanson CE, et al. (2010) Brain ventricular volume and cerebrospinal fluid biomarkers of Alzheimer's disease. J Alzheimers Dis 20: 647–657.

16. Fagan AM, Head D, Shah AR, Marcus D, Mintun M, et al. (2009) Decreased cerebrospinal fluid Abeta(42) correlates with brain atrophy in cognitively normal elderly. Ann Neurol 65: 176–183.

17. Basser PJ, Pierpaoli C (1996) Microstructural and physiological features of tissues elucidated by quantitative-diffusion-tensor MRI. J Magn Reson B 111: 209–219.

18. Hofling AA, Kim JH, Fantz CR, Sands MS, Song SK (2009) Diffusion tensor imaging detects axonal injury and demyelination in the spinal cord and cranial nerves of a murine model of globoid cell leukodystrophy. NMR Biomed.

19. Feng S, Hong Y, Zhou Z, Jinsong Z, Xiaofeng D, et al. (2009) Monitoring of acute axonal injury in the swine spinal cord with EAE by diffusion tensor imaging. J Magn Reson Imaging 30: 277–285.

20. Mac Donald CL, Dikranian K, Bayly P, Holtzman D, Brody D (2007) Diffusion tensor imaging reliably detects experimental traumatic axonal injury and indicates approximate time of injury. J Neurosci 27: 11869–11876.

21. Sun SW, Liang HF, Trinkaus K, Cross AH, Armstrong RC, et al. (2006) Noninvasive detection of cuprizone induced axonal damage and demyelination in the mouse corpus callosum. Magn Reson Med 55: 302–308.

22. Song SK, Yoshino J, Le TQ, Lin SJ, Sun SW, et al. (2005) Demyelination increases radial diffusivity in corpus callosum of mouse brain. Neuroimage 26: 132–140.

23. Song SK, Sun SW, Ramsbottom MJ, Chang C, Russell J, et al. (2002) Dysmyelination revealed through MRI as increased radial (but unchanged axial) diffusion of water. Neuroimage 17: 1429–1436.

24. Harsan LA, Poulet P, Guignard B, Steibel J, Parizel N, et al. (2006) Brain dysmyelination and recovery assessment by noninvasive in vivo diffusion tensor magnetic resonance imaging. J Neurosci Res 83: 392–402.

25. Budde MD, Kim JH, Liang HF, Russell JH, Cross AH, et al. (2007) Axonal injury detected by in vivo diffusion tensor imaging correlates with neurological disability in a mouse model of multiple sclerosis. NMR Biomed.

26. Wu Q, Butzkueven H, Gresle M, Kirchhoff F, Friedhuber A, et al. (2007) MR diffusion changes correlate with ultra-structurally defined axonal degeneration in murine optic nerve. Neuroimage 37: 1138–1147.

27. Bozzali M, Falini A, Franceschi M, Cercignani M, Zuffi M, et al. (2002) White matter damage in Alzheimer's disease assessed in vivo using diffusion tensor magnetic resonance imaging. J Neurol Neurosurg Psychiatry 72: 742–746.

28. Fellgiebel A, Schermuly I, Gerhard A, Keller I, Albrecht J, et al. (2008) Functional relevant loss of long association fibre tracts integrity in early Alzheimer's disease. Neuropsychologia 46: 1698–1706.

29. Hanyu H, Asano T, Sakurai H, Imon Y, Iwamoto T, et al. (1999) Diffusion-weighted and magnetization transfer imaging of the corpus callosum in Alzheimer's disease. J Neurol Sci 167: 37–44.

30. Huang J, Friedland RP, Auchus AP (2007) Diffusion tensor imaging of normal-appearing white matter in mild cognitive impairment and early Alzheimer disease: preliminary evidence of axonal degeneration in the temporal lobe. AJNR Am J Neuroradiol 28: 1943–1948.

31. Rose SE, Janke AL, Chalk JB (2008) Gray and white matter changes in Alzheimer's disease: a diffusion tensor imaging study. J Magn Reson Imaging 27: 20–26.

32. Salat DH, Tuch DS, van der Kouwe AJ, Greve DN, Pappu V, et al. (2008) White matter pathology isolates the hippocampal formation in Alzheimer's disease. Neurobiol Aging.

33. Stahl R, Dietrich O, Teipel SJ, Hampel H, Reiser MF, et al. (2007) White matter damage in Alzheimer disease and mild cognitive impairment: assessment with diffusion-tensor MR imaging and parallel imaging techniques. Radiology 243: 483–492.

34. Takahashi S, Yonezawa H, Takahashi J, Kudo M, Inoue T, et al. (2002) Selective reduction of diffusion anisotropy in white matter of Alzheimer disease brains measured by 3.0 Tesla magnetic resonance imaging. Neurosci Lett 332: 45–48.

35. Xie S, Xiao JX, Gong GL, Zang YF, Wang YH, et al. (2006) Voxel-based detection of white matter abnormalities in mild Alzheimer disease. Neurology 66: 1845–1849.

36. Duan JH, Wang HQ, Xu J, Lin X, Chen SQ, et al. (2006) White matter damage of patients with Alzheimer's disease correlated with the decreased cognitive function. Surg Radiol Anat 28: 150–156.

37. Medina D, deToledo-Morrell L, Urresta F, Gabrieli JDE, Moseley M, et al. (2006) White matter changes in mild cognitive impairment and AD: A diffusion tensor imaging study. Neurobiology of Aging 27: 663–672.

38. Canu E, McLaren DG, Fitzgerald ME, Bendlin BB, Zoccatelli G, et al. (2009) Microstructural Diffusion Changes are Independent of Macrostructural Volume Loss in Moderate to Severe Alzheimer's Disease. J Alzheimers Dis.

39. Stricker NH, Schweinsburg BC, Delano-Wood L, Wierenga CE, Bangen KJ, et al. (2009) Decreased white matter integrity in late-myelinating fiber pathways in Alzheimer's disease supports retrogenesis. Neuroimage 45: 10–16.

40. Cho H, Yang DW, Shon YM, Kim BS, Kim YI, et al. (2008) Abnormal integrity of corticocortical tracts in mild cognitive impairment: a diffusion tensor imaging study. J Korean Med Sci 23: 477–483.

41. Fellgiebel A, Wille P, Muller MJ, Winterer G, Scheurich A, et al. (2004) Ultrastructural hippocampal and white matter alterations in mild cognitive impairment: a diffusion tensor imaging study. Dement Geriatr Cogn Disord 18: 101–108.

42. Kantarci K, Jack CR, Jr., Xu YC, Campeau NG, O'Brien PC, et al. (2001) Mild cognitive impairment and Alzheimer disease: regional diffusivity of water. Radiology 219: 101–107.

43. Lovblad KO, Delavelle J, Wetzel S, Kelekis AD, Assal F, et al. (2004) ADC mapping of the aging frontal lobes in mild cognitive impairment. Neuroradiology 46: 282–286.

44. Rose SE, McMahon KL, Janke AL, O'Dowd B, de Zubicaray G, et al. (2006) Diffusion indices on magnetic resonance imaging and neuropsychological performance in amnestic mild cognitive impairment. J Neurol Neurosurg Psychiatry 77: 1122–1128.

45. Fellgiebel A, Muller MJ, Wille P, Dellani PR, Scheurich A, et al. (2005) Color-coded diffusion-tensor-imaging of posterior cingulate fiber tracts in mild cognitive impairment. Neurobiol Aging 26: 1193–1198.

46. Stenset V, Bjornerud A, Fjell AM, Walhovd KB, Hofoss D, et al. (2009) Cingulum fiber diffusivity and CSF T-tau in patients with subjective and mild cognitive impairment. Neurobiol Aging.

47. Nierenberg J, Pomara N, Hoptman MJ, Sidtis JJ, Ardekani BA, et al. (2005) Abnormal white matter integrity in healthy apolipoprotein E epsilon4 carriers. Neuroreport 16: 1369–1372.

48. Persson J, Lind J, Larsson A, Ingvar M, Cruts M, et al. (2006) Altered brain white matter integrity in healthy carriers of the APOE epsilon4 allele: a risk for AD? Neurology 66: 1029–1033.

49. Ryan L, Walther K, Bendlin BB, Lue LF, Walker DG, et al. (2011) Age-related differences in white matter integrity and cognitive function are related to APOE status. Neuroimage 54: 1565–1577.

50. Bendlin BB, Ries ML, Canu E, Sodhi A, Lazar M, et al. (2010) White matter is altered with parental family history of Alzheimer's disease. Alzheimers Dement 6: 394–403.

51. Xiong C, Roe CM, Buckles V, Fagan A, Holtzman D, et al. (2011) Role of Family History for Alzheimer Biomarker Abnormalities in the Adult Children Study. Arch Neurol 68: 1313–1319.

52. Smith CD, Chebrolu H, Andersen AH, Powell DA, Lovell MA, et al. (2010) White matter diffusion alterations in normal women at risk of Alzheimer's disease. Neurobiol Aging 31: 1122–1131.

53. Sager MA, Hermann B, La Rue A (2005) Middle-aged children of persons with Alzheimer's disease: APOE genotypes and cognitive function in the Wisconsin Registry for Alzheimer's Prevention. J Geriatr Psychiatry Neurol 18: 245–249.

54. Olsson B, Zetterberg H, Hampel H, Blennow K (2011) Biomarker-based dissection of neurodegenerative diseases. Prog Neurobiol.

55. Ashburner J, Friston KJ (2000) Voxel-based morphometry–the methods. Neuroimage 11: 805–821.

56. Morris JC, Heyman A, Mohs RC, Hughes JP, van Belle G, et al. (1989) The Consortium to Establish a Registry for Alzheimer's Disease (CERAD). Part I. Clinical and neuropsychological assessment of Alzheimer's disease. Neurology 39: 1159–1165.

57. McKhann G, Drachman D, Folstein M, Katzman R, Price D, et al. (1984) Clinical diagnosis of Alzheimer's disease: Report of the NINCDS-ADRDA workgroup under the auspices of the Department of Health and Human Services Task Force on Alzheimer's disease. Neurology 34: 939–944.

58. Folstein MF, Folstein SE, McHugh PR (1975) "Mini Mental State": a practical method for grading the cognitive state of patients for the clinician. Journal of Psychiatry Research 12: 189–198.

59. Benedict R (1997) Brief Visuospatial Memory Test-Revised. Lutz, FL: Psychological Assessment Resources Inc.

60. Benton AL, Hamsher K, Sivan AB (1983) Multilingual Aphasia Examination. Iowa City: AJA Associates.

61. Reitan RM, Wolfson D (1993) The Halstead-Reitan Neuropsychological Test Battery: Theory and clinical interpretation. Tucson: Neuropsychology Press.

62. Wechsler D (1997) Wechsler Adult Intelligence Scale-Third Edition. New York: Psych Corp.

63. Rey A (1964) L'examen clinique en psychologie. Paris: Presses Universitaires de France.

64. Carlsson CM, Gleason CE, Johnson SC, Xu G, Huang Y, et al. (2010) A randomized, double-blind placebo-controlled trial of simvastatin on CSF, MRI, and cognitive biomarkers in middle-aged adults at risk for Alzheimer's disease: The ESPRIT Study. Alzheimer's and Dementia 6: S151–S152.

65. Olsson A, Vanderstichele H, Andreasen N, De Meyer G, Wallin A, et al. (2005) Simultaneous measurement of beta-amyloid(1–42), total tau, and phosphorylated tau (Thr181) in cerebrospinal fluid by the xMAP technology. Clin Chem 51: 336–345.

66. Rosengren LE, Karlsson JE, Karlsson JO, Persson LI, Wikkelso C (1996) Patients with amyotrophic lateral sclerosis and other neurodegenerative diseases have increased levels of neurofilament protein in CSF. J Neurochem 67: 2013–2018.

67. Ashburner J, Friston KJ (2005) Unified segmentation. Neuroimage 26: 839–851.

68. Bendlin BB, Fitzgerald ME, Ries ML, Xu G, Kastman EK, et al. (2010) White matter in aging and cognition: a cross-sectional study of microstructure in adults aged eighteen to eighty-three. Dev Neuropsychol 35: 257–277.

69. Pfefferbaum A, Sullivan EV, Hedehus M, Lim KO, Adalsteinsson E, et al. (2000) Age-related decline in brain white matter anisotropy measured with spatially corrected echo-planar diffusion tensor imaging. Magn Reson Med 44: 259–268.

70. Salat DH, Tuch DS, Greve DN, van der Kouwe AJ, Hevelone ND, et al. (2005) Age-related alterations in white matter microstructure measured by diffusion tensor imaging. Neurobiol Aging 26: 1215–1227.

71. Menzler K, Belke M, Wehrmann E, Krakow K, Lengler U, et al. (2011) Men and women are different: diffusion tensor imaging reveals sexual dimorphism in the microstructure of the thalamus, corpus callosum and cingulum. Neuroimage 54: 2557–2562.

72. Genovese CR, Lazar NA, Nichols T (2002) Thresholding of statistical maps in functional neuroimaging using the false discovery rate. Neuroimage 15: 870–878.

73. Bartzokis G, Lu PH, Geschwind DH, Tingus K, Huang D, et al. (2007) Apolipoprotein E affects both myelin breakdown and cognition: implications for age-related trajectories of decline into dementia. Biol Psychiatry 62: 1380–1387.

74. Desai MK, Guercio BJ, Narrow WC, Bowers WJ (2011) An Alzheimer's disease-relevant presenilin-1 mutation augments amyloid-beta-induced oligodendrocyte dysfunction. Glia 59: 627–640.

75. Desai MK, Sudol KL, Janelsins MC, Mastrangelo MA, Frazer ME, et al. (2009) Triple-transgenic Alzheimer's disease mice exhibit region-specific

abnormalities in brain myelination patterns prior to appearance of amyloid and tau pathology. Glia 57: 54–65.

76. Herukka SK, Pennanen C, Soininen H, Pirttila T (2008) CSF Abeta42, tau and phosphorylated tau correlate with medial temporal lobe atrophy. J Alzheimers Dis 14: 51–57.

77. Sole-Padulles C, Llado A, Bartres-Faz D, Fortea J, Sanchez-Valle R, et al. (2011) Association between cerebrospinal fluid tau and brain atrophy is not related to clinical severity in the Alzheimer's disease continuum. Psychiatry Res 192: 140–146.

78. de la Monte SM (1989) Quantitation of cerebral atrophy in preclinical and end-stage Alzheimer's disease. Ann Neurol 25: 450–459.

79. Scheltens P, Barkhof F, Leys D, Wolters EC, Ravid R, et al. (1995) Histopathologic correlates of white matter changes on MRI in Alzheimer's disease and normal aging. Neurology 45: 883–888.

80. Bronge L, Bogdanovic N, Wahlund LO (2002) Postmortem MRI and histopathology of white matter changes in Alzheimer brains. A quantitative, comparative study. Dement Geriatr Cogn Disord 13: 205–212.

81. Roher AE, Weiss N, Kokjohn TA, Kuo YM, Kalback W, et al. (2002) Increased A beta peptides and reduced cholesterol and myelin proteins characterize white matter degeneration in Alzheimer's disease. Biochemistry 41: 11080–11090.

82. Li S, Pu F, Shi F, Xie S, Wang Y, et al. (2008) Regional white matter decreases in Alzheimer's disease using optimized voxel-based morphometry. Acta Radiol 49: 84–90.

83. Stout JC, Jernigan TL, Archibald SL, Salmon DP (1996) Association of dementia severity with cortical gray matter and abnormal white matter volumes in dementia of the Alzheimer type. Arch Neurol 53: 742–749.

84. Salat DH, Greve DN, Pacheco JL, Quinn BT, Helmer KG, et al. (2009) Regional white matter volume differences in nondemented aging and Alzheimer's disease. Neuroimage 44: 1247–1258.

85. Im K, Lee JM, Won Seo S, Hyung Kim S, Kim SI, et al. (2008) Sulcal morphology changes and their relationship with cortical thickness and gyral white matter volume in mild cognitive impairment and Alzheimer's disease. Neuroimage 43: 103–113.

86. Balthazar ML, Yasuda CL, Pereira FR, Pedro T, Damasceno BP, et al. (2009) Differences in grey and white matter atrophy in amnestic mild cognitive impairment and mild Alzheimer's disease. Eur J Neurol 16: 468–474.

87. Chaim TM, Duran FL, Uchida RR, Perico CA, de Castro CC, et al. (2007) Volumetric reduction of the corpus callosum in Alzheimer's disease in vivo as assessed with voxel-based morphometry. Psychiatry Res 154: 59–68.

88. Baxter LC, Sparks DL, Johnson SC, Lenoski B, Lopez JE, et al. (2006) Relationship of cognitive measures and gray and white matter in Alzheimer's disease. J Alzheimers Dis 9: 253–260.

89. Teipel SJ, Hampel H, Alexander GE, Schapiro MB, Horwitz B, et al. (1998) Dissociation between corpus callosum atrophy and white matter pathology in Alzheimer's disease. Neurology 51: 1381–1385.

90. Teipel SJ, Bayer W, Alexander GE, Zebuhr Y, Teichberg D, et al. (2002) Progression of corpus callosum atrophy in Alzheimer disease. Arch Neurol 59: 243–248.

91. Vermersch P, Scheltens P, Barkhof F, Steinling M, Leys D (1994) Evidence for atrophy of the corpus callosum in Alzheimer's disease. Eur Neurol 34: 83–86.

92. Wang PJ, Saykin AJ, Flashman LA, Wishart HA, Rabin LA, et al. (2006) Regionally specific atrophy of the corpus callosum in AD, MCI and cognitive complaints. Neurobiol Aging 27: 1613–1617.

93. Mielke MM, Kozauer NA, Chan KC, George M, Toroney J, et al. (2009) Regionally-specific diffusion tensor imaging in mild cognitive impairment and Alzheimer's disease. Neuroimage 46: 47–55.

94. Terry RD (1998) The cytoskeleton in Alzheimer disease. J Neural Transm Suppl 53: 141–145.

95. Stokin GB, Lillo C, Falzone TL, Brusch RG, Rockenstein E, et al. (2005) Axonopathy and transport deficits early in the pathogenesis of Alzheimer's disease. Science 307: 1282–1288.

96. Bartzokis G, Sultzer D, Lu PH, Nuechterlein KH, Mintz J, et al. (2004) Heterogeneous age-related breakdown of white matter structural integrity: implications for cortical "disconnection" in aging and Alzheimer's disease. Neurobiol Aging 25: 843–851.

97. Bartzokis G, Lu PH, Tishler TA, Fong SM, Oluwadara B, et al. (2007) Myelin breakdown and iron changes in Huntington's disease: pathogenesis and treatment implications. Neurochem Res 32: 1655–1664.

98. Bartzokis G (2004) Age-related myelin breakdown: a developmental model of cognitive decline and Alzheimer's disease. Neurobiol Aging 25: 5–18; author reply 49–62.

99. Friede RL, Samorajski T (1970) Axon caliber related to neurofilaments and microtubules in sciatic nerve fibers of rats and mice. Anat Rec 167: 379–387.

100. Sjogren M, Blomberg M, Jonsson M, Wahlund LO, Edman A, et al. (2001) Neurofilament protein in cerebrospinal fluid: a marker of white matter changes. J Neurosci Res 66: 510–516.

101. Norgren N, Rosengren L, Stigbrand T (2003) Elevated neurofilament levels in neurological diseases. Brain Res 987: 25–31.

102. Hu YY, He SS, Wang XC, Duan QH, Khatoon S, et al. (2002) Elevated levels of phosphorylated neurofilament proteins in cerebrospinal fluid of Alzheimer disease patients. Neurosci Lett 320: 156–160.

103. Rosengren LE, Karlsson JE, Sjogren M, Blennow K, Wallin A (1999) Neurofilament protein levels in CSF are increased in dementia. Neurology 52: 1090–1093.

104. Andreasen N, Gottfries J, Vanmechelen E, Vanderstichele H, Davidson P, et al. (2001) Evaluation of CSF biomarkers for axonal and neuronal degeneration, gliosis, and beta-amyloid metabolism in Alzheimer's disease. J Neurol Neurosurg Psychiatry 71: 557–558.

105. Vandermeeren M, Mercken M, Vanmechelen E, Six J, van de Voorde A, et al. (1993) Detection of tau proteins in normal and Alzheimer's disease cerebrospinal fluid with a sensitive sandwich enzyme-linked immunosorbent assay. J Neurochem 61: 1828–1834.

106. Fagan AM, Mintun MA, Mach RH, Lee SY, Dence CS, et al. (2006) Inverse relation between in vivo amyloid imaging load and cerebrospinal fluid Abeta42 in humans. Ann Neurol 59: 512–519.

107. Tapiola T, Alafuzoff I, Herukka SK, Parkkinen L, Hartikainen P, et al. (2009) Cerebrospinal fluid {beta}-amyloid 42 and tau proteins as biomarkers of Alzheimer-type pathologic changes in the brain. Arch Neurol 66: 382–389.

108. Richter-Landsberg C (2008) The cytoskeleton in oligodendrocytes. Microtubule dynamics in health and disease. J Mol Neurosci 35: 55–63.

109. Iwatsubo T, Hasegawa M, Ihara Y (1994) Neuronal and glial tau-positive inclusions in diverse neurologic diseases share common phosphorylation characteristics. Acta Neuropathol 88: 129–136.

110. Umahara T, Tsuchiya K, Ikeda K, Kanaya K, Iwamoto T, et al. (2002) Demonstration and distribution of tau-positive glial coiled body-like structures in white matter and white matter threads in early onset Alzheimer's disease. Neuropathology 22: 9–12.

111. Nishimura M, Tomimoto H, Suenaga T, Namba Y, Ikeda K, et al. (1995) Immunocytochemical characterization of glial fibrillary tangles in Alzheimer's disease brain. Am J Pathol 146: 1052–1058.

112. Gotz J, Chen F, Barmettler R, Nitsch RM (2001) Tau filament formation in transgenic mice expressing P301L tau. J Biol Chem 276: 529–534.

113. Higuchi M, Ishihara T, Zhang B, Hong M, Andreadis A, et al. (2002) Transgenic mouse model of tauopathies with glial pathology and nervous system degeneration. Neuron 35: 433–446.

114. Lin WL, Lewis J, Yen SH, Hutton M, Dickson DW (2003) Filamentous tau in oligodendrocytes and astrocytes of transgenic mice expressing the human tau isoform with the P301L mutation. Am J Pathol 162: 213–218.

115. Buerger K, Alafuzoff I, Ewers M, Pirttila T, Zinkowski R, et al. (2007) No correlation between CSF tau protein phosphorylated at threonine 181 with neocortical neurofibrillary pathology in Alzheimer's disease. Brain 130: e82.

116. Braak H, Braak E (1997) Frequency of stages of Alzheimer-related lesions in different age categories. Neurobiol Aging 18: 351–357.

117. Kester MI, Blankenstein MA, Bouwman FH, van Elk EJ, Scheltens P, et al. (2009) CSF biomarkers in Alzheimer's disease and controls: associations with APOE genotype are modified by age. J Alzheimers Dis 16: 601–607.

118. Sunderland T, Mirza N, Putnam KT, Linker G, Bhupali D, et al. (2004) Cerebrospinal fluid beta-amyloid1–42 and tau in control subjects at risk for Alzheimer's disease: the effect of APOE epsilon4 allele. Biol Psychiatry 56: 670–676.

119. Carlsson CM, Gleason CE, Hess TM, Moreland KA, Blazel HM, et al. (2008) Effects of simvastatin on cerebrospinal fluid biomarkers and cognition in middle-aged adults at risk for Alzheimer's disease. J Alzheimers Dis 13: 187–197.

120. Andersson C, Blennow K, Johansson SE, Almkvist O, Engfeldt P, et al. (2007) Differential CSF biomarker levels in APOE-epsilon4-positive and -negative patients with memory impairment. Dement Geriatr Cogn Disord 23: 87–95.

121. Herukka SK, Hallikainen M, Soininen H, Pirttila T (2005) CSF Abeta42 and tau or phosphorylated tau and prediction of progressive mild cognitive impairment. Neurology 64: 1294–1297.

122. Stomrud E, Hansson O, Zetterberg H, Blennow K, Minthon L, et al. (2010) Correlation of longitudinal cerebrospinal fluid biomarkers with cognitive decline in healthy older adults. Arch Neurol 67: 217–223.

123. Tournier JD, Mori S, Leemans A (2011) Diffusion tensor imaging and beyond. Magn Reson Med 65: 1532–1556.

Identification and Validation of Novel Cerebrospinal Fluid Biomarkers for Staging Early Alzheimer's Disease

Richard J. Perrin[1,2,3,9]*, Rebecca Craig-Schapiro[4,9], James P. Malone[5,6], Aarti R. Shah[4], Petra Gilmore[5,6], Alan E. Davis[5,6], Catherine M. Roe[3,4], Elaine R. Peskind[8,9], Ge Li[9], Douglas R. Galasko[10], Christopher M. Clark[11,12,13], Joseph F. Quinn[14], Jeffrey A. Kaye[14], John C. Morris[2,3,4], David M. Holtzman[3,4,5,6,7], R. Reid Townsend[5,6], Anne M. Fagan[3,4,7]

1 Division of Neuropathology, Washington University School of Medicine, St. Louis, Missouri, United States of America, 2 Department of Pathology and Immunology, Washington University School of Medicine, St. Louis, Missouri, United States of America, 3 Knight Alzheimer's Disease Research Center, Washington University School of Medicine, St. Louis, Missouri, United States of America, 4 Department of Neurology, Washington University School of Medicine, St. Louis, Missouri, United States of America, 5 Department of Medicine, Washington University School of Medicine, St. Louis, Missouri, United States of America, 6 Division of Metabolism and Proteomics Center, Washington University School of Medicine, St. Louis, Missouri, United States of America, 7 Hope Center for Neurological Disorders, Washington University School of Medicine, St. Louis, Missouri, United States of America, 8 Department of Veterans Affairs Northwest Network Mental Illness Research, Education, and Clinical Center, University of Washington School of Medicine, Seattle, Washington, United States of America, 9 Department of Psychiatry and Behavioral Sciences, University of Washington School of Medicine, Seattle, Washington, United States of America, 10 Department of Neurosciences, University of California at San Diego, San Diego, California, United States of America, 11 Department of Neurology, University of Pennsylvania, Philadelphia, Pennsylvania, United States of America, 12 Alzheimer's Disease Center, University of Pennsylvania, Philadelphia, Pennsylvania, United States of America, 13 Avid Radiopharmaceuticals, Philadelphia, Pennsylvania, United States of America, 14 Layton Aging and Alzheimer's Disease Center, Oregon Health Science University, Portland, Oregon, United States of America

Abstract

Background: Ideally, disease modifying therapies for Alzheimer disease (AD) will be applied during the 'preclinical' stage (pathology present with cognition intact) before severe neuronal damage occurs, or upon recognizing very mild cognitive impairment. Developing and judiciously administering such therapies will require biomarker panels to identify early AD pathology, classify disease stage, monitor pathological progression, and predict cognitive decline. To discover such biomarkers, we measured AD-associated changes in the cerebrospinal fluid (CSF) proteome.

Methods and Findings: CSF samples from individuals with mild AD (Clinical Dementia Rating [CDR] 1) (n = 24) and cognitively normal controls (CDR 0) (n = 24) were subjected to two-dimensional difference-in-gel electrophoresis. Within 119 differentially-abundant gel features, mass spectrometry (LC-MS/MS) identified 47 proteins. For validation, eleven proteins were re-evaluated by enzyme-linked immunosorbent assays (ELISA). Six of these assays (NrCAM, YKL-40, chromogranin A, carnosinase I, transthyretin, cystatin C) distinguished CDR 1 and CDR 0 groups and were subsequently applied (with tau, p-tau181 and Aβ42 ELISAs) to a larger independent cohort (n = 292) that included individuals with very mild dementia (CDR 0.5). Receiver-operating characteristic curve analyses using stepwise logistic regression yielded optimal biomarker combinations to distinguish CDR 0 from CDR>0 (tau, YKL-40, NrCAM) and CDR 1 from CDR<1 (tau, chromogranin A, carnosinase I) with areas under the curve of 0.90 (0.85–0.94 95% confidence interval [CI]) and 0.88 (0.81–0.94 CI), respectively.

Conclusions: Four novel CSF biomarkers for AD (NrCAM, YKL-40, chromogranin A, carnosinase I) can improve the diagnostic accuracy of Aβ42 and tau. Together, these six markers describe six clinicopathological stages from cognitive normalcy to mild dementia, including stages defined by increased risk of cognitive decline. Such a panel might improve clinical trial efficiency by guiding subject enrollment and monitoring disease progression. Further studies will be required to validate this panel and evaluate its potential for distinguishing AD from other dementing conditions.

Citation: Perrin RJ, Craig-Schapiro R, Malone JP, Shah AR, Gilmore P, Davis AE, et al. (2011) Identification and Validation of Novel Cerebrospinal Fluid Biomarkers for Staging Early Alzheimer's Disease. PLoS ONE 6(1): e16032. doi:10.1371/journal.pone.0016032

Editor: Mark P. Mattson, National Institute on Aging Intramural Research Program, United States of America

Received October 27, 2010; **Accepted** December 3, 2010; **Published** January 12, 2011

Funding: National Alzheimer's Coordinating Center (NACC) Grant U01 AG16976 (A.M.F.); P50 AG05681 (C.M.R., E.A.G.); P01 AG026276 (C.M.R., E.A.G.); P50 AG05136; P01 AG03991(J.C.M.); P30 NS057105 (D.M.H.); UL1 RR024992 (R.R.T.; C.M.R.); W.M. Keck Foundation (R.R.T.); P41 RR00954 (R.R.T); Dept. of Veterans Affairs (E.R.P.); AG020020 (G.L.); AG23185 (D.R.G.); AG08017 (J.F.Q.); AG08017 (J.A.K.); AG10124 (C.M.C); T32 NS007205 (R.J.P.); and the Charles and Joanne Knight Alzheimer Research Initiative (A.M.F.); Avid Radiopharmaceuticals (C.M.C., employment unrelated to this study). The funders had no role in study design, data collection and analysis, decision to publish, or preparation of the manuscript.

Competing Interests: D.M.H. co-founded C2N Diagnostics, is on the scientific advisory board of C2N Diagnostics, En Vivo, and Satori, consulted for Pfizer, and receives grants that did not support this work from Eli Lilly, Pfizer, and Astra-Zeneca. J.C.M. has consulted for Astra Zeneca, Genentech, and Merck, has received honoraria from ANA Soriano lecture, payment from Journal Watch for preparation of other manuscripts, royalties from Blackwell Publishers and Taylor and Francis, and travel funding for ANA meeting Baltimore. C.M.C. became emeritus at University of Pennsylvania on January 1, 2010, and now works for Avid Radiopharmaceuticals, which did not provide any funding for this study, and did not have any involvement or influence in data production, data analysis, decision to publish, or manuscript preparation. None of the above stated competing interests alter our adherence to all the PLoS ONE policies on sharing data and materials.

* E-mail: rperrin@path.wustl.edu

9 These authors contributed equally to this work.

Introduction

Clinicopathological studies suggest that Alzheimer's disease (AD) pathology (amyloid plaque formation, followed by gliosis and neurofibrillary tangle formation) begins 10–15 years before the onset of very mild dementia [1,2]. This period of 'preclinical AD' could provide an opportunity for disease modifying therapies to prevent or forestall the synaptic and neuronal losses associated with cognitive impairment [3–5]. However, before such interventions can be developed and judiciously administered, accurate tools must be in place to diagnose and monitor the pathophysiological condition of individuals with preclinical AD and very early stage AD dementia. Clinical examination cannot detect preclinical disease or measure cellular and molecular changes within the brain, and, in general, has limited accuracy when diagnosing the very earliest symptomatic stages of AD. Therefore, there is an urgent need to identify biomarkers that can do so. Because its composition is rapidly and directly influenced by the brain, the cerebrospinal fluid (CSF) proteome represents an appealing source for such biomarkers.

Indeed, a few CSF proteins have already shown promise as diagnostic biomarkers for clinical AD (dementia of the Alzheimer type [DAT]) and even preclinical AD. Lower mean levels of CSF $A\beta42$ and higher mean levels of tau and phosphorylated tau can distinguish groups with DAT from cognitively normal controls [6,7]. Unfortunately, value ranges for each biomarker show substantial overlap between groups.

Recently, using positron-emission tomography PET imaging with Pittsburgh Compound B (PIB) to measure brain amyloid in vivo, we and others have demonstrated that low CSF $A\beta42$ can serve as an indicator of amyloid deposition [8–13], and that CSF tau levels correlate positively with in vivo brain amyloid load [11,14]. Importantly, both of these associations are independent of clinical diagnosis [8–11], though CSF tau does correlate with more sensitive measures of cognition [14]. These findings suggest that the overlap of biomarker values between clinical groups may, in part, reflect "contamination" of control groups by cognitively normal individuals exhibiting amyloid plaques and early neurodegeneration (preclinical AD), low CSF $A\beta42$ and elevated CSF tau. Supporting this notion, elevated ratios of tau/$A\beta42$ and p-tau181/$A\beta42$ (consistent with the presence of amyloid plaques and neurodegeneration) have been associated with increased risk of converting from cognitive normalcy to mild cognitive impairment or dementia [9,15], and with increased rate of cognitive decline among those with very mild dementia [16]. Together, these findings suggest that CSF biomarkers can describe neuropathological state and trajectory. They also suggest that a pathological staging system based on biomarkers might be a favorable alternative or adjunct to clinical staging for guiding treatment decisions or designing clinical trials.

Beyond amyloid plaque formation, other features of AD pathophysiology might also be exploited as therapeutic targets, sources of diagnostic biomarkers, or measures of disease progression. In addition to $A\beta42$ and tau, many other candidate AD biomarkers have been identified by either targeted or unbiased proteomics screens [17–27]. Only a few of these studies have tested large, well-characterized cohorts, however. Even fewer have evaluated biomarkers for their ability to distinguish the very early stages of AD pathophysiology. Thus, there remains a critical need for validated AD biomarkers that can properly categorize individuals by early pathological stage; such markers may have potential for monitoring neuropathological decline and, thereby, for evaluating response to disease-modifying therapies.

The goal of this study, therefore, is to identify such CSF protein biomarkers for AD using the unbiased proteomic technique of two-dimensional difference-in-gel electrophoresis (2D-DIGE) coupled with liquid chromatography and tandem mass spectrometry (LC-MS/MS), and to evaluate them further in a larger independent cohort using quantitative enzyme-linked immunosorbent assays (ELISA). Our findings suggest that a small ensemble of novel biomarkers may be able to distinguish several stages of cognitive decline in early AD, and improve the ability of current leading biomarkers tau and $A\beta42$ to discriminate early symptomatic AD from cognitive normalcy.

Methods

Ethics Statement

The study protocols were approved by the institutional review boards of the University of Washington, the Oregon Health and Science University, the University of Pennsylvania, the University of California San Diego, and Washington University. Written informed consent was obtained from all participants at enrollment. All aspects of this study were conducted according to the principles expressed in the Declaration of Helsinki.

Participant Selection for Discovery Cohort

Participants (n = 48), community-dwelling volunteers from University of Washington [n = 18], Oregon Health and Science University [n = 11], University of Pennsylvania [n = 11], and University of California San Diego [n = 8], were 51–87 years of age and in good general health, having no other neurological, psychiatric, or major medical diagnoses that could contribute to dementia, nor use of exclusionary medications (e.g. anticoagulants) within 1–3 months of lumbar puncture (LP). Cognitive status was evaluated based on criteria from the National Institute of Neurological and Communicative Diseases and Stroke-Alzheimer's Disease and Related Disorders Association [28]. In the morning after overnight fasting, CSF was obtained by LP, collected and aliquoted in polypropylene tubes, and immediately frozen at $-80°C$. Participants who were cognitively normal (Clinical Dementia Rating [CDR] of 0 [n = 24]) [29], or had mild "probable AD" (CDR 1) (n = 24), were selected from a larger group of 120 individuals on the basis of CSF $A\beta42$ (relatively high and low values, respectively), and, when possible, CSF tau (relatively low and high values, respectively) to increase the likelihood of CDR 1 participants having and CDR 0 participants not having AD pathology. CSF $A\beta42$ and tau levels for the discovery cohort were all measured in a single laboratory using well-established ELISA assays ([30] and Innotest, Innogenetics, Ghent, Belgium). Although quantitative thresholds were not defined prior to sample selection, the lowest CDR 0 value and the highest CDR 1 value for CSF $A\beta42$ in this 'discovery cohort' were 609 and 361 pg/mL, respectively; ranges for CSF tau were 141–461 pg/mL for CDR 0 and 215–1965 pg/mL for CDR 1.

Participant Selection for Validation Cohort

Participants (n = 292), community-dwelling volunteers enrolled at the Knight Alzheimer Disease Research Center at Washington University (WU-ADRC), were ≥60 years of age and met the same exclusion criteria as the discovery cohort. The study protocol was approved by the Human Studies Committee at Washington University, and written and verbal informed consent was obtained from participants at enrollment. Cognitive status was determined as with the discovery cohort. Participants who were cognitively normal (CDR 0, n = 198), very mildly demented (CDR 0.5, n = 65) or mildly demented (CDR 1, n = 29) at the time of LP were selected without regard to previously measured biomarkers. Some CDR 0.5 participants met criteria for mild cognitive impairment (MCI) and some showed even milder impairment, and could be considered "pre-MCI" [31]. All CDR 1 individuals had received a diagnosis of DAT (See Table 1 for demographic characteristics). Apolipoprotein E (*APOE*) genotypes were determined by the WU-ADRC Genetics Core. Fasted CSF (20–30 mL) was collected, gently mixed, centrifuged, aliquoted and frozen at -80°C in polypropylene tubes [9].

Multi-Affinity Immunodepletion of CSF

A pooled CSF sample, containing an equivalent volume from every 'discovery' cohort sample, was prepared as an internal standard for 2D-DIGE to facilitate the matching of gel features, and to allow normalization of the intensity of each gel feature among different gels. To enrich for proteins of low-abundance prior to 2D-DIGE, each CSF sample was depleted of six highly-abundant proteins (albumin, IgG, IgA, haptoglobin, transferrin, and α-1-antitrypsin) by immunoaffinity chromatography (Agilent Technologies, Palo Alto, CA) according to the manufacturer's instructions and as described previously [32]. Depleted samples were then concentrated using 10 kDa exclusion filters to retain larger molecules. As a 'benchmark' of immunodepletion column performance, an aliquot of reference CSF was depleted after every group of seven experimental chromatographic depletions. Non-depleted reference CSF, depleted CSF and the proteins that were retained by the column were analyzed by 2D-DIGE as previously described [32,33]; gel images obtained from all reference CSF depletion analyses were similar (data not shown), indicating consistent column performance over time.

2D-DIGE

2D-DIGE was performed as described previously [32,33]. Briefly, CDR 0 and CDR 1 samples were randomly paired. 50 micrograms of protein from each paired sample and from an aliquot of the pooled CSF sample were labeled with one of three N-hydroxysuccinimide cyanine dyes. The labeled proteins and 100 micrograms of unlabeled protein from each sample were mixed and equilibrated with an immobilized pH gradient strip for isoelectric focusing (first dimension), after which the strip was treated with reducing and alkylating solutions prior to SDS-PAGE (second dimension). Cy2, Cy3 and Cy5-labeled images were

Table 1. Demographic, clinical, genotype characteristics of validation cohort.

Characteristic	CDR 0	CDR 0.5	CDR 1
Number of Participants	198	65	29
Gender (% Female)	63%	54%	52%
APOE genotype, % ε4 positive	35%	51%	59%
Mean MMSE score (SD)	28.9 (1.3)	26.3 (2.8)	22.3 (3.9)
Mean age at LP (SD), years	71.0 (7.3)	73.8 (6.8)	76.5 (6.2)
Mean CSF Aβ42 (SD), pg/mL	605 (240)	446 (230)	351 (118)
Mean CSF tau (SD), pg/mL	304 (161)	539 (276)	552 (263)
Mean CSF p-tau181 (SD), pg/mL	55 (25)	85 (44)	77 (38)

Abbreviations: CDR, Clinical Dementia Rating; CDR 0, cognitively normal; CDR 0.5, very mild dementia; CDR 1 mild dementia; APOE, apolipoprotein E; MMSE, Mini-Mental State Examination; LP, lumbar puncture; SD, standard deviation; CSF, cerebrospinal fluid; Aβ42, amyloid beta 42 peptide; p-tau181, tau phosphorylated at threonine 181.
doi:10.1371/journal.pone.0016032.t001

acquired on a Typhoon 9400 scanner (GE Healthcare, United Kingdom) at excitation/emission wavelengths of 488/520, 532/580, and 633/670 nm, respectively.

Gel Image and Statistical Analysis

The comparative two-dimensional gel analysis was performed using an established experimental design [34] in which the high variation between gels is minimized by including a common, labeled pooled sample in all gels. Intra-gel feature detection, quantification and inter-gel matching and quantification were performed using the Differential In-Gel Analysis (DIA) and Biological Variation Analysis (BVA) modules of DeCyder software v 6.5 (GE Healthcare), respectively, as described previously [32]. This process (DIA analysis) resulted in approximately 5,000 gel features per gel image. In five gels, one sample contained significant amounts of hemoglobin indicating possible blood contamination. Therefore, all images from gels with these hemoglobin-containing samples were removed from further analysis. Remaining gel images were separated into three sets: standard (pool of all samples), CDR 0 and CDR 1. The pooled sample image with the largest number of well-resolved gel features was chosen as a master image. Gel features in each remaining pooled sample image were hand matched to gel features in the master image. For each gel feature that was matched across >50% of the gels (n = 764), a Student's t-test ($\alpha = 0.05$) was performed to determine the statistical significance of CDR 0/CDR 1 ratios, using the DeCyder EDA (Extended Data Analysis) module. To maximize discovery rate and minimize type II error, no multiple test correction was applied. The image intensity data for the statistically significant gel features (n = 119) were then subjected to unsupervised hierarchical clustering (DeCyder EDA module).

Protein/Peptide Identification by LC-MS/MS

Gel features with significant intensity differences were targeted by a robotic gel sampling system (ProPic; Genomics Solutions, Ann Arbor, MI) and transferred into 96 well plates for in-gel digestion with trypsin using a modification of a method [35] described previously [33]. Aliquots of these digests were processed for and analyzed by LC-MS/MS using a capillary LC (Eksigent, Livermore CA) interfaced to a nano-LC-linear quadrupole ion trap Fourier transform ion cyclotron resonance mass spectrometer (nano-LC-FTMS) [36] QStar [37] or LTQ [36]. The tandem spectra were searched against the National Center for Biotechnology Information non-redundant protein database NR (downloaded on 02-18-2007) using MASCOT, version 2.2.04 (Matrix Sciences, London). The database searches were constrained by allowing for trypsin cleavage (with up to two missed cleavage sites), fixed modifications (carbamidomethylation of Cys residues) and variable modifications (oxidation of Met residues and N-terminal pyroglutamate formation). Protein identifications were considered genuine if at least two peptides were matched with individual MASCOT ion scores ≥ 40.

Using nano-LC-MS/MS, multiple proteins were identified in the majority of individual gel features. The frequent observation of multiple proteins in single gel features was attributed to the sensitivity and greater peptide coverage that can be achieved with nano-LC-MS methods as compared to, for example, MALDI-MS analysis of peptides from gel features. Assignment of the major protein(s) from each gel feature was achieved using quantitative proteomics from spectra counting [38]. The detection of multiple proteins within single gel features could also be attributed to artifacts and technical issues associated with 2D gel electrophoresis: 1) incomplete resolution of proteins by gel electrophoresis (due to similar charge and size characteristics, excessive abundance of

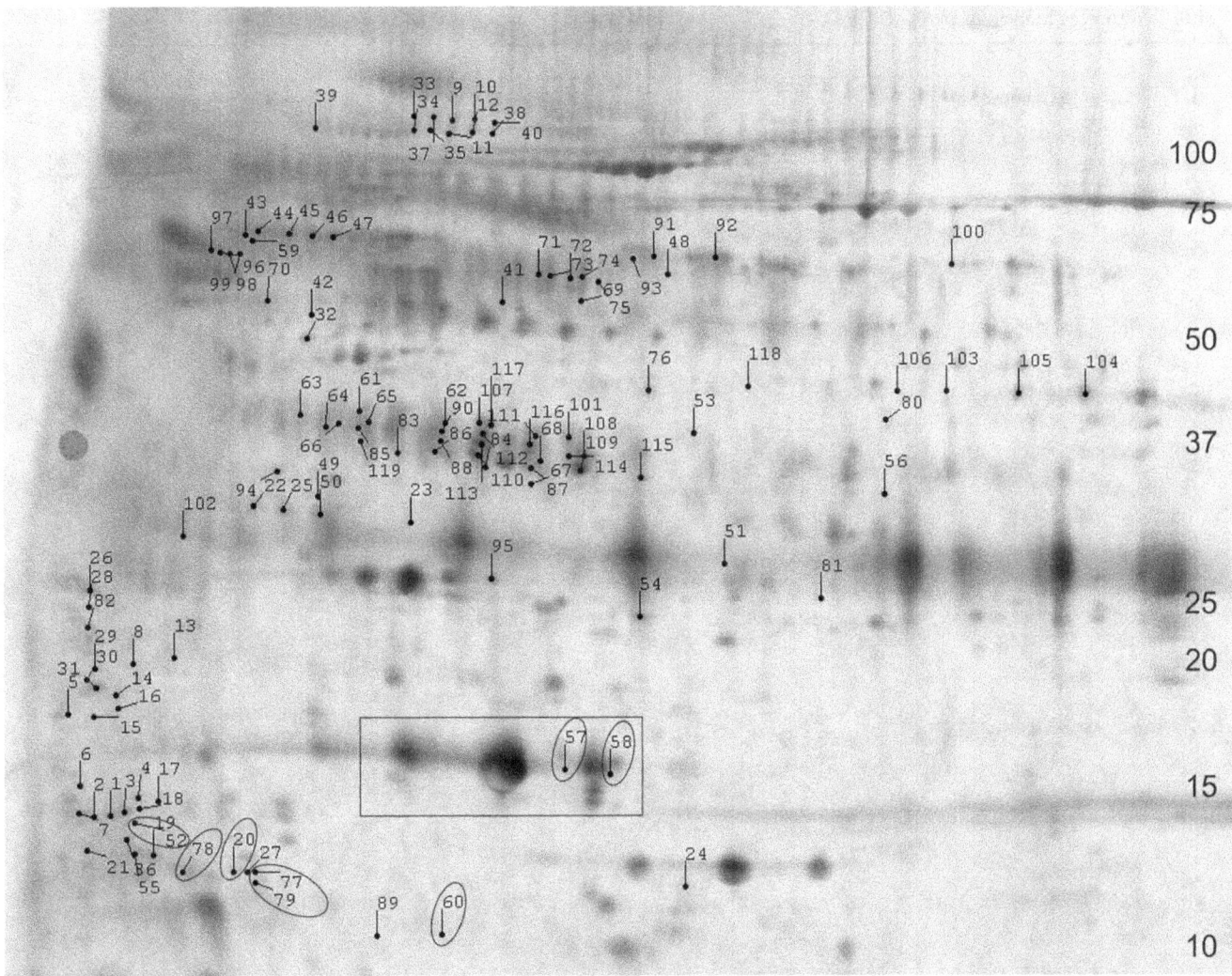

Figure 1. Two-dimensional difference in gel electrophoresis (2D-DIGE) of cerebrospinal fluid immunodepleted of six high abundance proteins. Representative 2D-DIGE (grayscale) image with labeled locations of 119 gel features that differed in intensity between CDR 0 and CDR 1 groups. Gel features are numbered 1 through 119, and relevant information about each is listed in Table 2 and in Table S1. Approximate molecular weight (in kilodaltons [kDa]) is indicated along the right border; isoelectric point ranges from 3 (left) to 11(right) and is non-linear (not shown). The large, intense, protein spots commonly attributed to transthyretin are boxed; a subset of the differentially abundant gel features in which transthyretin was identified by mass spectrometry is circled.
doi:10.1371/journal.pone.0016032.g001

neighboring proteins, or artifactual streaking); 2) changes in molecular weight associated with cyanine dye labeling, particularly for lower molecular weight proteins; and 3) sample 'carryover' during robotic gel sampling or during nano-LC-MS/MS.

All relevant proteomics data are detailed in Table S1.

Enzyme Linked Immunosorbent Assays (ELISAs) and Statistical Analyses

CSF samples were analyzed by ELISA in duplicate for Aβ42, total tau, and phospho-tau181 (Innotest, Innogenetics, Ghent, Belgium) after one freeze-thaw cycle, and in triplicate for all other ELISAs after two freeze-thaw cycles. Samples were evaluated using commercially available ELISAs for NrCAM (R&D Systems Inc., Minneapolis, MN), YKL-40 (Quidel Corporation, San Diego, CA), apolipoprotein E (Medical and Biological Laboratories Company, Ltd., Nagoya, Japan), clusterin/apolipoprotein J (ALPCO Diagnostics, Salem, NH), pigment epithelium-derived factor (PEDF)/serpin-F1 (Chemicon International Inc./ Millipore Corporation, Billerica, MA), beta-2 microglobulin (ALPCO

Diagnostics), ceruloplasmin (Assaypro, St. Charles, MO), chromogranin A (ALPCO Diagnostics, low binding capacity manufacturing protocol), transthyretin (Assaypro), and cystatin C (US Biological, Swampscott, MA), according to manufacturer's instructions, with adjustments for the analysis of CSF. A sandwich ELISA was developed for carnosinase I using goat anti-human carnosinase I antibody (2 μg/mL, R&D Systems Inc.) for capture, rabbit anti-human carnosinase I antibody (1 μg/mL, Sigma-Aldrich Corporation, St. Louis, MO) for detection, goat anti-rabbit:horseradish peroxidase (1:5000, Upstate Biologicals Inc./ Millipore Corporation) for reporting, and TMB (3,3′,5,5′-tetramethylbenzidine) Super Slow (Sigma-Aldrich Corporation) for color development; recombinant carnosinase I (R&D Systems Inc.) was used as standard.

Statistical analyses were performed using commercially available software: SAS 9.2 (SAS Institute Inc., Cary, NC) for Receiver Operating Characteristic (ROC)/area under curve (AUC) calculations and logistic regression analyses, and SPSS 18 (SPSS Inc., Chicago, IL) for all other analyses.

Table 2. Proteins identified by 2D-DIGE LC-MS/MS with differential abundance in CDR 1 vs. CDR 0 CSF.

Spot	BVA	GI number(s)	Protein	Change	p value	Protein
1	4709	31543193	hypothetical protein LOC146556	−1.36	7.02E-04	1
2	5659	4502807	chromogranin B	−1.31	1.18E-03	2
3	4683	4502101	annexin I	−1.31	9.54E-04	3
4	4608	62089004	chromogranin B	−1.24	6.49E-03	
		181387	cystatin C			4
		134464	secretogranin-2			5
5	4297	4502807	chromogranin B	−1.26	0.0157	
6	4545			−1.34	3.86E-03	
7	4695	4502807	chromogranin B	−1.27	0.0115	
8	4044	4502807	chromogranin B	−1.32	2.15E-03	
9	1314	1621283	neuronal cell adhesion molecule (NrCAM)	−1.22	0.0119	6
10	1320	1621283	neuronal cell adhesion molecule (NrCAM)	−1.33	6.31E-04	
11	1382	6651381	neuronal cell adhesion molecule (NrCAM)	−1.28	9.53E-04	
12	1383	6651381	neuronal cell adhesion molecule (NrCAM)	−1.25	6.64E-03	
13	4033	4502807	chromogranin B	−1.21	0.0419	
14	4191	4502807	chromogranin B	−1.23	0.0107	
15	4293	4502807	chromogranin B	−1.33	4.64E-03	
		825635	calmodulin			7
16	4266	62089004	chromogranin B	−1.22	0.0315	
17	4615			−1.22	0.0188	
18	4677			−1.3	9.63E-03	
19	4906	5454032	S100 calcium binding protein A1	−1.3	1.36E-04	8
		62898141	prosaposin			9
		627391	brain-associated small cell lung cancer antigen/NCAM-140/CD56			10
		17136078	VGF nerve growth factor inducible precursor			11
20	5014	443295	transthyretin	−1.3	2.10E-03	12
21	4884	224917	apolipoprotein CIII	−1.34	9.78E-04	13
		337760	prosaposin/cerebroside sulfate activator protein			
22	3423	39654998	chain A, Hr1b Domain From Prk1	−1.27	0.0133	14
		32171249	prostaglandin H2 D-isomerase/beta trace			15
23	3470	17402888	neuronal pentraxin receptor	−1.25	7.23E-03	16
		114593356	extracellular superoxide dismutase (SOD3)			17
24	4954	34616	beta-2 microglobulin	−1.3	4.15E-03	18
25	3436	32171249	prostaglandin H2 D-isomerase	−1.22	0.0266	
		178775	proapolipoprotein			19
		39654998	chain A, Hr1b Domain From Prk1			
26	3714			−1.27	0.03	
27	4922	39654998	chain A, Hr1b Domain From Prk1	−1.27	0.0194	
28	3786	2072129	chromogranin A	−1.38	8.96E-03	20
29	4076	7341255	brain acetylcholinesterase putative membrane anchor	−1.25	0.0375	21
30	4111	62089004	chromogranin B	−1.28	0.0206	
31	4167	4502807	chromogranin B	−1.29	0.0207	
32	2652	28373309	gelsolin	−1.23	0.0346	22
33	1313	6651381	neuronal cell adhesion molecule (NrCAM)	−1.19	8.08E-03	
34	1372	1620909	ceruloplasmin	−1.19	9.00E-03	23
		1483187	inter-alpha-trypsin inhibitor family heavy chain-related protein			24
		31874098	hypothetical protein (NrCAM)			
		6651381	neuronal cell adhesion molecule (NrCAM)			
35	1387	68534652	neuronal cell adhesion molecule (NrCAM)	−1.29	8.16E-05	
		1620909	ceruloplasmin			

Table 2. Cont.

Spot	BVA	GI number(s)	Protein	Change	p value	Protein
36	4808	337760	prosaposin/cerebroside sulfate activator protein	−1.22	0.0114	
37	1319	68534652	neuronal cell adhesion molecule (NrCAM)	−1.19	0.0198	
		1942284	ceruloplasmin			
38	1386	6651381	neuronal cell adhesion molecule (NrCAM)	−1.29	1.24E-03	
39	1353	21706696	calsyntenin 1	−1.22	0.0417	25
40	1329	1621283	neuronal cell adhesion molecule (NrCAM)	−1.22	4.61E-03	
41	2456	5802984	UDP-GlcNAc:betaGal beta-1,3-N-acetylglucosaminyltransferase 1	−1.13	0.0449	26
42	2550	20178323	pigment epithelium-derived factor precursor (PEDF)/Serpin-F1/EPC-1	−1.15	0.022	27
43	2125	21071039	carnosinase 1	−1.21	0.0245	28
44	2131	21071039	carnosinase 1	−1.19	0.049	
45	2152	21071039	carnosinase 1	−1.15	0.0366	
46	5614	21071039	carnosinase 1	−1.18	0.0109	
47	2166	21071039	carnosinase 1	−1.21	0.0122	
48	2328	416180	man9-mannosidase/α1,2-mannosidase IA	−1.16	0.0464	29
49	3360			−1.15	0.045	
50	3447	32171249	prostaglandin H2 D-isomerase/beta trace	−1.19	0.0334	
51	3546	1621283	neuronal cell adhesion molecule (NrCAM)	−1.17	0.0368	
		32171249	prostaglandin H2 D-isomerase/beta trace			
52	4745	443295	transthyretin	−1.26	0.0181	
53	3032	11056046	nectin-like molecule-1/SynCAM3/TSLL1	−1.13	0.0472	30
54	3718	39654998	chain A, Hr1b Domain From Prk1	−1.14	0.0455	
		32171249	prostaglandin H2 D-isomerase/beta trace			
55	4902	14277770	apolipoprotein C-Ii	−1.19	0.0495	31
		337760	prosaposin/cerebroside sulfate activator protein			
		2072129	chromogranin A			
56	3290	409725	carbonic anhydrase IV	−1.14	0.0141	32
57	4379	17942890	transthyretin	−1.15	0.0219	
		39654998	chain A, Hr1b Domain From Prk1			
		34999	cadherin 2 precursor			33
58	4388	32171249	prostaglandin H2 D-isomerase/beta trace	−1.14	0.0218	
		39654998	chain A, Hr1b Domain From Prk1			
		443295	transthyretin			
59	2192	21071039	carnosinase 1	−1.34	6.56E-03	
		532198	angiotensinogen			34
		5531817	secretogranin III			35
		9665262	EGF-containing fibulin-like extracellular matrix protein 1/Fibulin-3			36
		177933	alpha-1-antichymotrypsin			37
		4504893	kininogen 1			38
		36573	vitronectin			39
60	5336	443295	transthyretin	−1.17	0.0301	
61	3009	178855	apolipoprotein J/clusterin	−1.26	0.0288	40
		4557325	apolipoprotein E			41
62	3042	4557325/178853	apolipoprotein E	−1.21	0.047	
		338305	apolipoprotein J/clusterin			
63	3016	338305	apolipoprotein J/clusterin	−1.32	6.69E-05	
64	3050	4557325/178853	apolipoprotein E	−1.24	5.19E-04	
		178855	apolipoprotein J/clusterin			
65	3075	4557325/178853	apolipoprotein E	−1.42	5.59E-06	
		178855	apolipoprotein J/clusterin			
66	3038	4557325/178853	apolipoprotein E	−1.41	2.84E-05	

Table 2. Cont.

Spot	BVA	GI number(s)	Protein	Change	p value	Protein
		178855	apolipoprotein J/clusterin			
67	3301	178849	apolipoprotein E	−1.4	1.29E-05	
68	3182	4557325/178853	apolipoprotein E	−1.41	3.43E-04	
		178855	apolipoprotein J/clusterin			
69	2443	532198	angiotensinogen	−1.2	6.85E-03	
70	2493	4503009	carboxypeptidase E precursor	−1.23	6.09E-03	42
71	5621	532198	angiotensinogen	−1.17	0.0434	
72	5624	532198	angiotensinogen	−1.22	0.0147	
73	5622	553181	angiotensinogen	−1.17	0.04	
74	5625	532198	angiotensinogen	−1.16	0.0423	
75	5627			−1.22	0.0113	
76	2849	4557325	apolipoprotein E	−1.28	6.26E-03	
77	5009	443295	transthyretin	−1.24	0.0268	
78	5033	443295	transthyretin	−1.27	4.59E-03	
79	5078	443295	transthyretin	−1.2	0.0144	
80	2958	4504067	aspartate aminotransferase 1	−1.22	8.60E-03	43
81	3657	32171249	prostaglandin H2 D-isomerase/beta trace	−1.22	3.07E-03	
82	3867			−1.28	0.0437	
83	3176	4557325	apolipoprotein E	−1.63	3.03E-04	
84	3228	4557325	apolipoprotein E	−1.4	1.39E-03	
		443295	transthyretin			
85	3074	4557325/178853	apolipoprotein E	−2.36	4.41E-09	
86	5647	4557325	apolipoprotein E	−2.35	2.92E-07	
87	3224	4557325/178853	apolipoprotein E	−2.13	6.36E-07	
		443295	transthyretin			
88	3126	4557325/178853	apolipoprotein E	−1.93	7.55E-06	
89	5297			−1.44	0.0473	
90	3083	4557325	apolipoprotein E	−1.7	2.82E-05	
91	2218	112911	alpha-2-macroglobulin	1.22	0.0282	44
92	2226	6573461	apolipoprotein H	1.27	0.0305	45
93	2252	112911	alpha-2-macroglobulin	1.26	0.0267	
		4557327	apolipoprotein H			
94	3255			1.24	0.0315	
95	3630	178775	proapolipoprotein	1.24	0.0287	
		32171249	prostaglandin H2 D-isomerase/beta trace			
		39654998	chain A, Hr1b Domain From Prk1			
96	2229	177933	alpha-1-antichymotrypsin	1.42	3.09E-03	
97	2235	177933	alpha-1-antichymotrypsin	1.35	0.0388	
98	2261	177933	alpha-1-antichymotrypsin	1.3	6.04E-03	
99	2262	177933	alpha-1-antichymotrypsin	1.25	0.0294	
100	2220			1.29	0.0158	
101	3084			1.16	0.0211	
102	3508	32171249	prostaglandin H2 D-isomerase/beta trace	1.22	9.21E-03	
103	2825	23512215	chitinase 3-like 1/YKL-40/HC-gp39	1.41	0.0167	46
104	2863	4557018	chitinase 3-like 1/YKL-40/HC-gp39	1.5	0.0144	
105	2846	29726259	chitinase 3-like 1/YKL-40/HC-gp39	1.46	7.88E-03	
106	2843	23512215	chitinase 3-like 1/YKL-40/HC-gp39	1.32	0.0241	
107	3030	4557325	apolipoprotein E	2.46	3.70E-05	
108	3152	4557325/178853	apolipoprotein E	2.39	8.73E-07	
109	3203	178853	apolipoprotein E	3.23	3.13E-07	

Table 2. Cont.

Spot	BVA	GI number(s)	Protein	Change	p value	Protein
110	3185	4557325/178853	apolipoprotein E	1.9	9.72E-04	
		443295	transthyretin			
111	3069	338305	apolipoprotein J/clusterin	1.5	6.40E-04	
112	3079			1.64	4.47E-04	
113	3133	178853	apolipoprotein E	1.49	8.66E-04	
		338057	apolipoprotein J/clusterin			
114	3151	178853	apolipoprotein E	1.28	9.25E-03	
		338057	apolipoprotein J/clusterin			
115	3249	4557325	apolipoprotein E	1.37	2.46E-03	
		178855	apolipoprotein J/clusterin			
		443295	transthyretin			
116	3118	4557325/178853	apolipoprotein E	1.64	9.96E-04	
117	5698	178855	apolipoprotein J/clusterin	1.73	5.82E-04	
118	2819	40737343	C4B3	2	0.038	47
119	3137	4557325	apolipoprotein E	−2.5	8.52E-07	

Column 1, coded protein spot ID (as in Figure 1).
Column 2, biological variation analysis (BVA) number for spot generated by Decyder software.
Column 3, GI accession number(s) assigned to proteins identified by MASCOT.
Column 4, name of protein identified by MASCOT.
Column 5, fold-change in protein abundance; negative values indicate decreases in CDR 1 vs. CDR 0.
Column 6, p value of the CDR 1 versus CDR 0 comparison (Student's t test).
Column 7, consecutive numbering identifying proteins as unique.
doi:10.1371/journal.pone.0016032.t002

Comparisons between CDR 0 and CDR 1 groups of the 'discovery' cohort (one sample was unavailable for re-evaluation, n = 47) were performed using unpaired t-test. For the 'validation' cohort (n = 292), correlations with age and gender were evaluated using the Spearman rho correlation coefficient ($\alpha = 0.05$). Chi-square analyses were performed to evaluate need for adjustment for observed correlations. Comparisons between the three CDR groups were performed using one-way analysis of variance (ANOVA), with Bonferroni and LSD post-hoc tests for pair-wise group comparisons, with the following exceptions: one-way ANOVA with Welch's correction was applied for markers (transthyretin) demonstrating unequal variances (Levene <.05); markers correlating with age (tau, p-tau181, Aβ42, YKL-40) were evaluated by analysis of covariance (ANCOVA) adjusting for age, followed by Bonferroni and LSD post-hoc tests. Multiple post-hoc tests were applied in recognition of their different levels of stringency (Bonferroni > LSD), and their non-uniform popularity among statisticians. For CDR 0 vs >0 comparisons and CDR 1 vs <1 comparisons, unpaired t-test was used; Welch's correction for unequal variances was applied for YKL-40, p-tau181, tau, and Aβ42. For each biomarker measured in the larger 'validation' cohort, the ROC curve and the AUC were calculated for predicting CDR 0 versus CDR>0. A stepwise logistic regression analysis was used to identify an optimal combination of these biomarkers for this data set. These analyses were repeated for CDR 1 vs CDR<1.

Results

Sample Processing and 2D-DIGE Analysis

To identify new candidate biomarkers for AD, we utilized an unbiased proteomics approach, 2D-DIGE LC-MS/MS [32,33], to compare the relative concentrations of CSF proteins in individuals with mild "probable AD" (CDR 1, n = 24) to those in individuals with normal cognition (CDR 0, n = 24). The two clinical groups were selected on the basis of relative biomarker values for CSF Aβ42 and tau (see Methods), and differed somewhat with respect to age at LP and gender (CDR 0: 64.8±8.8 yrs, 38% female; CDR 1: 72.8 yrs ±7.9 yrs, 54% female). Five samples showed evidence of blood contamination by 2D-DIGE; the five gels containing these samples were excluded from subsequent image analyses. The remaining individual sample images (n = 38, from 19 gels) were aligned using the BVA module (described under Methods).

Among the 764 gel features that were present in >50% of the gels, 119 were found to have significant intensity differences between CDR 0 and CDR 1 groups (Student's t-test [$\alpha = 0.05$]) (Figure 1). The image intensity data for these 119 gel features were subjected to unsupervised hierarchical clustering (EDA module, DeCyder software) and the gel features themselves were analyzed for protein composition.

Protein Identification by LC-MS/MS

LC-MS/MS identified single dominant proteins in 78 of the 119 gel features (Table 2). In 29 gel features, our analyses identified two or more co-dominant proteins. The 12 remaining gel features were not annotated from the nano-LC-MS/MS data. Among the characterized gel features, there was considerable redundancy in protein identifications, with some proteins appearing in multiple gel features. Such 'redundant' gel features, likely representing a modified form or variant of the same 'parent' protein, generally migrated with some proximity on 2D-gel electrophoresis (Figure 1). Forty-seven unique proteins were identified (Table 2). Thirteen of these unique proteins had been identified in our previous studies [32,33] (including chromogranin B, cystatin C, prostaglandin H2 D-isomerase/beta trace, neuronal pentraxin receptor, gelsolin, beta-2 microglobulin, carnosinase I, angiotensinogen, apolipoprotein H, secretogranin III, alpha-1-antichymotrypsin, chitinase 3-like 1/YKL-40, and kininogen I) and others have been reported by other groups [17,19,20,23,25,27]. These previous reports provide supporting evidence that this list of proteins may contain viable candidate biomarkers for AD that are worthy of pursuit in validation experiments.

Unsupervised Clustering Analysis

The intensity data from the 119 gel features of interest were subjected to an unsupervised clustering analysis to evaluate their ability to segregate the CDR 0 and CDR 1 samples, and to assess their collective potential as a diagnostic biomarker panel (Figure 2). The 'heatmap' generated from this analysis appeared to segregate CDR 0 and CDR 1 individuals (indicated by green and red ovals, respectively) almost completely, with only four participants 'misclassified.' However, closer examination revealed an additional layer of segregation on the basis of *APOE* genotype (indicated by 'ApoE 4+ Cluster' and 'ApoE 4 – Cluster') which showed perfect

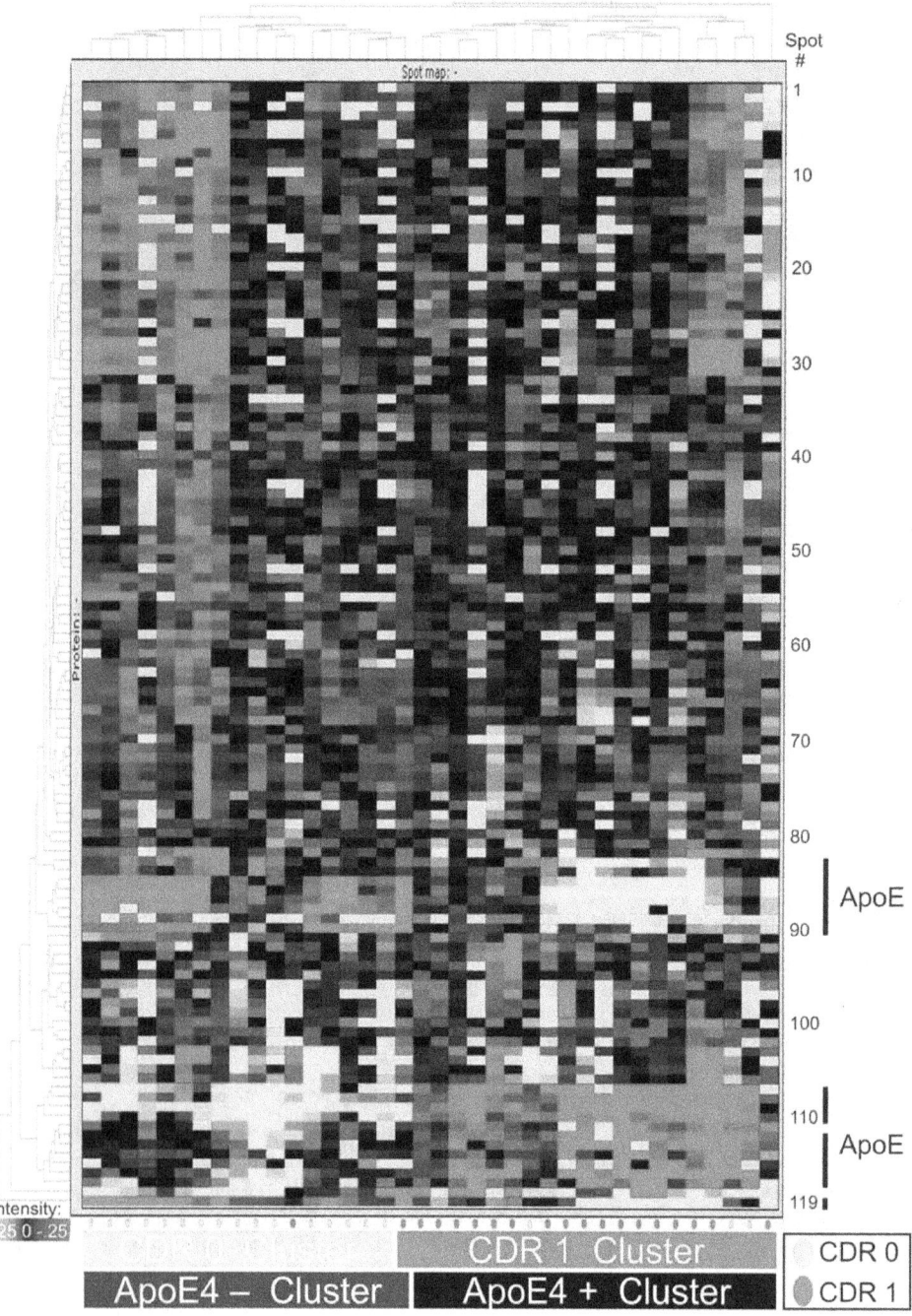

Figure 2. Unsupervised clustering of CSF samples by 2D-DIGE data from the 119 statistically significant gel features. (Student's t-test, $\alpha = 0.05$, present in >50% of images). Five gels containing hemoglobin (n = 10 samples) were excluded. Columns represent samples; rows, numbered 1 through 119 from top to bottom, represent gel features depicted in Figure 1. Gel feature intensity is encoded colorimetrically from red (low intensity) to green (high intensity); white indicates absent data. CDR status of individuals at time of CSF collection is encoded below by small green (CDR 0) and red (CDR 1) ovals; CDR 0 and CDR 1 clusters are indicated below by green and red bars, respectively. *APOE-ε4* allele status of individuals and groups, alike, is indicated by black (possessing ApoE4 protein, or one or two *APOE-ε4* alleles) or blue (possessing no ApoE4 protein, or no *APOE-ε4* alleles) bars. Rows representing gel features containing ApoE protein are indicated along the lower right border.

doi:10.1371/journal.pone.0016032.g002

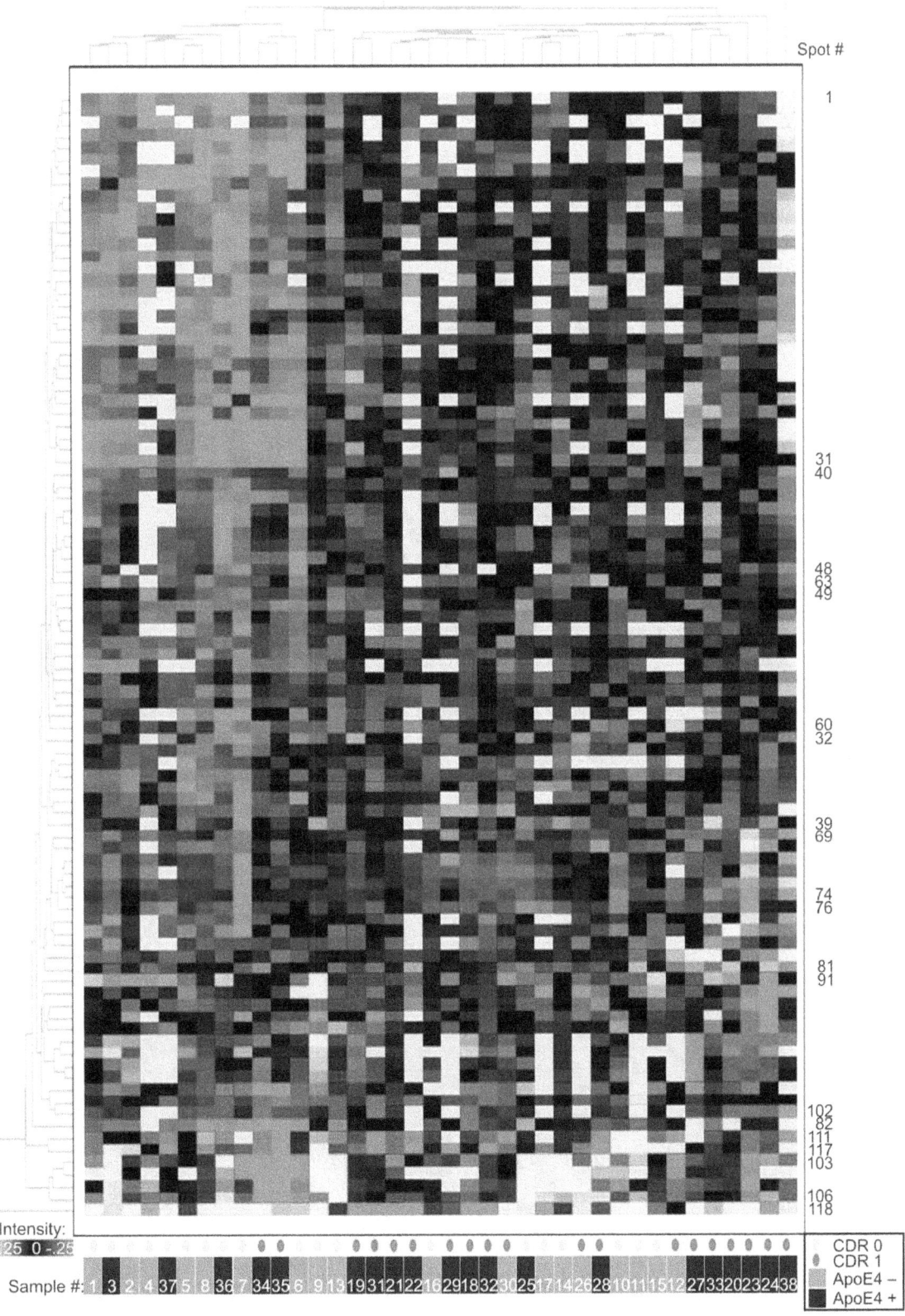

Figure 3. Unsupervised clustering of CSF samples by 2D-DIGE data, excluding gel features containing apoE protein. All other statistically significant gel features (Student's t-test α = 0.05, present in >50% of images) are retained. As in Figure 2, five gels containing hemoglobin (n = 10 samples) were excluded. Columns represent samples, numbered according to their original positions in Figure 2. Rows represent gel features, numbered as in Figure 2; unlabeled rows are in consecutive order from upper number to lower number, with interruptions in sequence indicated by labels. ApoE-containing features are removed. Gel feature intensity is encoded colorimetrically from red (low intensity) to green (high intensity); white indicates absent data. CDR status of participants at time of CSF collection is encoded below, by small green (CDR 0) and red (CDR 1) ovals. *APOE-ε4* status (as described for Figure 2) is indicated by blue (ApoE4 negative) or black (ApoE4 positive) bars, below. Clustering pattern of samples (numbered consecutively in order of appearance in Figure 2, from left to right) relative to Figure 2 is indicated by white numerals, below.
doi:10.1371/journal.pone.0016032.g003

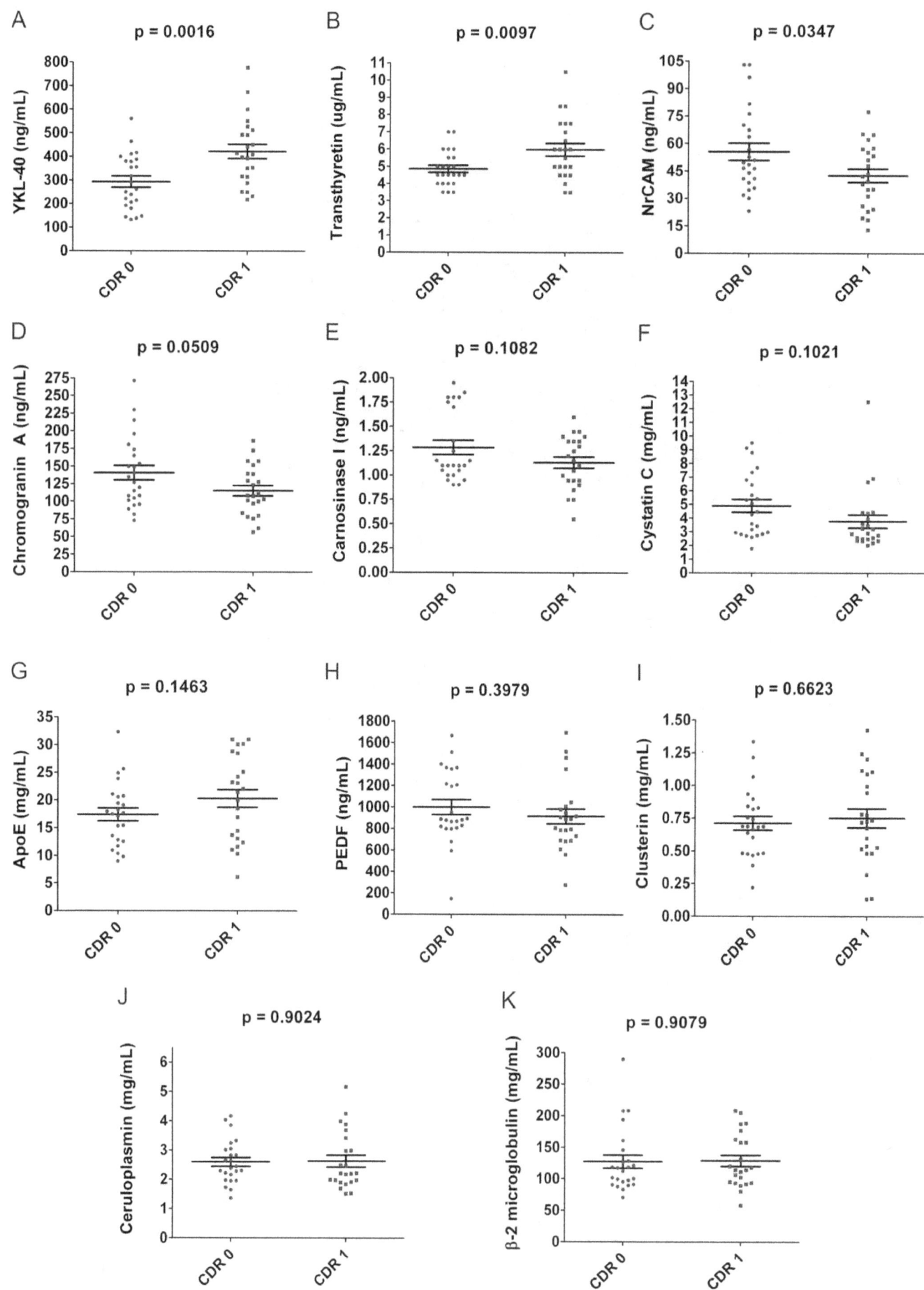

Figure 4. Quantitative ELISAs for 11 biomarker candidates applied to 'discovery' cohort CSF samples (n = 47). Each assay performed in triplicate; mean value reported for each sample. The six assays represented in the upper two rows (**A**. YKL-40, **B**. Transthyretin, **C**. NrCAM, **D**. Chromogranin A, **E**. Carnosinase I, and **F**. Cystatin C) measured differences between CDR 0 and CDR 1 groups (unpaired t-test); the five assays represented in the lower two rows (**G**. ApoE, **H**. PEDF, **I**. Clusterin, **J**. Ceruloplasmin, **K**. β-2 microglobulin) did not.
doi:10.1371/journal.pone.0016032.g004

sample segregation. Given that the *APOE-ε4* allele is a dominant genetic risk factor for AD, some clustering of individuals by *APOE* genotype might be expected simply from successful segregation of CDR 0 and CDR 1 individuals. However, we hypothesize that the apoE protein exerts a dominant clustering influence through the markedly different electrophoretic profiles of its different isoforms derived from *APOE-ε2*, *APOE-ε3* and *APOE- ε4* alleles (illustrated in Figure S1). ApoE was present in 24 of the 119 gel features found to differ in intensity between the CDR groups, and was found to be the primary protein in 12 of these gel features. This heterogeneous electrophoretic mobility of apoE results from the inherent charge differences of the three major apoE isoforms (-E2, -E3, -E4) and the appearance of each isoform as an array of multiple distinct gel features caused by post-translational modifications. These isoform-specific differences are reflected in the prominent red and green clusters, located within the lower third of Figure 2 (corresponding to gel features 83–90, 107–117, and 119), that correlate very closely with participant *APOE* genotypes. Recognizing this correlation, we hypothesized that *APOE* genotypes were in large part driving the clustering of participant samples in Figure 2. To test this hypothesis, we performed a second unsupervised clustering analysis, including only those gel features from the initial analysis that did not contain apoE protein (Figure 3). Although this 'apoE-free' analysis segregated CDR 1 and CDR 0 groups less completely, it appropriately re-clustered (by CDR status) several samples (#12, 36, 37) that were aberrantly segregated in Figure 2, potentially due to their *APOE* genotypes. Moreover, clustering of participant samples into *APOE* genotype subgroups in Figure 3 appears negligible. The underlying benefit of this 'apoE-free' analysis is that it reveals the sample-clustering potential of other gel features, which was previously obscured by the inclusion of apoE-containing gel features. As can now be better visualized in Figure 3, gel features appearing within the upper three-fourths of the heatmap appear to show greater intensity in CDR 1 samples; the converse is true of gel features within the lower fourth. It is important to note that measurements of Aβ42 and tau (two proteins measured by ELISA and not detected by 2D-DIGE) were not included in these clustering analyses; because these 'discovery' samples were selected for this study on the basis of CSF Aβ42 and tau levels, such inclusion would presumably yield perfect or near-perfect segregation by CDR status in this 'discovery' cohort. Therefore, this analysis reflects the potential of these candidate biomarkers to segregate CDR 0 and CDR 1 individuals *independent* of any contribution from current leading CSF biomarkers Aβ42 and tau. It does not address whether these biomarker candidates might improve upon the utility of Aβ42 and tau, however.

Validation of Candidate Biomarkers by ELISA

Before evaluating a subset of these candidate biomarkers in a larger independent sample set, we first assessed the capacity of protein-specific quantitative ELISAs to detect significant differences between the CDR 0 and CDR 1 groups of the original 'discovery' cohort. When possible, to facilitate future reproduction of our findings by other groups and potential translation to clinical use, we applied commercially available ELISA kits.

Of the eleven ELISAs applied to the 'discovery' cohort (n = 47, one sample was unavailable for validation), six (NrCAM, YKL-40,

chromogranin A, carnosinase I, transthyretin, cystatin C) showed statistically significant or near-significant differences between CDR 0 and CDR 1 groups (Figure 4); five others (PEDF, beta-2 microglobulin, clusterin/apoJ, ceruloplasmin, apoE) did not.

The six ELISAs that measured differences between the CDR 0 and CDR 1 CSF samples of the 'discovery' cohort were subsequently applied to a larger, independent set of CSF samples (n = 292) collected from volunteer participants studied by the WU-ADRC. This 'validation' cohort included a CDR 0.5 group in addition to CDR 0 and CDR 1 groups, allowing for biomarker assessment in the very early clinical stage of AD. Demographic, clinical, and genetic characteristics of these individuals at time of sample collection are presented in Table 1. Unlike the 'discovery' cohort, this 'validation' cohort was not preselected on the basis of prior biomarker values (CSF Aβ42 and tau), although assays for CSF Aβ42, tau and p-tau181 were performed.

Because the age and gender compositions differed among the clinical groups of the 'validation cohort,' we evaluated each of these 9 biomarkers (six novel candidates, Aβ42, tau, and p-tau181) for age and gender correlations in order to apply covariate analyses appropriately. Correlating with age were tau ($r = 0.318$, $p < 0.0001$), p-tau181 ($r = 0.2216$, $p < 0.001$), Aβ42 ($r = -0.2334$, $p < 0.0001$) and YKL-40 ($r = 0.4001$, $p < 0.001$); no biomarkers correlated with gender ($p > 0.05$).

As shown in Figure 5, statistically significant differences between clinically defined groups were measured for Aβ42, tau, p-tau181, NrCAM, YKL-40, chromogranin A, and carnosinase I; for transthyretin and cystatin C, non-significant trends were measured. These differences appeared in three patterns: Aβ42 showed a pronounced decrease from CDR 0 to CDR 0.5 and a lesser reduction from CDR 0.5 to CDR 1; tau, p-tau181, and YKL-40 showed increases that were equivalent in CDR 0.5 and CDR 1 relative to CDR 0; NrCAM, chromogranin A, and carnosinase I showed decreases relative to CDR 0 only in CDR 1, and not in CDR 0.5.

Diagnostic Utility of Validated Candidate Biomarkers

To evaluate and compare the potential of the validated candidate biomarkers and Aβ42, tau, and p-tau181 for identifying either very mild to mild dementia (combined CDR 0.5 and CDR 1) or mild dementia (CDR 1), ROC curves and AUCs were calculated for each biomarker using data from the 'validation' cohort (Figure 6A, B, Tables 3, 4). Stepwise logistic regression analyses indicated that, among the nine biomarkers under consideration, YKL-40, NrCAM and tau yielded the highest AUC (0.896) in discriminating cognitive normalcy (CDR 0) from very mild to mild dementia (CDR>0) (Figure 6C, Table 3); for discriminating mild dementia (CDR 1) from CDR<1, carnosinase I, chromogranin A and tau yielded the highest AUC (0.876) (Figure 6D, Table 4).

Discussion

Using an unbiased proteomics approach (2D-DIGE LC-MS/MS), this study identified 47 novel candidate CSF protein biomarkers for early AD. Subsequently, by evaluating a subset of these candidate biomarkers by ELISA, this study validated the

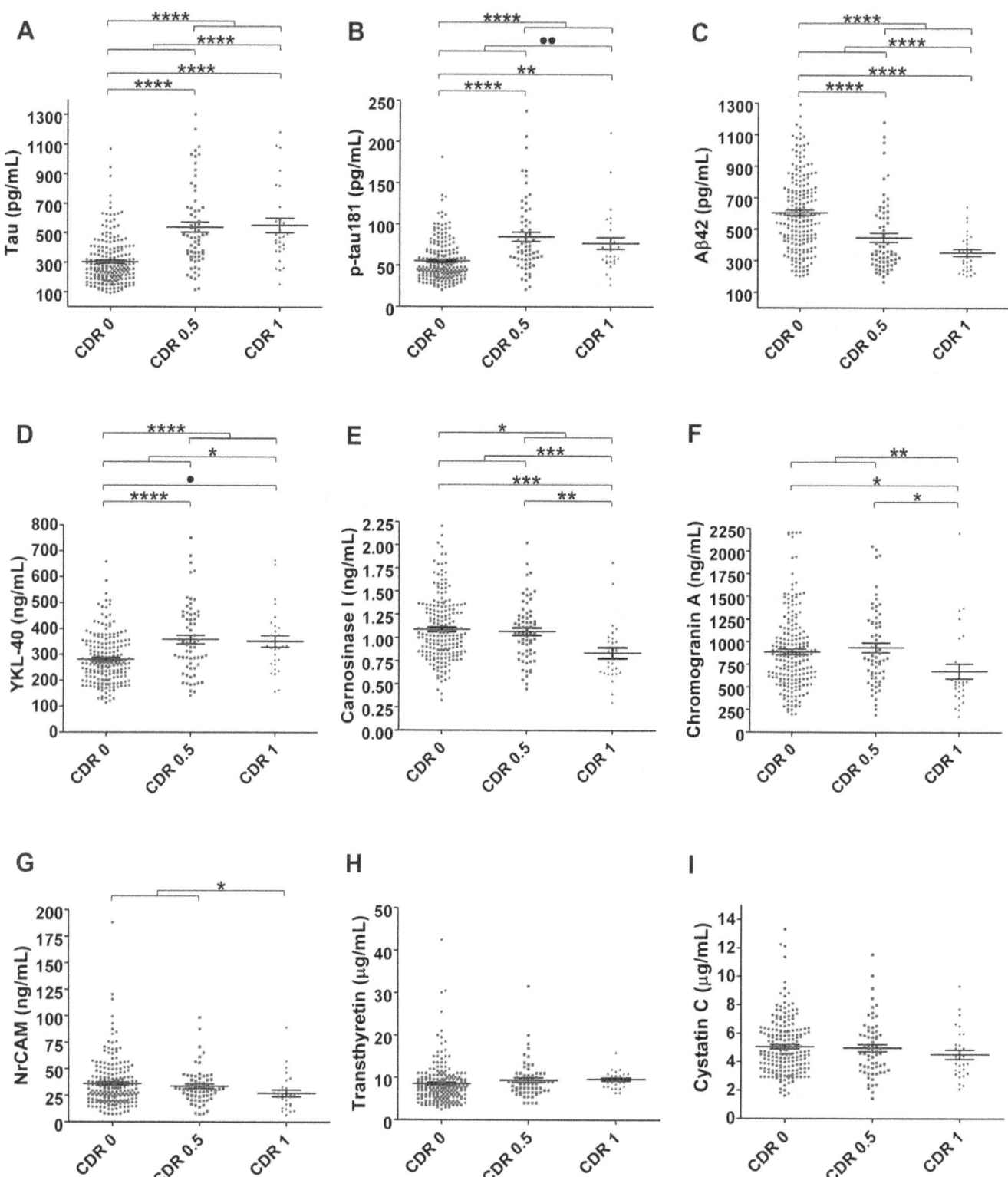

Figure 5. Six biomarker candidates and established biomarkers tau, p-tau181 and Aβ42 in 'validation' cohort CSF (n = 292). Each candidate biomarker assay was performed in triplicate, with one mean value reported for each sample; assays for tau, p-tau181 and Aβ42 were performed in duplicate. In addition to **A**. tau, **B**. p-tau181 and **C**. Aβ42 (top row), four assays (**D**. YKL-40, **E**. carnosinase I, **F**. chromogranin A, **G**. NrCAM) measured statistical differences between clinically defined groups, as indicated; **H**. transthyretin and **I**. cystatin C did not reach criterion ($\alpha = 0.05$) for any comparisons. *** p<0.05; * * p<0.01; * * * p< 0.001; * * * * p<0.0001; solid circle p<0.05** by LSD only; **double solid circle p<0.05** by unpaired t-test and Mann-Whitney, not by unpaired t-test with Welch's correction.
doi:10.1371/journal.pone.0016032.g005

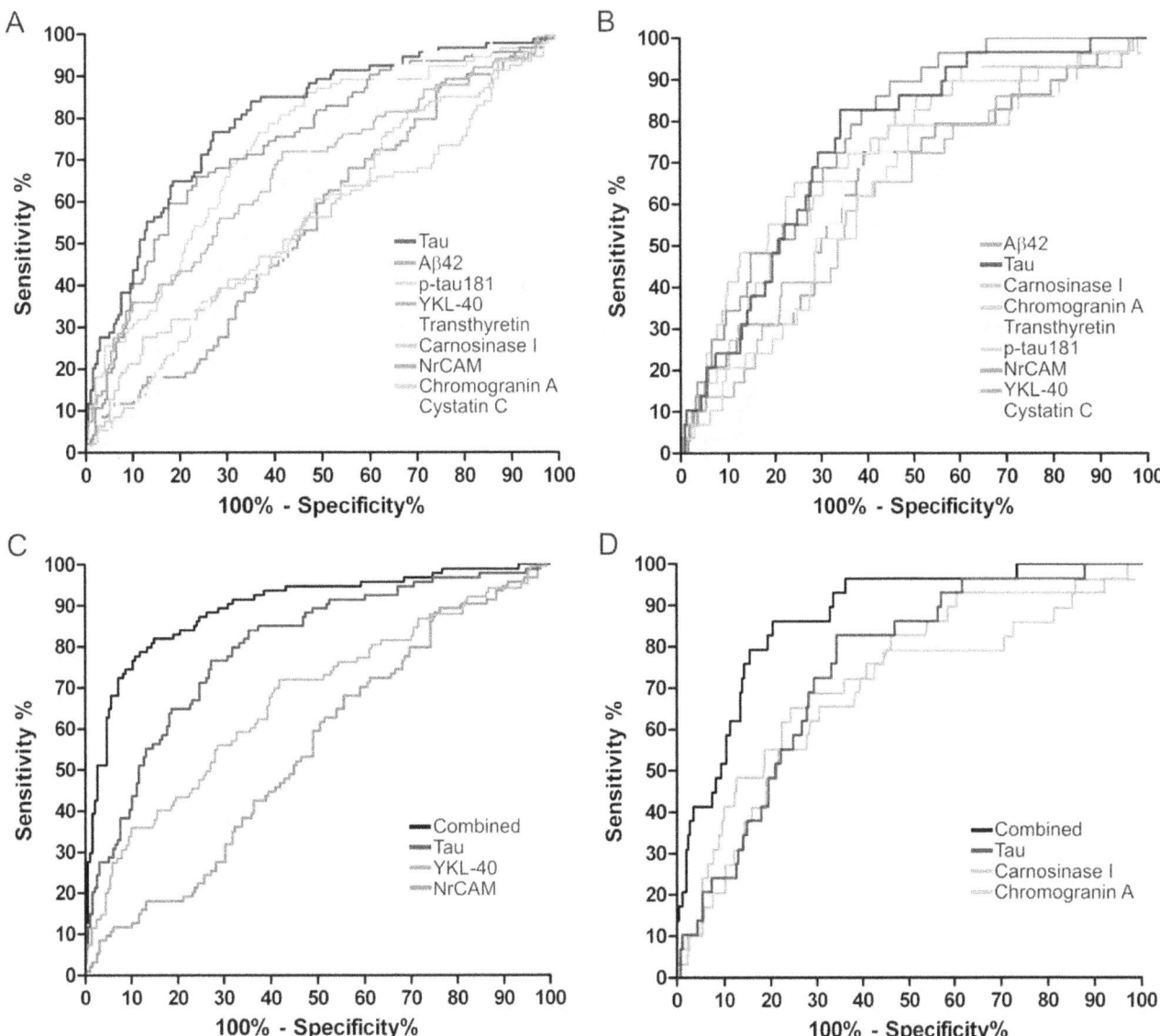

Figure 6. Receiver Operating Characteristic (ROC) curves of ELISA data from 'validation' cohort. Simple ROC analyses were performed for each biomarker to distinguish **A**. CDR>0 from CDR 0 ("earlier diagnosis") and **B**. CDR 1 from CDR<1 ("early diagnosis"). Stepwise logistic regression models were used to identify combinations of these biomarkers that would distinguish **C**. CDR>0 from CDR 0 ("earlier diagnosis"), AUC = 0.90 and **D**. CDR 1 from CDR<1 ("early diagnosis"), AUC = 0.88.
doi:10.1371/journal.pone.0016032.g006

utility of four candidate biomarkers for distinguishing groups with mild, very mild, or no dementia (CDR 1, 0.5, 0, respectively). Further statistical analyses demonstrated that these biomarkers could improve the accuracy of 'established' biomarkers Aβ42 and tau for the diagnosis of early AD.

The results from the 2D-DIGE LC-MS/MS portion of this study suggest that many of the recognized neuropathological changes of AD are represented by changes in the CSF proteome. Most of the 47 candidate biomarker proteins identified in this study can be placed into structural and/or functional categories (e.g. synaptic adhesion, synaptic function, dense core synaptic vesicle proteins, inflammation/complement, protease activity/inhibition, apolipo-proteins, etc.) associated with accepted neuropathophysiological changes in AD (Table 5). Unsupervised clustering analyses of these 2D-DIGE data, performed without the influence of CSF Aβ42, tau, p-tau181 and *APOE* genotype, additionally suggest that these biomarker candidates collectively show utility for discriminating groups with and without mild DAT (Figure 3).

In the second phase of this study, designed to measure a subset of candidate biomarker proteins in two independent sample sets by ELISA, four of the eleven candidate biomarkers that were tested showed capacity to distinguish clinical groups. However, seven candidate biomarkers did not show statistically significant differences between clinical groups in either the smaller 'discovery' cohort or the larger 'validation' cohort. Superficially, this 'failure rate' might cast doubt on the list of candidate biomarkers identified through 2D-DIGE. However, it is important to note that 2D-DIGE is sensitive to changes in concentrations of minor protein isoforms and post-translational modifications that may not significantly alter the global concentrations of a 'parent' protein, which would be measured by ELISA. Therefore, it is not surprising that some of the candidate biomarker ELISAs did not replicate the findings from 2D-DIGE. Transthyretin provides a prime example: all of the significant gel-features ascribed to transthyretin (gel features # 20, 52, 57, 58, 60, 77, 78, 79, 84, 87, 110, 115; Table 2) showed unusual electrophoretic patterns and

Table 3. Receiver Operating Characteristic Curve Areas for CDR 0 vs <0 Comparison.

Biomarker	Area Under Curve	Standard Error	95% Confidence Interval
Tau	0.8004	0.0279	0.7457–0.8551
Aβ42	0.7429	0.0315	0.6812–0.8046
p-tau181	0.7339	0.0315	0.6721–0.7956
YKL-40	0.6717	0.0349	0.6033–0.7401
Transthyretin	0.6190	0.0331	0.5541–0.6838
Carnosinase I	0.5735	0.0365	0.5020–0.6450
NrCAM	0.5422	0.0355	0.4726–0.6118
Chromogranin A	0.5303	0.0373	0.4572–0.6034
Cystatin C	0.5297	0.0366	0.4579–0.6014
Logistic Regression	0.8955	0.0212	0.8539–0.9372

ROC analyses of 'validation' cohort ELISA data were performed for each biomarker to distinguish CDR>0 from CDR 0 ("earlier diagnosis"). A stepwise logistic regression model, applied to identify a complementary combination of these biomarkers that would optimize accuracy (maximize area under the curve [AUC]) without including additional non-contributory biomarkers, accepted tau, YKL-40 and NrCAM and yielded an AUC of 0.8955 ("Logistic Regression," lowest row).
doi:10.1371/journal.pone.0016032.t003

were dwarfed by the canonical transthyretin gel features that did not individually show statistical differences (Figure 1). In fact, whereas most of the significant transthyretin 2D-DIGE gel features were decreased in AD, the global transthyretin levels measured by ELISA in the 'discovery' and 'validation' cohorts were actually mildly increased in groups with cognitive impairment (CDR>0) relative to those without (CDR 0) (Figures 4 and 5). To measure the sub-species of transthyretin that were identified by 2D-DIGE as decreasing in AD will require assays that specifically target relevant post-translational modifications and exclude other forms of transthyretin. Similarly, other 2D-DIGE biomarker candidates may also require specifically tailored assays for accurate, high-throughput measurement.

Nevertheless, four candidate biomarkers were successfully validated in both cohorts, and two others showed non-significant trends by ELISA in the larger 'validation' cohort (Figure 5). This larger cohort represented three different cognitive stages: normalcy, very mild dementia, and mild dementia (CDR 0, CDR 0.5, CDR 1, respectively), and revealed different patterns of CSF biomarker levels, vis-a-vis cognitive status. The CSF concentration of YKL-40, an astrocytic marker of plaque-associated neuroin-

flammation [137–148], is increased by the very earliest stage of clinical disease (CDR 0.5). Transthyretin [24,87,173,175,179–184] and cystatin C [22,173,185–188], two proteins with neuroprotective qualities that are implicated in preventing amyloidogenesis of Aβ peptide, show a similar pattern. In contrast, the concentrations of NrCAM, a synaptic adhesion molecule [19,46–49], chromogranin A, a dense core synaptic vesicle protein [19,20,22,59–62], and carnosinase I, a neuronal dipeptidase responsible for degradation of the anti-oxidant and metal-chelating dipeptide carnosine [33,107–111] do not decline until mild dementia ensues (CDR 1).

Like the current leading CSF biomarkers for AD (Aβ42, tau and p-tau181), all of these biomarker candidates show ranges with substantial overlap between clinically defined groups. This issue of overlapping values, common among candidate AD CSF biomarkers reported to date, suggests that any one biomarker will be insufficient to accurately identify early AD, and that an ensemble of complementary biomarkers will be required to provide adequate sensitivity and specificity. Therefore, to identify an optimal combination of these biomarkers that can distinguish the early clinical stages of AD from cognitive normalcy, we applied

Table 4. Receiver Operating Characteristic Curve Areas for CDR 1 vs <1 Comparison.

Biomarker	Area Under Curve	Standard Error	95% Confidence Interval
Aβ42	0.7690	0.0376	0.6953–0.8427
Tau	0.7502	0.0420	0.6679–0.8325
Carnosinase I	0.7277	0.0512	0.6273–0.8281
Chromogranin A	0.6879	0.0566	0.5771–0.7988
Transthyretin	0.6605	0.0380	0.5860–0.7350
p-tau181	0.6512	0.0483	0.5566–0.7458
NrCAM	0.6411	0.0553	0.5326–0.7495
YKL-40	0.6271	0.0532	0.5228–0.7313
Cystatin C	0.5752	0.0565	0.4645–0.6858
Logistic Regression	0.8762	0.0314	0.8147–0.9377

ROC analyses of 'validation' cohort ELISA data were performed for each biomarker to distinguish CDR 1 from CDR<1 ("early diagnosis"). A stepwise logistic regression model, applied to identify a complementary combination of these biomarkers that would optimize accuracy (maximize area under the curve [AUC]) without including additional non-contributory biomarkers, accepted tau, carnosinase I and chromogranin A, yielding an AUC of 0.8762 ("Logistic Regression," lowest row).
doi:10.1371/journal.pone.0016032.t004

Table 5. Candidate CSF biomarkers reflect AD-related pathophysiologic changes.

Functional/Structural Category	Protein	References
Adhesion molecules	N-Cadherin	[39-45]
	NrCAM	[19,46-49]
	Calsyntenin	[47,50-53]
	Neuronal Pentraxin Receptor	[47,54]
	Brain Associated Small Cell Lung Cancer Antigen (NCAM-140/CD56)	[55]
	Nectin-like molecule-1/TSLL1/SynCam3	[56-58]
Dense core vesicles	Chromogranin A	[19,20,22,59-62]
	Chromogranin B	[60,62]
	Secretogranin II	[60-63]
	Secretogranin III	[59,64,65]
	VGF NGF Inducible precursor	[20,22,23,66-69]
	Carboxypeptidase E	[70-75]
Synaptic/Neuronal metabolism	Aspartate aminotransferase I	[76-82]
Synaptic Function	S100A1	[83]
	Neuronal Pentraxin Receptor	[27,47,54]
	Brain Acetylcholinesterase Putative Membrane Anchor (CutA1)	[84,85]
	Calsyntenin	[47,50-53]
Neuroprotection	PEDF (Serpin-F1)	[86-96]
	Annexin I	[97-99]
	Prosaposin	[20,100-103]
	Secretogranin II	[104-106]
	Carnosinase I	[33,107-111]
	Extracellular superoxide dismutase (SOD3)	[112-114]
Apoptosis/Actin remodeling	Gelsolin	[115-121]
	Prk-1 (PKN)	[122-126]
Synaptic plasticity/Learning and memory	VGF NGF inducible precursor	[20,22,23,66-69]
	NrCAM	[19,46-49]
	β3GnT1	[49,127,128]
	Carnosinase I	[33,107-111]
	Carbonic Anhydrase IV	[129-131]
	S100A1	[132]
	Carboxypeptidase E	[70-75]
	Calmodulin	[133-136]
	Extracellular superoxide dismutase (SOD3)	[114]
Inflammation/Complement	*YKL-40/Chitinase 3-Like 1	[137-148]
	PEDF (Serpin-F1)	[86-96]
	Annexin I	[97-99]
	IHRP/ITIH4	[149,150]
	Vitronectin	[151-155]
	*Complement C4B3	[156-161]
	Kininogen I	[162,163]
	Chromogranin A	[19,20,22,59-62]
	Secretogranin III	[59,64,65]
	Apolipoprotein J	[27,152,156,157,164-167]
	Beta 2-microglobulin	[168-171]
	Extracellular superoxide dismutase (SOD3)	[172]
Prostaglandin metabolism	*Prostaglandin H2 D Isomerase/Beta-trace	[162,173-175]
Amyloid beta peptide binding/Amyloidogenesis	*Apolipoprotein A1 (proapolipoprotein)	[176,177]
	Apolipoprotein E	[178]
	Apolipoprotein J	[27,152,156,157,164-167]

Table 5. Cont.

Functional/Structural Category	Protein	References
	Transthyretin	[87,173,175,179-184]
	Gelsolin	[115-121]
	Vitronectin	[151-155]
	Cystatin C	[22,173,185-188]
	*Prostaglandin H2 D Isomerase/Beta-trace	[162,173-175]
	*α-2-macroglobulin	[19,189-194]
	*α-1-antichymotrypsin	[33,195-199]
Protease activity	*α-1-antichymotrypsin	[33,195-199]
	*α-2-macroglobulin	[19,189-194]
	Cystatin C	[22,173,185-188]
	Carboxypeptidase E	[70-75]
Matrix proteins	Fibulin 3 (EFEMP1)	[200-202]
	Vitronectin	[151-155]
Phospholipase activity	Annexin I (Lipocortin)	[97-99]
	Prosaposin	[20,100-103]
Apolipoproteins	*Apolipoprotein A1 (proapolipoprotein)	[24,165,166,176,177,203,204]
	Apolipoprotein CII	[25,166,205]
	Apolipoprotein CIII	[25,206,207]
	Apolipoprotein E	[24,27,165,204]
	Apolipoprotein J	[27,152,156,157,164-167]
	*Apolipoprotein H	[19,25,165,208,209]
Calcium binding/homeostasis	Calmodulin	[134-136]
	S100A1	[83,210]
	Annexin I (Lipocortin)	[97-99]
	Calsyntenin	[47,50-53]
	Gelsolin	[115-121]
Metal (Copper and Iron) Binding	Carnosinase I	[33,107-111]
	Ceruloplasmin	[211-217]
	Brain Acetylcholinesterase Putative Membrane Anchor (CutA1)	[84,85]
Chaperone complex/activity	S100A1	[218]
	Transthyretin (prealbumin)	[24,87,173,175,179-184]
Endoplasmic Reticulum - Associated Degradation	Man9-mannosidase	[219-221]
Extracellular and Intraneuronal pH	Carbonic Anhydrase IV	[129-131]
	Carnosinase I	[33,107-111]
Glycobiology (lactosamine synthesis)	β3GnT1	[49,127,128]
Hemodynamics	Angiotensinogen	[172,222]
	Extracellular superoxide dismutase (SOD3)	[172]
Thyroid hormone transport	Transthyretin (prealbumin)	[24,87,173,175,179-184]
Unknown	Hypothetical protein	

CSF biomarkers are grouped according to reported function(s) and, when appropriate, cellular locations. Asterisks (*) indicate those biomarkers found to be increased in AD CSF; the vast majority were decreased.
doi:10.1371/journal.pone.0016032.t005

stepwise logistic regression analyses to the ELISA data from our 'validation' cohort (Figure 6, Tables 3 and 4). These analyses suggest that four candidate AD biomarkers (YKL-40, NrCAM, chromogranin A, carnosinase I) can improve the ability of tau to classify individuals into CDR 0, CDR 0.5 and CDR 1 groups with appreciable accuracy.

It may appear counter-intuitive that Aβ42 and p-tau181, which individually discriminate very mild AD and mild AD from cognitively normal groups quite well, were not incorporated into either 'optimal' biomarker panel by the stepwise logistic regression analyses. Likewise, NrCAM was included in the optimal CDR 0 vs CDR>0 biomarker panel (AUC 0.896) even though its mean levels did not independently show a statistical difference between CDR 0 and CDR>0 groups. In considering this outcome, it may be worth noting that if NrCAM, transthyretin, chromogranin and cystatin C are removed from consideration, the stepwise logistic regression model for the CDR 0 vs CDR>0 comparison yields an 'optimal' biomarker panel that includes only tau, Aβ42 and carnosinase I, with an AUC of 0.849 (not shown). In this restricted analysis, the paired contribution of Aβ42 and carnosinase I to tau is apparently greater than that of YKL-40. These analyses illustrate how 'unpredictable' and context-dependent optimal biomarker combinations can be, and suggest that biomarker complementarity may be more important to consider than each biomarker's independent performance, when choosing a biomarker panel. Of course, it will be necessary to replicate these findings in additional independent cohorts. It will also be essential to evaluate a greater number of candidate biomarkers in similar fashion, in order to construct a biomarker panel with even greater accuracy.

Another worthwhile feature to consider when evaluating and selecting CSF biomarkers is relative concentration in the blood (plasma, serum), because biomarker measurements in CSF can be artifactually influenced by subtle blood contamination at the time of lumbar puncture; from this perspective, ideal CSF biomarkers show CSF concentrations that are equal to or greater than those in blood. An additional reason to assess plasma/serum concentrations of candidate CSF biomarkers is to determine if venipuncture, which is more easily performed than lumbar puncture, might yield equivalent information. Among the six CSF biomarkers identified by stepwise logistic regression analysis in the current study, Aβ42 and tau [8–11], YKL-40 [137], and chromogranin A [223] show higher levels in CSF than in plasma; carnosinase I levels appear similar in CSF and serum [110]; NrCAM levels appear higher in

serum than in CSF, although the forms of NrCAM present in these fluids may differ [224]. Concerning independent utility as biomarkers for AD, only plasma YKL-40 and serum NrCAM have shown promise [137,225], albeit inferior to that of CSF YKL-40 and NrCAM demonstrated here. Plasma tau concentrations in AD and controls are below the level of detection of the most commonly used tau assays, and plasma Aβ42 [8–11] and plasma chromogranin A (R.Perrin et al., unpublished data) concentrations show no significant differences among CDR groups. Serum carnosinase *activity* likewise has not shown significant differences between AD and controls in one small study [111], though a difference between AD and mixed dementia (including vascular dementia) has been reported [111]. To our knowledge, an evaluation of plasma or serum carnosinase I *concentrations* in the context of AD has not yet been performed or reported. Further assessment of the potential of these and other proteins as candidate AD biomarkers in plasma or serum, complete with evaluation of their performance as ensembles, remains an important task for future studies. Currently, however, this panel of six biomarkers appears likely to show much greater promise in its application to CSF.

Indeed, by providing proof of concept, this study outlines a scheme to categorize the early stages of AD using CSF protein biomarkers that reflect established features of the pathophysiological evolution of the disease (Figure 7). Building upon previous findings that low CSF Aβ42 can identify cognitively normal individuals with plaques (preclinical AD) [8,11], and that tau/Aβ42 and YKL-40/Aβ42 ratios can predict risk of developing

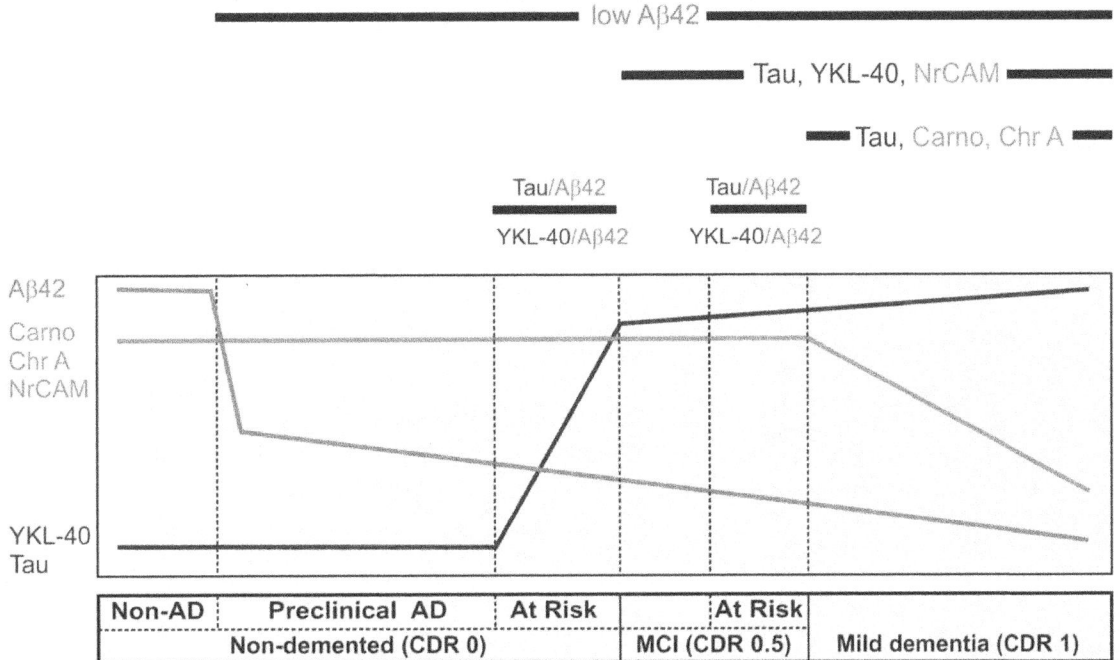

Figure 7. Hypothetical model defines early stages of AD by temporal pattern of CSF protein biomarker levels. The horizontal bar (below) describes the early clinicopathological progression from cognitive normalcy without AD pathology ('**Non-AD**') to mild dementia in six stages. As depicted by the curves above, **Non-AD** CSF has high Aβ42 (red line), high chromogranin A (Chr A), carnosinase I (Carno I) and NrCAM (green line), and low YKL-40 and tau (blue line). Reduced CSF Aβ42 correlates with amyloid plaque deposits, the first sign of neuropathologically identifiable AD ('**preclinical AD**') [8]. CSF Aβ42 appears to decrease further as cognition declines from normal (Clinical Dementia Rating [CDR] 0) to very mild cognitive impairment (**MCI, CDR 0.5**) to mild dementia (**CDR 1**). When considered as ratios with Aβ42, CSF markers of neuroinflammation (e.g. YKL-40) and neurofibrillary tangle pathology (e.g. tau) appear to increase before and predict the onset of very mild cognitive impairment (**MCI, CDR 0.5**), defining a **CDR 0** group '**At Risk**' for cognitive decline [9,15,137]; YKL-40 and tau also appear to be higher among who progress rapidly from very mild to mild dementia, defining a **CDR 0.5** group '**At Risk**' for impending cognitive decline [137,230]. Reductions in synapse-associated (NrCAM, chromogranin A) and neuronal (carnosinase I) proteins, and increases in YKL-40 and tau mirror the progression and anatomical spread of synaptic and neuronal losses, gliosis and tau pathology associated with cognitive decline, and can be used to define **CDR 0.5** and **CDR 1**.
doi:10.1371/journal.pone.0016032.g007

cognitive impairment [9,15,137], this minimal panel of six CSF biomarkers (YKL-40, NrCAM, chromogranin A, carnosinase I, tau and Aβ42) begins to segregate individuals into six clinico-pathological categories: normal cognition without amyloid plaques, normal cognition with amyloid plaques (preclinical AD), normal cognition at increased risk to develop dementia (converters), very mild dementia (CDR 0.5), very mild dementia at increased risk for progression, and mild dementia (CDR 1) (Figure 7).

We acknowledge that this minimal panel of biomarkers currently has insufficient sensitivity and specificity for clinical application, particularly because it has not been fully evaluated for its ability to discriminate AD from non-AD causes of dementia (although Aβ42, p-tau181, tau, and specific fragments of chromogranin A and cystatin C have shown some ability to distinguish AD from frontotemporal lobar degeneration [FTLD]) [22,226,227]. The incorporation of additional biomarkers that are likely to discriminate early AD from cognitive normalcy, such as those identified in the first phase of this study, or other biomarkers that have already shown promise for distinguishing AD from other leading causes of dementia (e.g. agouti related peptide, eotaxin-3, and hepatocyte growth factor [19], complement C3a des-arg and integral membrane protein 2B CT [22], for FTLDs; and alpha-synuclein [228], apoH and vitamin D binding protein [25] for Lewy body disorders), would likely improve the panel's diagnostic utility. However, even in its current form, this initial panel might show value if applied in the context of clinical trial design, wherein simple enrichment of study populations for characteristics of interest would increase efficiency and power and reduce duration and cost. A biomarker panel like this one might also allow clinical trials to evaluate stage-specific responses to treatment, which may differ. Finally, because most of these biomarkers reflect underlying pathological changes in real time, it is appealing to speculate that these biomarkers may have additional utility for evaluating clinically imperceptible treatment responses (as in [229]) and for monitoring neuropathological – rather than cognitive – decline.

Supporting Information

Figure S1 ApoE protein isoforms appear in different gel features on 2D-DIGE. Overlays of fluorescent 2D-DIGE images from gels representing CSF from two individuals with homozygosity for *APOE-ε2* (green) or *APOE-ε3* (red) (panel **A**) and for *APOE-ε3* (green) or *APOE-ε4* (red) (panel **B**) illustrate the heterogeneity of signal distribution by isoelectric point and molecular weight among apoE protein isoforms derived from different alleles. In panels **C, D, E, F, G, H**, signal intensities of individual CSF samples, grouped by genotype (2/2, 3/3 and 4/4 represent homozygotes; 2/3, 3/4 represent heterozygotes) are indicated for six apoE gel features (labeled C, D, E, F, G, H in panels **A** and **B**), illustrating that gel features C and D represent apoE2; gel feature E represents multiple forms; gel feature F represents apoE3; and gel features G and H, apoE4. (TIF)

Table S1 Mass spectrometry and protein identification data for 2D-DIGE gel features that differ in AD CSF. Results are ordered sequentially by "heat map #" [column A], corresponding to the 'heat map' row numbers in Figure 2. "Spot" [column B] refers to BVA number (see Methods). "(Accession) primary protein name" [column C] provides the gi number and protein name from the NCBI database. "Protein molecular weight" [column D] is the gene product molecular weight in Daltons. "Protein score" [column E] is the MASCOT-generated protein score. "Protein ID probability" [column F] indicates Scaffold's percent probability that the protein identification is correct. "Spectral count" [column G] is the number of spectra assigned to the protein by Scaffold. "Unique proteins" [column H] refers to the number of recognized tryptic peptides attributed to the protein by MASCOT. "Peptide sequence" [column I] indicates the amino acid sequence of the tryptic peptide predicted by MASCOT. "MASCOT ion score" [column J] is the MASCOT quality assessment of the peptide sequence assignment. "M/Z (observed)" [column K] is mass/charge ratio. "Mass (observed)" [column L] of peptide is indicated in Daltons. "Mass (theoretical)" [column M] is idealized tryptic peptide mass as predicted by NCBI. "Mass error (ppm)" [column N] is the error in parts per million determined through comparison of theoretical peptide mass to data generated by mass spectrometry. "MS source" [column O] reflects the mass spectrometer that produced the observed data (Q-STAR or LTQ-FT). "Modifications" [column P] lists variable post-translational modifications identified by mass spectrometry peptide sequence analysis. (XLS)

Acknowledgments

The authors would like to express our appreciation to the Biomarker Core, Clinical Core, Data Management and Statistics Core, Genetics Core, lumbar puncture physicians, and volunteer participants of the Knight ADRC of Washington University in St. Louis, and to the volunteer participants of the University of Washington, the Oregon Health and Science University, the University of Pennsylvania, and the University of California San Diego.

Author Contributions

Conceived and designed the experiments: RJP RC-S DMH JCM AMF RRT. Performed the experiments: RJP RC-S JPM AED PG RRT ARS. Analyzed the data: RJP RC-S JPM AED PG RRT ARS CMR DMH AMF. Contributed reagents/materials/analysis tools: RRT ERP GL DRG CMC JFQ JAK DMH JCM AMF. Wrote the paper: RJP RC-S JPM RRT. All authors revised the manuscript for important intellectual content and gave final approval of the version to be published.

References

1. Braak H, Braak E (1997) Frequency of stages of Alzheimer-related lesions in different age categories. Neurobiol Aging 18: 351–357.
2. Morris J, Price J (2001) Pathologic correlates of nondemented aging, mild cognitive impairment, and early stage Alzheimer's disease. J Mol Neurosci 17: 101–118.
3. Price J, Ko A, Wade M, Tsou S, McKeel D, et al. (2001) Neuron number in the entorhinal cortex and CA1 in preclinical Alzheimer's disease. Arch Neurol 58: 1395–1402.
4. Barnes LL, Schneider JA, Boyle PA, Bienias JL, Bennett DA (2006) Memory complaints are related to Alzheimer disease pathology in older persons. Neurology 67: 1581–1585.
5. Markesbery W, Schmitt F, Kryscio R, Davis D, Smith C, et al. (2006) Neuropathologic substrate of Mild Cognitive Impairment. Arch Neurol 63: 38–46.
6. Motter R, Vigo-Pelfrey C, Kholodenko D, Barbour R, Johnson-Wood J, et al. (1995) Reduction of β-amyloid peptide$_{42}$ in the cerebrospinal fluid of patients with Alzheimer's disease. Ann Neurol 38: 643–648.
7. Sunderland T, Linker G, Mirza N, Putnam K, Friedman D, et al. (2003) Decreased β-amyloid$_{1-42}$ and increased tau levels in cerebrospinal fluid of patients with Alzheimer's disease. JAMA 289: 2094–2103.
8. Fagan A, Mintun M, Mach R, Lee S-Y, Dence C, et al. (2006) Inverse relation between in vivo amyloid imaging load and CSF Aβ42 in humans. Ann Neurol 59: 512–519.

9. Fagan A, Roe C, Xiong C, Mintun M, Morris J, et al. (2007) Cerebrospinal fluid tau/Aβ42 ratio as a prediction of cognitive decline in nondemented older adults. Arch Neurol 64: 343–349.

10. Fagan AM, Head D, Shah AR, Marcus D, Mintun M, et al. (2009) Decreased cerebrospinal fluid Abeta(42) correlates with brain atrophy in cognitively normal elderly. Ann Neurol 65: 176–183.

11. Fagan AM, Mintun MA, Shah AR, Aldea P, Roe CM, et al. (2009) Cerebrospinal fluid tau and ptau(181) increase with cortical amyloid deposition in cognitively normal individuals: implications for future clinical trials of Alzheimer's disease. EMBO Mol Med 1: 371–380.

12. Tolboom N, van der Flier WM, Yaqub M, Boellaard R, Verwey NA, et al. (2009) Relationship of cerebrospinal fluid markers to 11C-PiB and 18F-FDDNP binding. J Nucl Med 50: 1464–1470.

13. Grimmer T, Riemenschneider M, Forstl H, Henriksen G, Klunk WE, et al. (2009) Beta amyloid in Alzheimer's disease: increased deposition in brain is reflected in reduced concentration in cerebrospinal fluid. Biol Psychiatry 65: 927–934.

14. Jagust WJ, Landau SM, Shaw LM, Trojanowski JQ, Koeppe RA, et al. (2009) Relationships between biomarkers in aging and dementia. Neurology 73: 1193–1199.

15. Li G, Sokal I, Quinn J, Leverenz J, Brodey M, et al. (2007) CSF tau/Aβ42 ratio for increased risk of mild cognitive impairment: A follow-up study. Neurology 69: 631–639.

16. Snider BJ, Fagan AM, Roe C, Shah AR, Grant EA, et al. (2009) Cerebrospinal fluid biomarkers and rate of cognitive decline in very mild dementia of the Alzheimer type. Arch Neurol 66: 638–645.

17. Zhang J, Goodlett DR, Quinn JF, Peskind E, Kaye JA, et al. (2005) Quantitative proteomics of cerebrospinal fluid from patients with Alzheimer disease. J Alzheimers Dis 7: 125–133; discussion 173–180.

18. Ray S, Britschgi M, Herbert C, Takeda-Uchimura Y, Boxer A, et al. (2007) Classification and prediction of clinical Alzheimer's diagnosis based on plasma signaling proteins. Nat Med 13: 1359–1362.

19. Hu WT, Chen-Plotkin A, Arnold SE, Grossman M, Clark CM, et al. (2010) Novel CSF biomarkers for Alzheimer's disease and mild cognitive impairment. Acta Neuropathol 119: 669–678.

20. Simonsen AH, McGuire J, Podust VN, Davies H, Minthon L, et al. (2008) Identification of a novel panel of cerebrospinal fluid biomarkers for Alzheimer's disease. Neurobiol Aging 29: 961–968.

21. Simonsen A, McGuire J, Hansson O, Zetterberg H, Podust V, et al. (2007) Novel panel of cerebrospinal fluid biomarkers for the prediction of progression to Alzheimer dementia in patients with mild cognitive impairment. Arch Neurol 64: 366–370.

22. Simonsen AH, McGuire J, Podust VN, Hagnelius NO, Nilsson TK, et al. (2007) A novel panel of cerebrospinal fluid biomarkers for the differential diagnosis of Alzheimer's disease versus normal aging and frontotemporal dementia. Dement Geriatr Cogn Disord 24: 434–440.

23. Carrette O, Demalte I, Scherl A, Yalkinoglu O, Corthals G, et al. (2003) A panel of cerebrospinal fluid potential biomarkers for the diagnosis of Alzheimer's disease. Proteomics 3: 1486–1494.

24. Davidsson P, Westman-Brinkmalm A, Nilsson CL, Lindbjer M, Paulson L, et al. (2002) Proteome analysis of cerebrospinal fluid proteins in Alzheimer patients. Neuroreport 13: 611–615.

25. Abdi F, Quinn J, Jankovic J, McIntosh M, Leverenz J, et al. (2006) Detection of biomarkers with a multiplex quantitative proteomic platform in cerebrospinal fluid of patients with neurodegenerative disorders. J Alzheimers Dis 9: 293–348.

26. Choe L DAM, Relkin NR, Pappin D, Ross P, Williamson B, Guertin S, Pribil P, Lee KH (2007) 8-plex quantitation of changes in cerebrospinal fluid protein expression in subjects undergoing intravenous immunoglobulin treatment for Alzheimer's disease. Proteomics 7: 3651–3660.

27. Finehout EJ, Franck Z, Choe LH, Relkin N, Lee KH (2007) Cerebrospinal fluid proteomic biomarkers for Alzheimer's disease. Ann Neurol 61: 120–129.

28. McKhann G, Drachman D, Folstein M, Katzman R, Price D, et al. (1984) Clinical diagnosis of Alzheimer's disease: report of the NINCDS-ADRDA Work Group under the auspices of Department of Health and Human Services Task Force on Alzheimer's Disease. Neurology 34: 939–944.

29. Morris JC (1993) The Clinical Dementia Rating (CDR). Current version and scoring rules. Neurology 43: 2412–2414.

30. Suzuki N, Cheung TT, Cai XD, Odaka A, Otvos L, Jr., et al. (1994) An increased percentage of long amyloid beta protein secreted by familial amyloid beta protein precursor (beta APP717) mutants. Science 264: 1336–1340.

31. Storandt M, Grant E, Miller J, Morris J (2006) Longitudinal course and neuropathologic outcomes in original vs revised MCI and in pre-MCI. Neurology 67: 467–473.

32. Hu Y, Malone J, Fagan A, Townsend R, Holtzman D (2005) Comparative proteomic analysis of intra- and interindividual variation in human cerebrospinal fluid. Mol & Cell Proteom 4: 2000–2009.

33. Hu Y, Hosseini A, Kauwe J, Gross J, Cairns N, et al. (2007) Identification and validation of novel CSF biomarkers for early stages of Alzheimer's disease. Proteomics - Clin Appl 1: 1373–1384.

34. Alban A, David SO, Bjorkesten L, Andersson C, Sloge E, et al. (2003) A novel experimental design for comparative two-dimensional gel analysis: two-dimensional difference gel electrophoresis incorporating a pooled internal standard. Proteomics 3: 36–44.

35. Havlis J TH, Sebela M, Shevchenko A (2003) Fast-response proteomics by accelerated in-gel digestion of proteins. Anal Chem 75: 1300–1306.

36. King J, Gross J, Lovly C, Rohrs H, Piwnica-Worms H, et al. (2006) Accurate mass-driven analysis for the characterization of protein phosphorylation. Study of the human chk2 protein kinase Anal Chem 78: 2171–2181.

37. Bredemeyer A, Lewis R, Malone J, Davis A, Gross J, et al. (2004) A proteomic approach for the discovery of protease substrates. Proc Natl Acad Sci USA 101: 11785–11790.

38. Liu H, Sadygov RG, Yates JR, 3rd (2004) A model for random sampling and estimation of relative protein abundance in shotgun proteomics. Anal Chem 76: 4193–4201.

39. Uemura K, Lill CM, Banks M, Asada M, Aoyagi N, et al. (2009) N-cadherin-based adhesion enhances Abeta release and decreases Abeta42/40 ratio. J Neurochem 108: 350–360.

40. Mysore SP, Tai CY, Schuman EM (2007) Effects of N-cadherin disruption on spine morphological dynamics. Front Cell Neurosci 1: 1.

41. Bekirov IH NV, Svoronos A, Huntley GW, Benson DL (2008) Cadherin-8 and N-cadherin differentially regulate pre- and postsynaptic development of the hippocampal mossy fiber pathway. Hippocampus 18: 349–363.

42. Jang YN, Jung YS, Lee SH, Moon CH, Kim CH, et al. (2009) Calpain-mediated N-cadherin proteolytic processing in brain injury. J Neurosci 29: 5974–5984.

43. Kubota K, Inoue K, Hashimoto R, Kumamoto N, Kosuga A, et al. (2009) Tumor necrosis factor receptor-associated protein 1 regulates cell adhesion and synaptic morphology via modulation of N-cadherin expression. J Neurochem 110: 496–508.

44. Latefi NS, Pedraza L, Schohl A, Li Z, Ruthazer ES (2009) N-cadherin prodomain cleavage regulates synapse formation in vivo. Dev Neurobiol 69: 518–529.

45. Schrick C, Fischer A, Srivastava DP, Tronson NC, Penzes P, et al. (2007) N-cadherin regulates cytoskeletally associated IQGAP1/ERK signaling and memory formation. Neuron 55: 786–798.

46. Kalus I, Bormann U, Mzoughi M, Schachner M, Kleene R (2006) Proteolytic cleavage of the neural cell adhesion molecule by ADAM17/TACE is involved in neurite outgrowth. J Neurochem 98: 78–88.

47. Yin GN, Lee HW, Cho JY, Suk K (2009) Neuronal pentraxin receptor in cerebrospinal fluid as a potential biomarker for neurodegenerative diseases. Brain Res 1265: 158–170.

48. Aisa B, Gil-Bea FJ, Solas M, García-Alloza M, Chen CP, et al. (2010) Altered NCAM Expression Associated with the Cholinergic System in Alzheimer's Disease. J Alzheimers Dis 20: 659–668.

49. Storan MJ, Magnaldo T, Biol-N'Garagba MC, Zick Y, Key B (2004) Expression and putative role of lactoseries carbohydrates present on NCAM in the rat primary olfactory pathway. J Comp Neurol 475: 289–302.

50. Konecna A, Frischknecht R, Kinter J, Ludwig A, Steuble M, et al. (2006) Calsyntenin-1 docks vesicular cargo to kinesin-1. Mol Biol Cell 17: 3651–3663.

51. Ludwig A, Blume J, Diep TM, Yuan J, Mateos JM, et al. (2009) Calsyntenins Mediate TGN Exit of APP in a Kinesin-1-Dependent Manner. Traffic 10: 572–589.

52. Vogt L, Schrimpf SP, Meskenaite V, Frischknecht R, Kinter J, et al. (2001) Calsyntenin-1, a proteolytically processed postsynaptic membrane protein with a cytoplasmic calcium-binding domain. Mol Cell Neurosci 17: 151–166.

53. Hintsch G, Zurlinden A, Meskenaite V, Steuble M, Fink-Widmer K, et al. (2002) The calsyntenins—a family of postsynaptic membrane proteins with distinct neuronal expression patterns. Mol Cell Neurosci 21: 393–409.

54. Cho RW, Park JM, Wolff SB, Xu D, Hopf C, et al. (2008) mGluR1/5-dependent long-term depression requires the regulated ectodomain cleavage of neuronal pentraxin NPR by TACE. Neuron 57: 858–871.

55. Umezawa Y, Kuge S, Kikyo N, Shirai T, Watanabe J, et al. (1991) Identity of brain-associated small cell lung cancer antigen and the CD56 (NKH-1/Leu-19) leukocyte differentiation antigen and the neural cell adhesion molecule. Jpn J Clin Oncol 21: 251–255.

56. Kakunaga S, Ikeda W, Itoh S, Deguchi-Tawarada M, Ohtsuka T, et al. (2005) Nectin-like molecule-1/TSLL1/SynCAM3: a neural tissue-specific immuno-globulin-like cell-cell adhesion molecule localizing at non-junctional contact sites of presynaptic nerve terminals, axons and glia cell processes. J Cell Sci 118: 1267–1277.

57. Gao J, Chen T, Hu G, Gong Y, Qiang B, et al. (2008) Nectin-like molecule 1 is a glycoprotein with a single N-glycosylation site at N290KS which influences its adhesion activity. Biochim Biophys Acta 1778: 1429–1435.

58. Fogel AI, Akins MR, Krupp AJ, Stagi M, Stein V, et al. (2007) SynCAMs organize synapses through heterophilic adhesion. J Neurosci 27: 12516–12530.

59. Hosaka M, Suda M, Sakai Y, Izumi T, Watanabe T, et al. (2004) Secretogranin III binds to cholesterol in the secretory granule membrane as an adapter for chromogranin A. J Biol Chem 279: 3627–3634.

60. Lechner T, Adlassnig C, Humpel C, Kaufmann WA, Maier H, et al. (2004) Chromogranin peptides in Alzheimer's disease. Exp Gerontol 39: 101–113.

61. Lassmann H, Weiler R, Fischer P, Bancher C, Jellinger K, et al. (1992) Synaptic pathology in Alzheimer's disease: immunological data for markers of synaptic and large dense-core vesicles. Neuroscience 46: 1–8.

62. Eder U, Leitner B, Kirchmair R, Pohl P, Jobst KA, et al. (1998) Levels and proteolytic processing of chromogranin A and B and secretogranin II in cerebrospinal fluid in neurological diseases. J Neural Transm 105: 39–51.

63. Kaufmann WA, Barnas U, Humpel C, Nowakowski K, DeCol C, et al. (1998) Synaptic loss reflected by secretoneurin-like immunoreactivity in the human hippocampus in Alzheimer's disease. Eur J Neurosci 10: 1084–1094.

64. Paco S, Pozas E, Aguado F (2010) Secretogranin III is an astrocyte granin that is overexpressed in reactive glia. Cereb Cortex 20: 1386–1397.

65. Hosaka M, Watanabe T (2010) Secretogranin III: a bridge between core hormone aggregates and the secretory granule membrane. Endocr J 57: 275–286.

66. Bozdagi O, Rich E, Tronel S, Sadahiro M, Patterson K, et al. (2008) The neurotrophin-inducible gene Vgf regulates hippocampal function and behavior through a brain-derived neurotrophic factor-dependent mechanism. J Neurosci 28: 9857–9869.

67. Rüetschi U, Zetterberg H, Podust VN, Gottfries J, Li S, et al. (2005) Identification of CSF biomarkers for frontotemporal dementia using SELDI-TOF. Exp Neurol 196: 273–281.

68. Levi A, Ferri GL, Watson E, Possenti R, Salton SR (2004) Processing, distribution, and function of VGF, a neuronal and endocrine peptide precursor. Cell Mol Neurobiol 24: 517–533.

69. Alder J, Thakker-Varia S, Bangasser DA, Kuroiwa M, Plummer MR, et al. (2003) Brain-derived neurotrophic factor-induced gene expression reveals novel actions of VGF in hippocampal synaptic plasticity. J Neurosci 23: 10800–10808.

70. Steiner DF (1998) The proprotein convertases. Curr Opin Chem Biol 2(1): 31–39.

71. Zhu X, Wu K, Rife L, Cawley NX, Brown B, et al. (2005) Carboxypeptidase E is required for normal synaptic transmission from photoreceptors to the inner retina. J Neurochem 95: 1351–1362.

72. Hosaka M, Watanabe T, Sakai Y, Kato T, Takeuchi T (2005) Interaction between secretogranin III and carboxypeptidase E facilitates prohormone sorting within secretory granules. J Cell Sci 118: 4785–4795.

73. Park JJ, Koshimizu H, Loh YP (2009) Biogenesis and transport of secretory granules to release site in neuroendocrine cells. J Mol Neurosci 37: 151–159.

74. Woronowicz A, Koshimizu H, Chang SY, Cawley NX, Hill JM, et al. (2008) Absence of carboxypeptidase E leads to adult hippocampal neuronal degeneration and memory deficits. Hippocampus 18: 1051–1063.

75. Woronowicz A, Cawley NX, Chang SY, Koshimizu H, Phillips AW, et al. (2010) Carboxypeptidase E knockout mice exhibit abnormal dendritic arborization and spine morphology in central nervous system neurons. J Neurosci Res 88: 64–72.

76. Arun P, Moffett JR, Namboodiri AM (2009) Evidence for mitochondrial and cytoplasmic N-acetylaspartate synthesis in SH-SY5Y neuroblastoma cells. Neurochem Int 55: 219–225.

77. Schmidbaur JM, Kugler P, Horvath E (1990) Glutamate producing aspartate aminotransferase in glutamatergic perforant path terminals of the rat hippocampus. Cytochemical and lesion studies. Histochemistry 94: 427–433.

78. Würdig S, Kugler P (1991) Histochemistry of glutamate metabolizing enzymes in the rat cerebellar cortex. Neurosci Lett 130: 165–168.

79. Riemenschneider M, Buch K, Schmolke M, Kurz A, Guder WG (1997) Diagnosis of Alzheimer's disease with cerebrospinal fluid tau protein and aspartate aminotransferase. Lancet 351: 63–64.

80. D'Aniello A, Fisher G, Migliaccio N, Cammisa G, D'Aniello E, et al. (2005) Amino acids and transaminases activity in ventricular CSF and in brain of normal and Alzheimer patients. Neurosci Lett 388: 49–53.

81. Jansen Steur E, Vermes I, de Vos RA (1998) Cerebrospinal-fluid tau protein and aspartate aminotransferase in Parkinson's disease. Lancet 351: 1105–1106.

82. Tapiola T, Lehtovirta M, Pirttilä T, Alafuzoff I, Riekkinen P, et al. (1998) Increased aspartate aminotransferase activity in cerebrospinal fluid and Alzheimer's disease. Lancet 352: 287.

83. Wright NT, Cannon BR, Zimmer DB, Weber DJ (2009) S100A1: Structure, Function, and Therapeutic Potential. Curr Chem Biol 3: 138–145.

84. Liang D, Nunes-Tavares N, Xie HQ, Carvalho S, Bon S, et al. (2009) Protein CutA undergoes an unusual transfer into the secretory pathway and affects the folding, oligomerization, and secretion of acetylcholinesterase. J Biol Chem 284: 5195–5207.

85. Perrier AL, Cousin X, Boschetti N, Haas R, Chatel JM, et al. (2000) Two distinct proteins are associated with tetrameric acetylcholinesterase on the cell surface. J Biol Chem 275: 34260–34265.

86. Ablonczy Z, Prakasam A, Fant J, Fauq A, Crosson C, et al. (2009) Pigment epithelium-derived factor maintains retinal pigment epithelium function by inhibiting vascular endothelial growth factor-R2 signaling through gamma-secretase. J Biol Chem 284: 30177–30186.

87. Castano E, Roher A, Esh C, Kokjohn T, Beach T (2006) Comparative proteomics of cerebrospinal fluid in neuropathologically-confirmed Alzheimer's disease and non-demented elderly subjects. Neurol Res 28: 155–163.

88. Yamagishi S, Inagaki Y, Takeuchi M, Sasaki N (2004) Is pigment epithelium-derived factor level in cerebrospinal fluid a promising biomarker for early diagnosis of Alzheimer's disease? Med Hypotheses 63: 115–117.

89. Takanohashi A, Yabe T, Schwartz JP (2005) Pigment epithelium-derived factor induces the production of chemokines by rat microglia. Glia 51: 266–278.

90. Bilak MM, Corse AM, Bilak SR, Lehar M, Tombran-Tink J, et al. (1999) Pigment epithelium-derived factor (PEDF) protects motor neurons from chronic glutamate-mediated neurodegeneration. J Neuropathol Exp Neurol 58: 719–728.

91. Davidsson P, Sjögren M, Andreasen N, Lindbjer M, Nilsson CL, et al. (2002) Studies of the pathophysiological mechanisms in frontotemporal dementia by proteome analysis of CSF proteins. Brain Res Mol Brain Res 109: 128–133.

92. Kuncl RW, Bilak MM, Bilak SR, Corse AM, Royal W, et al. (2002) Pigment epithelium-derived factor is elevated in CSF of patients with amyotrophic lateral sclerosis. J Neurochem 81: 178–184.

93. Yabe T, Sanagi T, Yamada H (2010) The neuroprotective role of PEDF: implication for the therapy of neurological disorders. Curr Mol Med 10: 259–266.

94. Sanagi T, Yabe T, Yamada H (2005) The regulation of pro-inflammatory gene expression induced by pigment epithelium-derived factor in rat cultured microglial cells. Neurosci Lett 380: 105–110.

95. Sanagi T, Yabe T, Yamada H (2008) Gene transfer of PEDF attenuates ischemic brain damage in the rat middle cerebral artery occlusion model. J Neurochem 106: 1841–1854.

96. Pang IH, Zeng H, Fleenor DL, Clark AF (2007) Pigment epithelium-derived factor protects retinal ganglion cells. BMC Neurosci 8: 11.

97. Perretti M, D'Acquisto F (2009) Annexin A1 and glucocorticoids as effectors of the resolution of inflammation. Nat Rev Immunol 9: 62–70.

98. Lim LH, Pervaiz S (2007) Annexin 1: the new face of an old molecule. FASEB Journal 21: 968–975.

99. Eberhard DA, Brown MD, VandenBerg SR (1994) Alterations of annexin expression in pathological neuronal and glial reactions. Immunohistochemical localization of annexins I, II (p36 and p11 subunits), IV, and VI in the human hippocampus. Am J Pathol 145: 640–649.

100. Misasi R, Hozumi I, Inuzuka T, Capozzi A, Mattei V, et al. (2009) Biochemistry and neurobiology of prosaposin: a potential therapeutic neuro-effector. Cent Nerv Syst Agents Med Chem 9: 119–131.

101. Ochiai T, Takenaka Y, Kuramoto Y, Kasuya M, Fukuda K, et al. (2008) Molecular mechanism for neuro-protective effect of prosaposin against oxidative stress: its regulation of dimeric transcription factor formation. Biochim Biophys Acta 1780: 1441–1447.

102. Sikora J, Harzer K, Elleder M (2007) Neurolysosomal pathology in human prosaposin deficiency suggests essential neurotrophic function of prosaposin. Acta Neuropathol 113: 163–175.

103. O'Brien JS, Carson GS, Seo HC, Hiraiwa M, Kishimoto Y (1994) Identification of prosaposin as a neurotrophic factor. Proc Natl Acad Sci U S A 91: 9593–9596.

104. Li L, Hung AC, Porter AG (2008) Secretogranin II: a key AP-1-regulated protein that mediates neuronal differentiation and protection from nitric oxide-induced apoptosis of neuroblastoma cells. Cell Death Differ 15: 879–888.

105. Shyu WC, Lin SZ, Chiang MF, Chen DC, Su CY, et al. (2008) Secretoneurin promotes neuroprotection and neuronal plasticity via the Jak2/Stat3 pathway in murine models of stroke. J Clin Invest 118: 133–148.

106. Gasser MC, Berti I, Hauser KF, Fischer-Colbrie R, Saria A (2003) Secretoneurin promotes pertussis toxin-sensitive neurite outgrowth in cerebellar granule cells. J Neurochem 85: 662–669.

107. Hipkiss AR (2007) Could carnosine or related structures suppress Alzheimer's disease? J Alzheimers Dis 11: 229–240.

108. Guiotto A, Calderan A, Ruzza P, Borin G (2005) Carnosine and carnosine-related antioxidants: a review. Curr Med Chem 12: 2293–2315.

109. Yin GN, Lee HW, Cho JY, Suk K (2009) Neuronal pentraxin receptor in cerebrospinal fluid as a potential biomarker for neurodegenerative diseases. Brain Res 1265: 158–170.

110. Teufel M, Saudek V, Ledig JP, Bernhardt A, Boularand S, et al. (2003) Sequence identification and characterization of human carnosinase and a closely related non-specific dipeptidase. J Biol Chem 278: 6521–6531.

111. Balion CM, Benson C, Raina PS, Papaioannou A, Patterson C, et al. (2007) Brain type carnosinase in dementia: a pilot study. BMC Neurol 7: 38.

112. Zelko IN, Mariani TJ, Folz RJ (2002) Superoxide dismutase multigene family: a comparison of the CuZn-SOD (SOD1), Mn-SOD (SOD2), and EC-SOD (SOD3) gene structures, evolution, and expression. Free Radic Biol Med 33: 337–349.

113. Folz RJ, Crapo JD (1994) Extracellular superoxide dismutase (SOD3): tissue-specific expression, genomic characterization, and computer-assisted sequence analysis of the human EC SOD gene. Genomics 22: 162–171.

114. Levin ED (2005) Extracellular superoxide dismutase (EC-SOD) quenches free radicals and attenuates age-related cognitive decline: opportunities for novel drug development in aging. Curr Alzheimer Res 2: 191–196.

115. Kothakota S, Azuma T, Reinhard C, Klippel A, Tang J, et al. (1997) Caspase-3-generated fragment of gelsolin: effector of morphological change in apoptosis. Science 278: 294–298.

116. Nag S, Ma Q, Wang H, Chumnarnsilpa S, Lee WL, et al. (2009) Ca2+ binding by domain 2 plays a critical role in the activation and stabilization of gelsolin. Proc Natl Acad Sci U S A 106: 13713–13718.

117. Chauhan VP, Ray I, Chauhan A, Wisniewski HM (1999) Binding of gelsolin, a secretory protein, to amyloid beta-protein. Biochem Biophys Res Commun 258: 241–246.

118. Ray I, Chauhan A, Wegiel J, Chauhan VP (2000) Gelsolin inhibits the fibrillization of amyloid beta-protein, and also defibrillizes its preformed fibrils. Brain Res 853: 344–351.

119. Ji L, Chauhan A, Wegiel J, Essa MM, Chauhan V (2009) Gelsolin is proteolytically cleaved in the brains of individuals with Alzheimer's disease. J Alz Dis 18: 105–111.

120. Slee EA, Adrain C, Martin SJ (2001) Executioner caspase-3, -6, and -7 perform distinct, non-redundant roles during the demolition phase of apoptosis. J Biol Chem 276: 7320–7326.

121. Antequera D, Vargas T, Ugalde C, Spuch C, Molina JA, et al. (2009) Cytoplasmic gelsolin increases mitochondrial activity and reduces Abeta burden in a mouse model of Alzheimer's disease. Neurobiol Dis 36: 42–50.

122. Owen D, Lowe PN, Nietlispach D, Brosnan CE, Chirgadze DY, et al. (2003) Molecular dissection of the interaction between the small G proteins Rac1 and RhoA and protein kinase C-related kinase 1 (PRK1). J Biol Chem 278: 50578–50587.

123. Palmer RH, Parker PJ (1995) Expression, purification and characterization of the ubiquitous protein kinase C-related kinase 1. Biochem J 309: 315–320.

124. Okii N, Amano T, Seki T, Matsubayashi H, Mukai H, et al. (2007) Fragmentation of protein kinase N (PKN) in the hydrocephalic rat brain. Acta Histochem Cytochem 40: 113–121.

125. Takahashi M, Mukai H, Toshimori M, Miyamoto M, Ono Y (1998) Proteolytic activation of PKN by caspase-3 or related protease during apoptosis. Proc Natl Acad Sci U S A 95: 11566–11571.

126. Ueyama T, Ren Y, Sakai N, Takahashi M, Ono Y, et al. (2001) Generation of a constitutively active fragment of PKN in microglia/macrophages after middle cerebral artery occlusion in rats. J Neurochem 79: 903–913.

127. Henion TR, Raitcheva D, Grosholz R, Biellmann F, Skarnes WC, et al. (2005) Beta1,3-N-acetylglucosaminyltransferase 1 glycosylation is required for axon pathfinding by olfactory sensory neurons. J Neurosci 25: 1894–1903.

128. Puche AC, Bartlett PF, Key B (1997) Substrate-bound carbohydrates stimulate signal transduction and neurite outgrowth in an olfactory neuron cell line. Neuroreport 8: 3183–3188.

129. Svichar N, Esquenazi S, Waheed A, Sly WS, Chesler M (2006) Functional demonstration of surface carbonic anhydrase IV activity on rat astrocytes. Glia 53: 241–247.

130. Svichar N, Waheed A, Sly WS, Hennings JC, Hubner CA, et al. (2009) The Carbonic Anhydrases CA4 and CA14 Both Enhance AE3-Mediated Cl–HCO3 Exchange in Hippocampal Neurons. J Neurosci 29: 3252–3258.

131. Shah GN, Ulmasov B, Waheed A, Becker T, Makani S, et al. (2005) Carbonic anhydrase IV and XIV knockout mice: roles of the respective carbonic anhydrases in buffering the extracellular space in brain. Proc Natl Acad Sci U S A 102: 16771–16776.

132. Benfenati F, Ferrari R, Onofri F, Arcuri C, Giambanco I, et al. (2004) S100A1 codistributes with synapsin I in discrete brain areas and inhibits the F-actin-bundling activity of synapsin I. J Neurochem 89: 1260–1270.

133. Redondo RL, Okuno H, Spooner PA, Frenguelli BG, Bito H, et al. (2010) Synaptic tagging and capture: differential role of distinct calcium/calmodulin kinases in protein synthesis-dependent long-term potentiation. J Neurosci 30: 4981–4989.

134. Zhong L, Cherry T, Bies CE, Florence MA, Gerges NZ (2009) Neurogranin enhances synaptic strength through its interaction with calmodulin. EMBO J 28: 3027–3039.

135. Liu X, Yang PS, Yang W, Yue DT (2010) Enzyme-inhibitor-like tuning of Ca(2+) channel connectivity with calmodulin. Nature 463: 968–972.

136. Supnet C, Bezprozvanny I (2010) Neuronal calcium signaling, mitochondrial dysfunction, and Alzheimer's disease. J Alzheimers Dis 20(Suppl 2): S487–498.

137. Craig-Schapiro R, Perrin RJ, Roe CM, Xiong C, Carter D, et al. (2010) YKL-40: A Novel Prognostic Fluid Biomarker for Preclinical Alzheimer's Disease. Biol Psychiatry 68: 903–12.

138. Colton CA, Mott RT, Sharpe H, Xu Q, Van Nostrand WE, et al. (2006) Expression profiles for macrophage alternative activation genes in AD and in mouse models of AD. J Neuroinflammation 3: 27.

139. Kolson DL (2008) YKL-40: a candidate biomarker for simian immunodeficiency virus and human immunodeficiency virus encephalitis? Am J Pathol 173: 25–29.

140. Bonneh-Barkay D, Bissel SJ, Wang G, Fish KN, Nicholl GC, et al. (2008) YKL-40, a marker of simian immunodeficiency virus encephalitis, modulates the biological activity of basic fibroblast growth factor. Am J Pathol 173: 130–143.

141. Ostergaard C, Johansen JS, Benfield T, Price PA, Lundgren JD (2002) YKL-40 is elevated in cerebrospinal fluid from patients with purulent meningitis. Clin Diagn Lab Immunol 9: 598–604.

142. Kaynar MY, Tanriverdi T, Kafadar AM, Kacira T, Yurdakul F, et al. (2005) YKL-40 levels in the cerebrospinal fluid and serum of patients with aneurysmal subarachnoid hemorrhage: preliminary results. J Clin Neurosci 12: 754–757.

143. Junker N, Johansen JS, Hansen LT, Lund EL, Kristjansen PE (2005) Regulation of YKL-40 expression during genotoxic or microenvironmental stress in human glioblastoma cells. Cancer Sci 96: 183–190.

144. Hakala BE, White C, Recklies AD (1993) Human cartilage gp-39, a major secretory product of articular chondrocytes and synovial cells, is a mammalian member of a chitinase protein family. J Biol Chem 268: 25803–25810.

145. Chupp GL, Lee CG, Jarjour N, Shim YM, Holm CT, et al. (2007) A chitinase-like protein in the lung and circulation of patients with severe asthma. N Engl J Med 357: 2016–2027.

146. Ling H, Recklies AD (2004) The chitinase 3-like protein human cartilage glycoprotein 39 inhibits cellular responses to the inflammatory cytokines interleukin-1 and tumour necrosis factor-alpha. Biochem J 380: 651–659.

147. Létuvé S, Kozhich A, Arouche N, Grandsaigne M, Reed J, et al. (2008) YKL-40 is elevated in patients with chronic obstructive pulmonary disease and activates alveolar macrophages. J Immunol 181: 5167–5173.

148. Roberts ES, Zandonatti MA, Watry DD, Madden LJ, Henriksen SJ, et al. (2003) Induction of pathogenic sets of genes in macrophages and neurons in NeuroAIDS. Am J Pathol 162: 2041–2057.

149. Choi-Miura NH, Takahashi K, Yoda M, Saito K, Hori M, et al. (2000) The novel acute phase protein, IHRP, inhibits actin polymerization and phagocytosis of polymorphonuclear cells. Inflamm Res 49: 305–310.

150. Choi-Miura NH (2004) Novel human plasma proteins, IHRP (acute phase protein) and PHBP (serine protease), which bind to glycosaminoglycans. Curr Med Chem Cardiovasc Hematol Agents 2: 239–248.

151. Akiyama H, Kawamata T, Dedhar S, McGeer PL (1991) Immunohistochemical localization of vitronectin, its receptor and beta-3 integrin in Alzheimer brain tissue. J Neuroimmunol 32: 19–28.

152. McGeer PL, Kawamata T, Walker DG (1992) Distribution of clusterin in Alzheimer brain tissue. Brain Res 579: 337–341.

153. Shin TM, Isas JM, Hsieh CL, Kayed R, Glabe CG, et al. (2008) Formation of soluble amyloid oligomers and amyloid fibrils by the multifunctional protein vitronectin. Mol Neurodegener 3: 16.

154. Milner R, Campbell IL (2003) The extracellular matrix and cytokines regulate microglial integrin expression and activation. J Immunol 170: 3850–3858.

155. Milner R, Crocker SJ, Hung S, Wang X, Frausto RF, et al. (2007) Fibronectin-and vitronectin-induced microglial activation and matrix metalloproteinase-9 expression is mediated by integrins alpha5beta1 and alphavbeta5. J Immunol 178: 8158–8167.

156. Lambert JC, Heath S, Even G, Campion D, Sleegers K, et al. (2009) Genome-wide association study identifies variants at CLU and CR1 associated with Alzheimer's disease. Nat Genet 41: 1094–1099.

157. Zanjani H, Finch CE, Kemper C, Atkinson J, McKeel D, et al. (2005) Complement activation in very early Alzheimer disease. Alzheimer Dis Assoc Disord 19: 55–66.

158. Stoltzner SE, Grenfell TJ, Mori C, Wisniewski KE, Wisniewski TM, et al. (2000) Temporal accrual of complement proteins in amyloid plaques in Down's syndrome with Alzheimer's disease. Am J Pathol 156: 489–499.

159. Loeffler DA, Camp DM, Schonberger MB, Singer DJ, LeWitt PA (2004) Early complement activation increases in the brain in some aged normal subjects. Neurobiol Aging 25: 1001–1007.

160. Finehout EJ, Franck Z, Lee KH (2005) Complement protein isoforms in CSF as possible biomarkers for neurogenerative disease. Dis Markers 21: 93–101.

161. Masaki T, Matsumoto M, Nakanishi I, Yasuda R, Seya T (1992) Factor I-dependent inactivation of human complement C4b of the classical pathway by C3b/C4b receptor (CR1, CD35) and membrane cofactor protein (MCP, CD46). J Biochem 111: 573–578.

162. Puchades M, Hansson S, Nilsson C, Andreasen N, Blennow K, et al. (2003) Proteomic studies of potential cerebrospinal fluid protein markers for Alzheimer's disease. Mol Brain Res 118: 140–146.

163. Bergamaschini L, Donarini C, Gobbo G, Parnetti L, Gallai V (2001) Activation of complement and contact system in Alzheimer's disease. Mech Ageing Dev 122: 1971–1983.

164. Murphy BF, Saunders JR, O'Bryan MK, Kirszbaum L, Walker ID, et al. (1989) SP-40 is an inhibitor of C5b-6-initiated haemolysis. Int Immunol 1: 551–554.

165. Koch S, Donarski N, Goetze K, Kreckel M, Stuerenburg HJ, et al. (2001) Characterization of four lipoprotein classes in human cerebrospinal fluid. J Lipid Res 42: 1143–1151.

166. Harr SD, Uint L, Hollister R, Hyman BT, Mendez AJ (1996) Brain expression of apolipoproteins E, J, and A-I in Alzheimer's disease. J Neurochem 66: 2429–2435.

167. Harold D, Abraham R, Hollingworth P, Sims R, Gerrish A, et al. (2009) Genome-wide association study identifies variants at CLU and PICALM associated with Alzheimer's disease. Nat Genet 41: 1088–1093.

168. Perarnau B, Siegrist CA, Gillet A, Vincent C, Kimura S, et al. (1990) Beta 2-microglobulin restriction of antigen presentation. Nature 346: 751–754.

169. Vitiello A, Potter TA, Sherman LA (1990) The role of beta 2-microglobulin in peptide binding by class I molecules. Science 250: 1423–1426.

170. Berggard I, Bearn AG (1968) Isolation and properties of a low molecular weight beta-2-globulin occurring in human biological fluids. J Biol Chem 243: 4095–4103.

171. Nissen MH, Roepstorff P, Thim L, Dunbar B, Fothergill JE (1990) Limited proteolysis of beta 2-microglobulin at Lys-58 by complement component C1s. Eur J Biochem 189: 423–429.

172. Lob HE, Marvar PJ, Guzik TJ, Sharma S, McCann LA, et al. Induction of hypertension and peripheral inflammation by reduction of extracellular superoxide dismutase in the central nervous system. Hypertension 55: 277–283, 276p following 283.

173. Hansson SF, Andréasson U, Wall M, Skoog I, Andreasen N, et al. (2009) Reduced levels of amyloid-beta-binding proteins in cerebrospinal fluid from Alzheimer's disease patients. J Alzheimers Dis 16: 389–397.

174. Kanekiyo T, Ban T, Aritake K, Huang ZL, Qu WM, et al. (2007) Lipocalin-type prostaglandin D synthase/beta-trace is a major amyloid beta-chaperone in human cerebrospinal fluid. Proc Natl Acad Sci U S A 104: 6412–6417.

175. Lovell MA, Lynn BC, Xiong S, Quinn JF, Kaye J, et al. (2008) An aberrant protein complex in CSF as a biomarker of Alzheimer disease. Neurology 70: 2212–2218.

176. Paula-Lima AC, Tricerri MA, Brito-Moreira J, Bomfim TR, Oliveira FF, et al. (2009) Human apolipoprotein A-I binds amyloid-beta and prevents Abeta-induced neurotoxicity. Int J Biochem Cell Biol 41: 1361–1370.

177. Wisniewski T, Golabek AA, Kida E, Wisniewski KE, Frangione B (1995) Conformational mimicry in Alzheimer's disease. Role of apolipoproteins in amyloidogenesis. Am J Pathol 147: 238–244.

178. Kim J, Basak JM, Holtzman DM (2009) The role of apolipoprotein E in Alzheimer's disease. Neuron 63: 287–303.

179. Biroccio A, Del Boccio P, Panella M, Bernardini S, Di Ilio C, et al. (2006) Differential post-translational modifications of transthyretin in Alzheimer's disease: a study of the cerebral spinal fluid. Proteomics 6: 2305–2313.

180. Wati H, Kawarabayashi T, Matsubara E, Kasai A, Hirasawa T, et al. (2009) Transthyretin accelerates vascular Abeta deposition in a mouse model of Alzheimer's disease. Brain Pathol 19: 48–57.

181. Buxbaum JN, Ye Z, Reixach N, Friske L, Levy C, et al. (2008) Transthyretin protects Alzheimer's mice from the behavioral and biochemical effects of Abeta toxicity. Proc Natl Acad Sci U S A 105: 2681–2686.

182. Buxbaum JN, Reixach N (2009) Transthyretin: the servant of many masters. Cell Mol Life Sci 66: 3095–3101.

183. Costa R, Ferreira-da-Silva F, Saraiva MJ, Cardoso I (2008) Transthyretin protects against A-beta peptide toxicity by proteolytic cleavage of the peptide: a mechanism sensitive to the Kunitz protease inhibitor. PLoS One 3: e2899.

184. Choi SH, Leight SN, Lee VM, Li T, Wong PC, et al. (2007) Accelerated Abeta deposition in APPswe/PS1deltaE9 mice with hemizygous deletions of TTR (transthyretin). J Neurosci 27: 7006–7010.

185. Kaeser SA, Herzig MC, Coomaraswamy J, Kilger E, Selenica ML, et al. (2007) Cystatin C modulates cerebral beta-amyloidosis. Nat Genet 39: 1437–1439.

186. Sun B, Zhou Y, Halabisky B, Lo I, Cho SH, et al. (2008) Cystatin C-cathepsin B axis regulates amyloid beta levels and associated neuronal deficits in an animal model of Alzheimer's disease. Neuron 60: 247–257.

187. Mi W, Pawlik M, Sastre M, Jung SS, Radvinsky DS, et al. (2007) Cystatin C inhibits amyloid-beta deposition in Alzheimer's disease mouse models. Nat Genet 39: 1440–1442.

188. Selenica ML, Wang X, Ostergaard-Pedersen L, Westlind-Danielsson A, Grubb A (2007) Cystatin C reduces the in vitro formation of soluble Abeta1-42 oligomers and protofibrils. Scand J Clin Lab Invest 67: 179–190.

189. Wood JA, Wood PL, Ryan R, Graff-Radford NR, Pilapil C, et al. (1993) Cytokine indices in Alzheimer's temporal cortex: no changes in mature IL-1 beta or IL-1RA but increases in the associated acute phase proteins IL-6, alpha 2-macroglobulin and C-reactive protein. Brain Res 629: 245–252.

190. Narita M, Holtzman DM, Schwartz AL, Bu G (1997) α2-Macroglobulin complexes with and mediates the endocytosis of β-amyloid peptide via cell surface low-density lipoprotein receptor-related protein. J Neurochem 69: 1904–1911.

191. Hye A, Lynham S, Thambisetty M, Causevic M, Campbell J, et al. (2006) Proteome-based plasma biomarkers for Alzheimer's disease. Brain 129: 3042–3050.

192. Kovacs DM (2000) alpha2-macroglobulin in late-onset Alzheimer's disease. Exp Gerontol 35: 473–479.

193. French K, Yerbury JJ, Wilson MR (2008) Protease activation of alpha2-macroglobulin modulates a chaperone-like action with broad specificity. Biochemistry 47: 1176–1185.

194. Hughes SR, Khorkova O, Goyal S, Knaeblein J, Heroux J, et al. (1998) Alpha2-macroglobulin associates with beta-amyloid peptide and prevents fibril formation. Proc Natl Acad Sci U S A 95: 3275–3280.

195. Abraham C, Selkoe D, Potter H (1988) Immunochemical identification of the serine protease inhibitor alpha 1-antichymotrypsin in the brain amyloid deposits of Alzheimer's disease. Cell 52: 487–501.

196. Harigaya Y, Shoji M, Nakamura T, Matsubara E, Hosoda K, et al. (1995) Alpha 1-antichymotrypsin level in cerebrospinal fluid is closely associated with late onset Alzheimer's disease. Intern Med 34: 481–484.

197. Abraham CR, McGraw WT, Slot F, Yamin R (2000) Alpha 1-antichymotrypsin inhibits A beta degradation in vitro and in vivo. Ann N Y Acad Sci 920: 245–248.

198. DeKosky S, Ikonomovic MD, Wang X, Farlow M, Wisniewski S, et al. (2003) Plasma and cerebrospinal fluid 1-Antichymotrypsin levels in Alzheimer's disease: correlation with cognitive impairment. Ann Neurol 53: 81–90.

199. Nielsen HM, Minthon L, Londos E, Blennow K, Miranda E, et al. (2007) Plasma and CSF serpins in Alzheimer disease and dementia with Lewy bodies. Neurology 69: 1569–1579.

200. Vukovic J, Marmorstein LY, McLaughlin PJ, Sasaki T, Plant GW, et al. (2009) Lack of fibulin-3 alters regenerative tissue responses in the primary olfactory pathway. Matrix Biol 28: 406–415.

201. Hu B, Thirtamara-Rajamani KK, Sim H, Viapiano MS (2009) Fibulin-3 is uniquely upregulated in malignant gliomas and promotes tumor cell motility and invasion. Mol Cancer Res 7: 1756–1770.

202. Klenotic PA, Munier FL, Marmorstein LY, Anand-Apte B (2004) Tissue inhibitor of metalloproteinases-3 (TIMP-3) is a binding partner of epithelial growth factor-containing fibulin-like extracellular matrix protein 1 (EFEMP1). Implications for macular degenerations. J Biol Chem 279: 30469–30473.

203. Vollbach H, Heun R, Morris CM, Edwardson JA, McKeith IG, et al. (2005) APOA1 polymorphism influences risk for early-onset nonfamilar AD. Ann Neurol 58: 436–441.

204. Montine TJ, Montine KS, Swift LL (1997) Central nervous system lipoproteins in Alzheimer's disease. Am J Path 151: 1571–1575.

205. Gunzburg MJ, Perugini MA, Howlett GJ (2007) Structural basis for the recognition and cross-linking of amyloid fibrils by human apolipoprotein E. J Biol Chem 282: 35831–35841.

206. Sun Y, Shi J, Zhang S, Tang M, Han H, et al. (2005) The APOC3 SstI polymorphism is weakly associated with sporadic Alzheimer's disease in a Chinese population. Neurosci Lett 380: 219–222.

207. Houlden H, Crook R, Duff K, Hutton M, Collinge J, et al. (1995) Apolipoprotein E alleles but neither apolipoprotein B nor apolipoprotein AI/CIII alleles are associated with late onset, familial Alzheimer's disease. Neurosci Lett 188: 202–204.

208. Pan S, Rush J, Peskind ER, Galasko D, Chung K, et al. (2008) Application of targeted quantitative proteomics analysis in human cerebrospinal fluid using a liquid chromatography matrix-assisted laser desorption/ionization time-of-flight tandem mass spectrometer (LC MALDI TOF/TOF) platform. J Proteome Res 7: 720–730.

209. Katzav A, Faust-Socher A, Kvapil F, Michaelson DM, Blank M, et al. (2009) Antiphospholipid syndrome induction exacerbates a transgenic Alzheimer disease model on a female background. Neurobiol Aging.

210. Zimmer DB, Chaplin J, Baldwin A, Rast M (2005) S100-mediated signal transduction in the nervous system and neurological diseases. Cell Mol Biol (Noisy-le-grand) 51: 201–214.

211. Loeffler DA, LeWitt PA, Juneau PL, Sima AA, Nguyen HU, et al. (1996) Increased regional brain concentrations of ceruloplasmin in neurodegenerative disorders. Brain Res 738: 265–274.

212. Castellani RJ, Smith MA, Nunomura A, Harris PL, Perry G (1999) Is increased redox-active iron in Alzheimer disease a failure of the copper-binding protein ceruloplasmin? Free Radic Biol Med 26: 1508–1512.

213. Kaneko K, Yoshida K, Arima K, Ohara S, Miyajima H, et al. (2002) Astrocytic deformity and globular structures are characteristic of the brains of patients with aceruloplasminemia. J Neuropathol Exp Neurol 61: 1069–1077.

214. Kessler H, Pajonk FG, Meisser P, Schneider-Axmann T, Hoffmann KH, et al. (2006) Cerebrospinal fluid diagnostic markers correlate with lower plasma copper and ceruloplasmin in patients with Alzheimer's disease. J Neural Transm 113: 1763–1769.

215. Capo CR, Arciello M, Squitti R, Cassetta E, Rossini PM, et al. (2008) Features of ceruloplasmin in the cerebrospinal fluid of Alzheimer's disease patients. Biometals 21: 367–372.

216. Squitti R, Quattrocchi CC, Salustri C, Rossini PM (2008) Ceruloplasmin fragmentation is implicated in 'free' copper deregulation of Alzheimer's disease. Prion 2: 23–27.

217. Squitti R, Bressi F, Pasqualetti P, Bonomini C, Ghidoni R, et al. (2009) Longitudinal prognostic value of serum "free" copper in patients with Alzheimer disease. Neurology 72: 50–55.

218. Okada M, Hatakeyama T, Itoh H, Tokuta N, Tokumitsu H, et al. (2004) S100A1 is a novel molecular chaperone and a member of the Hsp70/Hsp90 multichaperone complex. J Biol Chem 279: 4221–4233.

219. Lein ES, Callaway EM, Albright TD, Gage FH (2005) Redefining the boundaries of the hippocampal CA2 subfield in the mouse using gene expression and 3-dimensional reconstruction. J Comp Neurol 485: 1–10.

220. Hosokawa N, You Z, Tremblay LO, Nagata K, Herscovics A (2007) Stimulation of ERAD of misfolded null Hong Kong alpha1-antitrypsin by Golgi alpha1,2-mannosidases. Biochem Biophys Res Commun 362: 626–632.

221. Schweden J, Bause E (1989) Characterization of trimming Man9-mannosidase from pig liver. Purification of a catalytically active fragment and evidence for the transmembrane nature of the intact 65 kDa enzyme. Biochem J 264: 347–355.

222. Kehoe PG, Miners S, Love S (2009) Angiotensins in Alzheimer's disease - friend or foe? Trends Neurosci 32: 619–628.

223. Blennow K, Davidsson P, Wallin A, Ekman R (2004) Chromogranin A in cerebrospinal fluid: a biochemical marker for synaptic degeneration in Alzheimer's disease? Dementia 6: 306–11.

224. Massaro AR, De Pascalis D, Carnevale A, Carbone G (2009) The neural cell adhesion molecule (NCAM) present in the cerebrospinal fluid of multiple sclerosis patients is unsialylated. Eur Rev Med Pharmacol Sci 13: 397–9.

225. Todaro L, Puricelli L, Gioseffi H, Pallotta MG, Lastiri J, et al. (2004) Neural cell adhesion molecule in human serum. Increased levels in dementia of the Alzheimer type. Neurobiol Dis 15: 387–393.

226. Kapaki E, Paraskevas GP, Papageorgiou SG, Bonakis A, Kalfakis N, et al. (2008) Diagnostic value of CSF biomarker profile in frontotemporal lobar degeneration. Alzheimer Dis Assoc Disord 22: 47–53.

227. Bian H, Van Swieten JC, Leight S, Massimo L, Wood E, et al. (2008) CSF biomarkers in frontotemporal lobar degeneration with known pathology. Neurology 70: 1827–1835.

228. Mollenhauer B, Cullen V, Kahn I, Krastins B, Outeiro TF, et al. (2008) Direct quantification of CSF alpha-synuclein by ELISA and first cross-sectional study in patients with neurodegeneration. Exp Neurol 213: 315–325.

229. Bateman RJ, Siemers ER, Mawuenyega KG, Wen G, Browning KR, et al. (2009) A gamma-secretase inhibitor decreases amyloid-beta production in the central nervous system. Ann Neurol 66: 48–54.

230. Hansson O, Zetterberg H, Buchhave P, Londos E, Blennow K, et al. (2006) Association between CSF biomarkers and incipient Alzheimer's disease in patients with mild cognitive impairment: A follow-up study. Lancet Neurol 5: 228–234.

Evaluating Amyloid-β Oligomers in Cerebrospinal Fluid as a Biomarker for Alzheimer's Disease

Mikko Hölttä[1]*, Oskar Hansson[2], Ulf Andreasson[1], Joakim Hertze[2], Lennart Minthon[2], Katarina Nägga[2], Niels Andreasen[3], Henrik Zetterberg[1,4], Kaj Blennow[1]

1 Institute of Neuroscience and Physiology, Department of Psychiatry and Neurochemistry, The Sahlgrenska Academy at University of Gothenburg, Mölndal, Sweden, 2 Clinical Memory Research Unit, Department of Clinical Sciences Malmö, Lund University, Malmö, Sweden, 3 Department of Clinical Neurosciences and Family Medicine, Section of Geriatric Medicine, Karolinska University Hospital, Stockholm, Sweden, 4 UCL Institute of Neurology, University College London, London, United Kingdom

Abstract

The current study evaluated amyloid-β oligomers (Aβo) in cerebrospinal fluid as a clinical biomarker for Alzheimer's disease (AD). We developed a highly sensitive Aβo ELISA using the same N-terminal monoclonal antibody (82E1) for capture and detection. CSF samples from patients with AD, mild cognitive impairment (MCI), and healthy controls were examined. The assay was specific for oligomerized Aβ with a lower limit of quantification of 200 fg/ml, and the assay signal showed a tight correlation with synthetic Aβo levels. Three clinical materials of well characterized AD patients (n = 199) and cognitively healthy controls (n = 148) from different clinical centers were included, together with a clinical material of patients with MCI (n = 165). Aβo levels were elevated in the all three AD-control comparisons although with a large overlap and a separation from controls that was far from complete. Patients with MCI who later converted to AD had increased Aβo levels on a group level but several samples had undetectable levels. These results indicate that presence of high or measurable Aβo levels in CSF is clearly associated with AD, but the overlap is too large for the test to have any diagnostic potential on its own.

Citation: Hölttä M, Hansson O, Andreasson U, Hertze J, Minthon L, et al. (2013) Evaluating Amyloid-β Oligomers in Cerebrospinal Fluid as a Biomarker for Alzheimer's Disease. PLoS ONE 8(6): e66381. doi:10.1371/journal.pone.0066381

Editor: Sergio T. Ferreira, Federal University of Rio de Janeiro, Brazil

Received December 18, 2012; **Accepted** May 4, 2013; **Published** June 14, 2013

Funding: This work was supported by Stiftelsen Gamla tjänarinnor, Gun och Bertil Stohnes stiftelse, Demensfonden, Kungliga och Hvitfeldtska stiftelsen, Stiftelsen Greta Johansson och Brita Anderssons Minnesfond, Adlerbertska stiftelsen. The funders had no role in study design, data collection and analysis, decision to publish, or preparation of the manuscript.

Competing Interests: The authors have declared that no competing interests exist.

* E-mail: mikko.holtta@neuro.gu.se

Introduction

Alzheimer's disease (AD) is the most common form of dementia affecting more than 15 million people in the world and is characterized by progressive neuronal degeneration with depositions of amyloid plaques and neurofibrillary tangles [1]. The amyloid plaques have been shown to mainly consist of aggregated amyloid-β (Aβ) 1–42, while the neurofibrillary tangles consist of aggregated phosphorylated tau [2,3]. The pathological process is believed to begin 10–20 years before the first clinical symptoms arise, with amyloid plaque formation starting in the neocortex and can later on be seen throughout the brain [4]. As an intermediate state before Aβ forms plaques, small soluble aggregates called Aβ oligomers (Aβo) are believed to be formed [5,6,7]. Animal studies in rodents have shown that small soluble Aβo impair memory [8], affect long term potentiation [9], and lead to cognitive deficits [10]. The neurotoxic effects of Aβo appear to involve modulation of the NMDA receptor and metabotropic glutamate receptors and possibly also pore formation in membranes [11,12,13,14]. The neurotoxic effect can be reversed in rodents by using immunotherapy against Aβ and by inhibiting Aβ oligomerization with peptides [15,16,17,18].

Today, three established cerebrospinal fluid (CSF) biomarkers are used to aid the diagnosis of AD; increased phosphorylated tau (P-tau$_{181}$), increased total tau (T-tau), and decreased Aβ$_{1-42}$, for review see [19]. Several studies have demonstrated that Aβ$_{1-42}$ levels are decreased in AD patients compared to healthy controls,

and this is also reported in patients with prodromal AD [20,21,22]. Amyloid plaques in the brain can be visualized by positron emission tomography (PET), using the ligand ^{11}C-PIB, which binds to fibrillar Aβ [23]. The belief is that the lowering of Aβ$_{1-42}$ is caused by its incorporation into plaques, which is consistent with studies showing that high ^{11}C-PIB binding correlates with lower levels of Aβ$_{1-42}$ in CSF [24,25]. If this lowering is caused by Aβ oligomerization and aggregation, Aβo would potentially be an early biomarker for AD reflecting an ongoing pathology.

In CSF, Aβo has been measured with various techniques [26,27,28,29]. Fukumoto and co-workers recently showed high CSF levels of Aβo in AD patients using and assay based on the monoclonal antibody BAN50 both for capture and detection and synthetic Aβo as standard [30]. Using flow cytometry, Santos and co-workers [31] showed that there was a trend of elevated Aβo levels in AD patients compared to controls and Gao and co-workers [32] also found increased levels of oligomeric Aβ$_{1-40}$ in CSF using a novel misfolded protein assay. Using nanoparticle detection an increase in amyloid-β-derived diffusible ligands has also been reported [29].

In this study, we developed a sandwich ELISA using the same N-terminally specific Aβ antibody as both capture and detection antibody to measure Aβo in CSF. N-terminally specific antibodies have been demonstrated to have higher affinity against fibrillar Aβ than antibodies with an epitope against the more C-terminal part of the Aβ sequence [33,34], indicating that the N-terminal part of the Aβ sequence is the most likely one to be exposed in Aβ aggregates. We compared four patient materials with AD patients to healthy controls, and also a longitudinal mild cognitive impairment (MCI) cohort, to evaluate whether Aβo measured with this type of assay could be used as a clinical biomarker.

Materials and Methods

Participants

Four study populations were recruited at three specialized and coordinated memory clinics in Sweden within the Swedish Brain Power network (Malmö, Stockholm and Piteå). The Piteå and Stockholm centers are run by the same clinician with identical sampling and storage protocols and are hence considered as one center. Demographics and biochemical characteristics are given in Table 1. A set of nine younger controls from the Malmö clinic, median age 42, were included to study possible age effects. All subjects underwent an extensive clinical examination, also including cognitive evaluations with mini-mental state examination (MMSE) [35]. All patients also underwent imaging of the brain and lumbar puncture for CSF collection.

Controls had no history or clinical signs of neurological or psychiatric disease or cognitive symptoms. AD was diagnosed following the criteria for probable AD according to the National Institute of Neurological and Communicative Disorders and Stroke- Alzheimer's Disease and Related Disorders Association (NINCDS-ADRDA) [36]. Disease severity was evaluated using MMSE scores and mild patients had a MMSE of 25–30; moderate AD patients had a MMSE of 17–24, and severe AD patients had a MMSE of 16 or lower. MCI was diagnosed in patients with cognitive impairment that did not fulfill the criteria for dementia [37]. During clinical follow-up of the patients with MCI at baseline, 35% developed AD and 30% developed other forms dementia disorders, but 47% were cognitively stable for a median time of 6.3 years (range 3.0y to 9.6y).

CSF collection was conducted following standardized operating procedures [19]. Lumbar puncture was performed in the L3–L4 or L4–L5 interspace. The first 12 mL of CSF was collected in a polypropylene tube and was centrifuged at 2000×g at 4°C for 10 min. The supernatant was pipetted off, gently mixed to avoid possible gradient effects, and aliquoted in polypropylene tubes that were stored at −80°C pending biochemical analyses.

Ethics Statement

The studies were approved by the ethics committees at Lund University, Umeå University and Karolinska Institute. The participants provided their verbal informed consent for research, documented in the patient journals, which is the standard procedure in Sweden and approved by the ethics committees.

Amyloid-β Oligomer ELISA

For the Aβo ELISA the Aβ N-terminal specific antibody 82E1 [38] (IBL international, Hamburg, Germany) was used both for capture and detection. The use of the same monoclonal antibody for capture and detection has been demonstrated in previous studies to specifically detect aggregated forms of Aβ without detecting monomers [30,39,40,41]. A synthetic dimer consisting of two $A\beta_{1-11}$ peptides with an added C-terminal cysteine through which the peptides were coupled via a disulfide bridge (Caslo, Denmark) was used to create the standard curve. A schematic outline of the Aβo ELISA is presented in Figure 1A.

An ELISA plate (Black MaxiSorp FluoroNunc, Nunc, Denmark) was coated with 82E1 diluted in 50 mM $NaHCO_3$, pH 9.6 to a concentration of 1 μg/ml, 100 μl/well, over night in +4°C. The plate was washed 5 times with 350 μl phosphate buffered saline containing 0.05% Tween20 (Bio-Rad) (PBST). Blocking was done using 2% bovine serum albumin (BSA) (Sigma Aldrich) dissolved in PBST, 300 μl/well at room temperature (RT) for 1 h. The plate was then washed 5 times with PBST. The standard was prepared by dilution of the synthetic dimer in 0.1% BSA-PBST, 200–102,000 fg/ml. CSF samples and standards were added in duplicates, 100 μl/well and incubated for 1 h at RT, where after the plate was washed 5 times with PBST. Detection antibody, biotinylated 82E1, diluted in 0.1% BSA-PBST to a concentration of 750 ng/ml, was added, 100 μl/well, and incubated for 1 h in RT. The plate was washed 5 times with PBST. NeutrAvidin horseradish peroxidase conjugate (Thermo Scientific), diluted

Table 1. Demographics and biomarker concentrations for all AD patients, MCI patients and controls.

Study	Diagnosis	Nr	Sex (M/F)	Age (years)	$A\beta_{1-42}$ (pg/ml)	P-tau$_{181}$ (pg/ml)	T-tau (pg/ml)	MMSE	Aβo (fg/ml)
I	Control	31	16/15	61 (52, 67)	690 (466, 898)	47 (33, 61)	285 (188, 365)	29 (28, 29)	522 (339, 781)
	AD	42	10/32	79 (74, 81)***	370 (318, 415)***	92 (80, 116)***	770 (640, 895)***	21 (19, 23)***	1040 (773, 1,303)***
II	Control	22	10/12	69 (66, 72)	780 (645, 1,060)	–	405 (178, 500)	30 (30, 30)	0 (0, 0)
	AD	51	22/29	79 (75, 81)***	440 (326, 508)***	–	623 (465, 858)***	23 (20, 26)***	717 (0, 1,490)***
III	Control	62	17/45	74 (68, 78)	298 (237, 342)	33 (23, 41)	79 (56, 97)	29 (28, 30)	0 (0, 0)
	MCI-AD	58	21/37	78 (73, 81)	146 (119, 177)***	49 (36, 67)***	129 (93, 181)**	26 (25, 27)***	0 (0, 313)**
	MCI-Stable	77	34/43	67 (62, 75)***	266 (217, 298)**	27 (19, 36)*	71 (50, 90)	28 (28, 29)**	0 (0, 295)
IV	Control	33	13/20	69 (62, 72)	867 (737, 1060)	–	383 (250, 502)	30 (30, 30)	1538 (504, 2408)
	Severe	11	7/4	79 (68, 82)**	398 (366, 400)***	–	937 (648, 1270)***	12 (13, 16)***	1250 (576, 2082)
	Moderate	51	21/30	80 (75, 83)***	435 (370, 494)***	–	760 (595, 886)***	21 (20, 23)***	2647 (1395, 3451)***
	Mild	44	18/26	77 (74, 81)***	473 (440, 524)***	–	848 (631, 899)***	27 (26, 28)***	2467 (1250, 3387)**

Data are given as medians with 25th and 75th percentiles.
*p<0.05,
**p<0.01,
***p<0.001 vs. control group.
The analyses of $A\beta_{1-42}$, P-tau$_{181}$ and T-tau have been performed with ELISA earlier [22,48,49,50].
doi:10.1371/journal.pone.0066381.t001

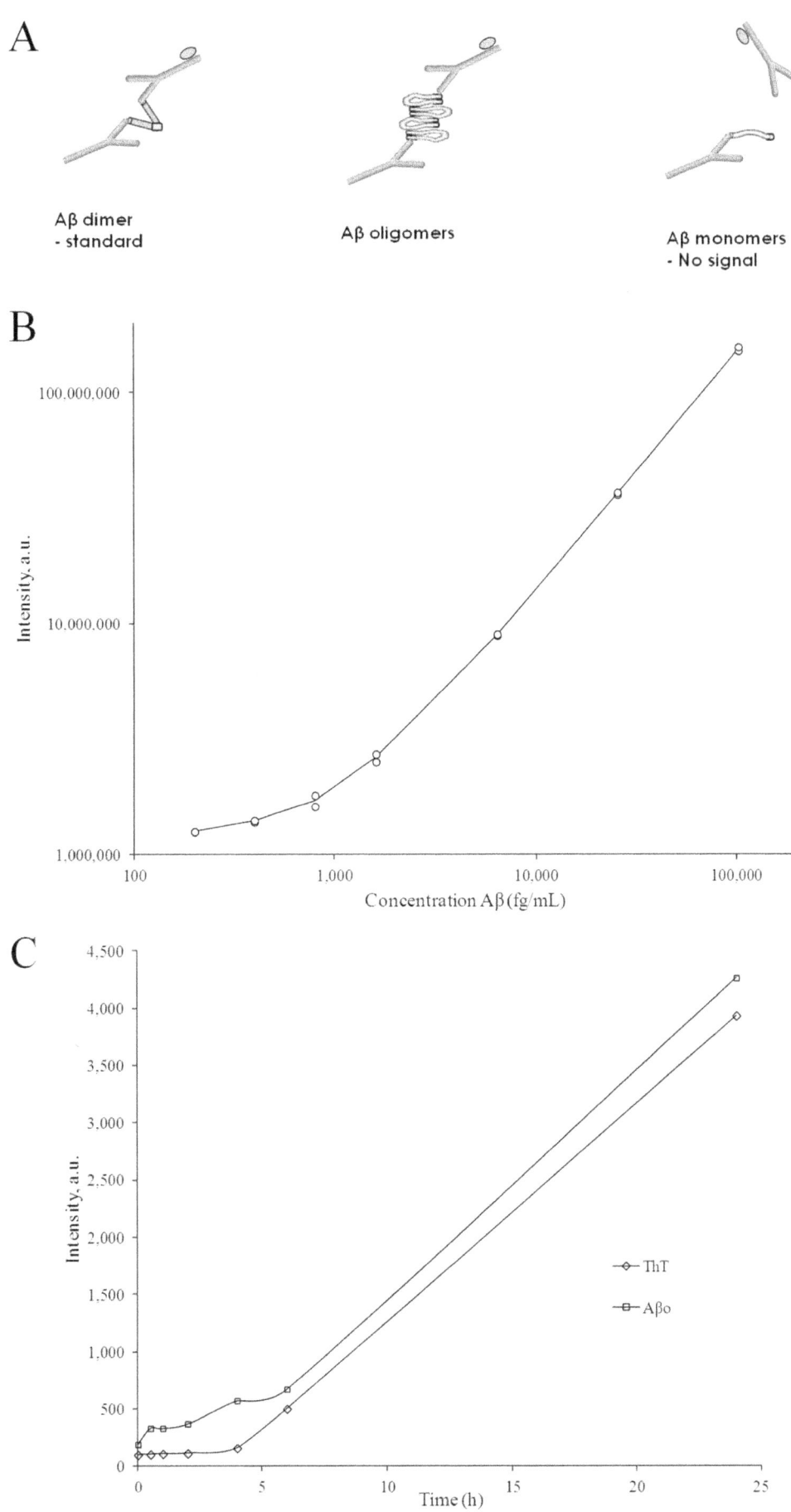

Figure 1. ELISA method for Aβ oligomers in cerebrospinal fluid. A) Schematic drawing of the principle for the method. Left: The Aβo ELISA is based on the use of the same N-terminal anti-Aβ monoclonal antibody twice. The ELISA plate is coated with 82E1 to capture all forms of Aβ, while biotinylated 82E1 is used for detection. A synthetic Aβ dimer, with two N-termini, is used as standard. Middle: Aβos, with several free N-terminals, are detected in the assay. Right: monomeric Aβ will have their epitopes blocked by the capture antibody and are thus not detected by the detection antibody. B) Example of a typical standard curve from the Aβo assay. The standard curve ranges from 200–102,400 fg/mL. The assay has a lower limit of quantification of 200 fg/mL. C) Measurement of synthetic Aβo formation by the Aβo ELISA. Synthetic Aβ$_{1-42}$ was allowed to aggregate into Aβ oligomers. The signal in the Aβo ELISA was compared with a Thioflavin-T (ThT) assay for aggregated Aβ. The Aβo ELISA detects the formation of synthetic Aβo at an earlier stage than the ThT assay, while following the increase of oligomerization in parallel with the ThT assay after 5 hours.
doi:10.1371/journal.pone.0066381.g001

1:5,000 in 0.1% BSA-PBST, was added, 100 µl/well, and incubated for 1 h at RT, and the plate was washed 5 times with PBST. For detection SuperSignal Femto maximum sensitivity substrate (Thermo Scientific, Pierce Biotechnology, Rockford, Illinois, USA) 100 µl/well was used, read 1 s/well on a Victor X4 (Perkin Elmer). The read-out data from Victor X4 were analyzed with SoftMax Pro 4.7.1 (Molecular Devices).

The detection was done using a colorimetric method for the oligomerization study and on the analyses of brain tissue. TMB substrate (Bio-Rad), 100 µl/well was incubated at RT for 15 min, and the reaction was stopped with 100 µl of 2 M H_2SO_4. Absorbance was measured at 450 nm using a V-Max microplate reader (Molecular Devices).

All samples for each individual study were analyzed on the same day.

ThT Oligomerization Assay

To initiate the oligomerization, a buffer solution containing ThT (Sigma-Aldrich) was added to synthetic Aβ$_{1-42}$ (Anaspec), reconstituted in 10 mM NaOH. The final concentrations were 200 mM HEPES, pH 8, 40 µM ThT, and 40 µM Aβ$_{1-42}$. The mixture was transferred to a black 384-well microtiter plate (Nunc, Denmark) and overlaid with mineral oil (Sigma-Aldrich) to prevent evaporation. Fluorescence was measured at 37°C in kinetic mode every 30 min using a SpectraMax Gemini XPS (Molecular Devices) with excitation and emission wavelengths of 450 nm and 485 nm, respectively. One vial with the exact same reagents was in parallel kept in 37°C from which samples were taken at given time points, quickly frozen, and stored at −80°C pending the Aβo ELISA analysis.

Cross Reactivity

To test the cross reactivity to monomeric Aβ in the Aβo ELISA, Aβ$_{1-16}$ was diluted in 0.1% BSA-PBST in concentrations up to 100,000 pg/ml, while Aβ$_{1-40}$ was diluted up to 5,000 pg/ml and measured with the Aβo ELISA.

Brain Tissue from AD Patients and Tg2576 Mice

Cortical tissue from Tg2576 mice were prepared as described previously [42]. In brief the brain cortices were homogenized in a Tris buffer and centrifuged at 16.000×g where after the supernatants were collected and analyzed. Human AD brain was homogenized in Tris buffer containing Complete Proteasinhibitor (Roche, Protease Inhibitor Cocktail tablets) and 0.5% Triton x-100, and centrifuged at 30,000×g for 60 min at 4°C. The supernatant was analyzed.

Freeze/thawing Experiments

CSF samples (n = 4) were thawed and kept in room temperature and then re-frozen at −80°C in 5 cycles. An identical sample was kept in −80°C that did not undergo the freeze/thaw cycles to be used as control.

Heterophilic Antibodies

A set of eight CSF samples, with Aβo concentration range of 600–4800 fg/mL, were used to evaluate whether heterophilic antibodies interfere with the assay. The CSF samples were mixed with mouse IgG (Sigma-Aldrich, I5381) to a concentration of 10 µg/mL and incubated for 30 minutes before being analyzed together with the same samples without added mouse IgG.

Molecular Weight Filtration of Oligomers

Synthetic Aβo generated according to Berghorn et al [43] were sequentially spun through different sized molecular weight cut-off filters (Amicon ultra, Millipore), 50 kDa, 30 kDa, and 10 kDa and the fractions from these were analyzed.

Statistics

Statistical analyses were performed with SPSS PASW 18 (SPSS Inc, Chicago, Illinois, USA), using nonparametric tests because of skewed distribution in the variables. For comparisons between groups Mann Whitney U-test was used, and data are presented as median with interquartile range. Correlation analyses were done using the Spearman correlation coefficient. Scatter plots were done using GraphPad Prism v5.02 (GraphPad Software Inc, La Jolla, California, USA).

Results

Aβo ELISA Characteristics

The standard curve used in the Aβo assay ranged from 200 fg/mL to 102,400 fg/mL, Figure 1B. The limit of quantification was determined to 200 fg/mL by calculating the Aβo concentration at 10 standard deviations above the blank.

The specificity for the assay was tested using oligomerized Aβ$_{1-42}$, generated according to the protocol developed by Berghorn et al [43], which followed a titration curve. In contrast, spiking with monomeric Aβ$_{1-16}$ up to 100,000 pg/ml or monomeric Aβ$_{1-40}$ up to 5,000 pg/ml did not result in any detectable concentration. The specificity for oligomerized Aβ was also seen when a ThT assay was performed in parallel to the Aβo ELISA. As can be seen in Figure 1C there is no reaction at time point zero, with a dramatic increase between 2–24 hours. The Aβo ELISA also showed an earlier detection of Aβo formation than the ThT assay (Figure 1C). The assay was also tested for interference from heterophilic antibodies by mixing CSF with mouse IgG, allowing potential heterophilic antibodies to react with the mouse IgG and thus block their ability to cross-react with the capture and detection antibody. This showed no significant decrease in the Aβo signal.

With the Aβo assay, it was possible to measure Aβo in brain extracts from transgenic mice. The concentrations of soluble Aβo in brain cortex tissue from Tg2576 mice extracted with TBS were 106 pg Aβo/mg protein at the age of 7 days and decreased to 67 pg Aβo/mg protein at the age of 90 days. In human AD brain an Aβo concentration of 826 pg/mg protein was measured. The assay reacts with synthetic oligomers with a molecular weight above 10 kDa, showing reactivity for Aβo with a molecular weight of 10–30 kDa, 30–50 kDa, and >50 kDa.

The measured values of the freeze/thawed samples did not significantly diverge from samples that did not undergo these cycles. The coefficient of variation (CV) of the freeze/thawed sample compared to the control samples where in the range 1–18%. The intra-assay CV was less than 7% determined by measuring 7 CSF samples in duplicate. The inter-assay CV was less than 20%.

Clinical Studies on the Diagnostic Performance of CSF Aβ Oligomers

In the first clinical study, we found a significant (p<0.0001) increase in AD CSF Aβo compared to the control group (Figure 2a), 1040 fg/mL and 522 fg/mL respectively. However, there was a marked overlap between the two groups, 64% of AD patients had a CSF level of Aβo higher than the optimal cut-off of 835 fg/mL (84% specificity).

For this reason, we analyzed a second clinical study of AD patients with dementia from another clinical center. We could verify a significant (p<0.001) increase in the CSF levels of Aβo compared to the control group (Figure 2b), 717 fg/mL and <200 fg/mL respectively. However, again there was a marked overlap between the two groups, 67% of AD patients had CSF levels of Aβo higher than the optimal cut-off of 215 fg/mL (86% specificity).

We then hypothesized that there may be a more marked release of Aβo into CSF during the earlier stages of the disease. We therefore analyzed an independent clinical study including patients with MCI. In this clinical study (Figure 2C), we found that MCI patients who later converted to AD (MCI-AD) had increased levels of Aβo compared to controls, p<0.01, <200 fg/mL and 210 fg/mL respectively, while patients with stable MCI did not differ from controls, <200 fg/ml and <200 fg/mL respectively. However, there was a marked overlap between MCI-AD and controls, with only 44% of MCI-AD patients having CSF Aβo levels above the cut-off of 230 fg/mL (85% specificity).

Last, we tested the reverse hypothesis, that there may be a more marked release of Aβo into CSF during the very last stages of the disease. The basis for this hypothesis was that plaques may act as a reservoir for aggregated Aβ, which in the later stages of the disease might have reached their maximal capacity, causing Aβo to leak

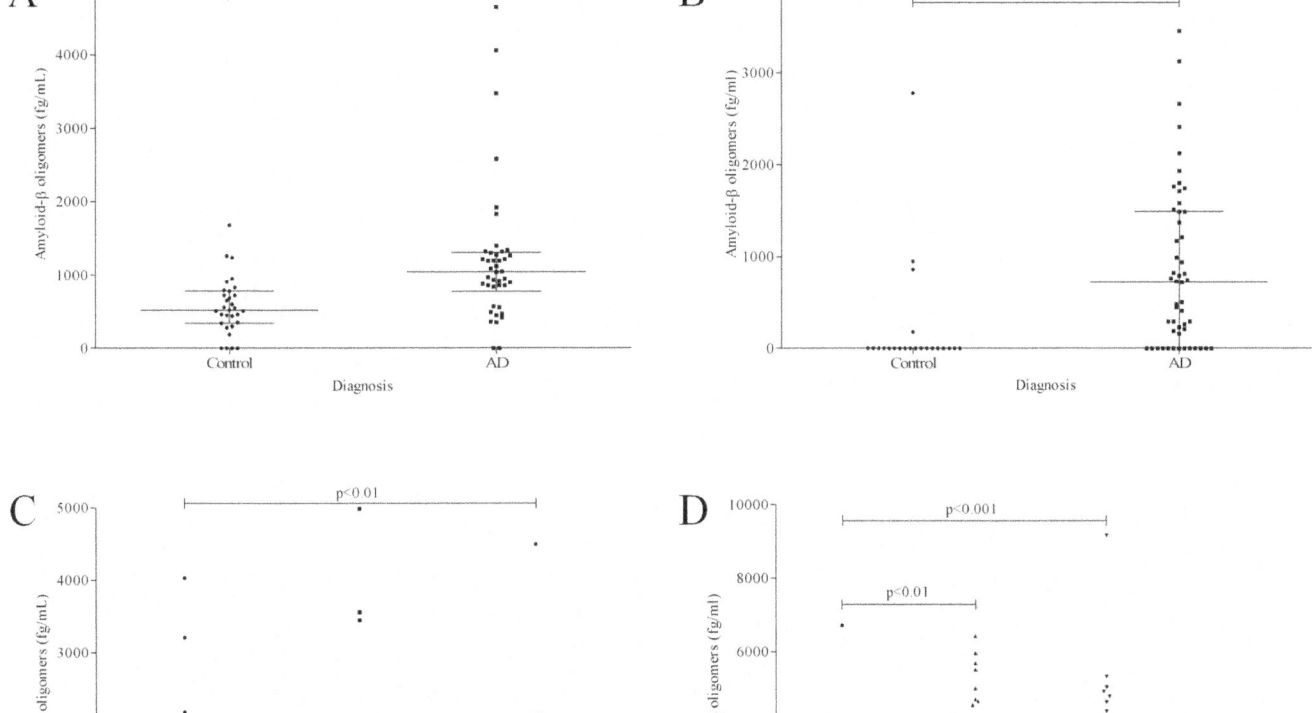

Figure 2. Cerebrospinal fluid Aβ oligomers in independent clinical samples. A) First AD study (Malmö). Increased CSF levels of Aβo in the AD group (n = 42) compared to the control group (n = 31), p<0.0001. Bars indicate median with interquartile range. B) Second AD study (Piteå and Stockholm). Increased CSF levels of Aβo in the group of patients with AD (n = 51) compared to the control group (n = 22), p<0.001. Bars indicate median with interquartile range. C) MCI study. Increased CSF levels of Aβo in the group of MCI patients who converted to AD during the follow-up period (n = 58) as compared to the control group (n = 62), p<0.01. No significant difference in CSF Aβo between stable MCI (p = 0.059) and controls. Bars indicate median with interquartile range. D) Clinical study on AD with different severity of dementia. Increased CSF levels of Aβo in the group of AD patients with mild (n = 44, p<0.01) and moderate (n = 51, p<0.001) dementia as compared to the control group (n = 33). No significant change was found in the AD group with severe dementia (n = 11) compared to the control group. Bars indicate median with interquartile range.

doi:10.1371/journal.pone.0066381.g002

out from the brain into the CSF. We therefore analyzed an independent clinical study with AD patients with different severity of dementia (mild – moderate – severe) based on their MMSE scores. In this clinical study (Figure 2D) we found that AD patients with mild (2467 fg/mL) and moderate (2647 fg/mL) dementia had significantly higher levels of Aβo compared to healthy controls (1538 fg/mL), $p < 0.01$ and $p < 0.001$ respectively, while AD patients with severe dementia (1250 fg/mL) did not significantly differ from the control group (Figure 2d).

Aβo in Relation to Established Biomarkers for AD

In all four studies, the levels of the three established biomarkers were significantly changed in the AD vs. control population, with decreased $A\beta_{1-42}$, increased $P\text{-tau}_{181}$, and increased T-tau in the AD group (Table 1). This was also seen in the MCI patients who later converted to AD (Table 1).

No significant correlations were found between Aβo and the biomarkers in any of the control, AD or MCI groups.

Influence of Age on Aβo

The age of the subjects did not correlate with Aβo levels in any of the groups. A comparison between younger healthy controls against the healthy controls in study I, both sampled at the same clinic, did not show any significant age difference between the Aβo levels, 1160 fg/mL vs. 580 fg/mL respectively, $p = 0.277$.

Discussion

In this study we evaluated if CSF Aβo could be used as a clinical biomarker for AD by analyzing four different patient materials from different clinical centers. Three patient materials were analyzed, where AD patients consistently had significantly increased levels of Aβo compared to controls. In one study stable MCI and MCI-AD patients were analyzed, which showed an increase in Aβo in MCI-AD patients but not in stable MCI patients.

We developed a highly sensitive and specific CSF Aβo ELISA, similar to the one used by Xia et al [44], where we used a synthetic Aβ dimer with two free N-terminals, instead of a preparation of aggregated $A\beta_{1-42}$ used in earlier studies [30,32] to create the standard curve and a chemiluminescent substrate for detection. The use of a synthetic dimer enables quantification and comparisons of results longitudinally since the dimer is stable and at known concentrations. This gives an Aβo concentration which is relative to the dimer, and the signal from a synthetic oligomer mixture correlates with the dimer concentration when titrated in parallel, why differences in Aβo levels between AD and controls won't be affected by the use of a dimer instead of a mixture of synthetic oligomers. The Aβo ELISA was run in parallel with a ThT assay showing that the oligomerization of $A\beta_{1-42}$ measured by the Aβo ELISA followed the results from the ThT assay. The assay detects Aβo larger than 10 kDa which includes slightly smaller Aβo than Fukumoto et al [30] detect with their assay, but the clinical relevance of these are unknown. No correlation was found between age and Aβo levels in the patient groups, and there was no significant difference in Aβo levels between younger and older healthy controls. A relatively high amount of Aβo was detected in human brain tissue from AD patients confirming that it could also detect naturally occurring Aβo. Aβo was also detected in the brains from transgenic Tg2576 mice, overexpressing human Aβ, where the Aβo levels decreased with age, which is the opposite to findings on the same mice with a different type of Aβo assay [42]. This might reflect that the two assays detect different populations of Aβo, where the assay used in

this paper seems to detect oligomers that are present at highest concentration early in the disease. A potential risk with these kinds of assays is the presence of heterophilic antibodies which could cause a false positive signal, although mainly affecting plasma samples [45]. To show that the Aβo signals was not caused by heterophilic antibodies, a set of CSF samples were spiked with a high concentration of irrelevant mouse IgG, to quench potential heterophilic antibodies, and then measured with the Aβo ELISA. This did not show a decrease in the Aβo levels indicating that the signals were not caused by heterophilic antibodies.

Patients with AD would be expected to have increased concentrations of Aβo since this would reflect the AD pathogenesis with aggregation of Aβ in the brain leading to amyloid plaques. Although it has been reported that the amyloid plaque burden in the brain weakly correlates with the severity of dementia in AD patients [46]. We found higher levels of CSF Aβo in AD patients, although we could not find any correlation between $A\beta_{1-42}$ and Aβo in any of the studies. This would indicate that the lowering of CSF $A\beta_{1-42}$ is not, at least solely, explained by its incorporation into oligomeric forms. The same has been suggested for plasma Aβ and Aβo [44]. Only a small fraction of $A\beta_{1-40}$ and $A\beta_{1-42}$, which are in the high pg/mL to low ng/mL range, seems to be in oligomeric form in CSF, perhaps because the oligomers are stuck in the brain.

We detected that patients with MCI who later converted to AD had increased levels of Aβo compared to controls, while this increase in Aβo was not seen in patients with stable MCI. Although this difference was seen on a group level, many of the samples had lower Aβo levels than could be measured using our Aβo ELISA. The overlap of the Aβo values between the MCI-AD group and control group was substantial and should thus be interpreted with caution. When comparing AD patients that were divided according to their MMSE scores to study how oligomers varied at different stages of AD, we found that AD patients with mild and moderate AD had significantly higher levels of Aβo than controls, while AD patients with severe AD did not differ significantly from the control group. It almost seems as if Aβo levels increase at the onset of the disease when the clinical symptoms appear, and then rises as the disease progresses to later fall back down as the disease gets severe.

To our knowledge no previous study has measured CSF Aβo on several patient materials spanning different stages of AD. In some of the patient materials many of the samples had undetectable or very low levels of Aβo. We cannot explain why the number of patients who had undetectable levels of Aβo varied among the different studies, although there could be some differences in the materials used for sampling CSF at the different centers. There were also some controls in our study who had relatively high levels of Aβo for unknown reason. The controls have been followed up to ensure that they did not develop AD in the near future, minimizing the risk of them having incipient AD although it cannot be fully excluded given that the disease has an onset many years before clinical symptoms [21,22]. The differences in the patients materials are not likely due to freeze/thawing since we could not detect any loss or gain in Aβo levels when CSF samples were freeze/thawed in five cycles. It has been shown that Aβ is not affected by long term storage [47], although it cannot be completely ruled out that storage conditions might affect the levels of oligomeric forms of the protein. The samples for each study were sampled at one clinical centre and stored in the same way, minimizing possible artifacts from long term storage or differences in sample handling. Even though various techniques have been used to measure CSF Aβo [26,27,28,29,30,31,32], and what was seen in our study, the results seem to remain the same with an increase of Aβo in AD and MCI-AD patients, although with a marked overlap to the controls, resulting in a too weak separation to be considered as a clinical biomarker at this stage. However, as a marker in clinical studies, Aβo can be monitored within patients to measure if CSF Aβo are reduced as an effect of these treatments. This would indicate that the compounds reach their target and reduce the levels of the neurotoxic Aβo.

Acknowledgments

We thank Christina Unger for providing brain extracts from Tg2576 mice.

Author Contributions

Conceived and designed the experiments: MH KB HZ. Performed the experiments: MH OH JH NA UA KN LM. Analyzed the data: MH HZ KB. Contributed reagents/materials/analysis tools: KB HZ OH JH NA KN LM. Wrote the paper: MH.

References

1. Blennow K, de Leon MJ, Zetterberg H (2006) Alzheimer's disease. Lancet 368: 387–403.
2. Jarrett JT, Berger EP, Lansbury PT Jr (1993) The carboxy terminus of the beta amyloid protein is critical for the seeding of amyloid formation: implications for the pathogenesis of Alzheimer's disease. Biochemistry 32: 4693–4697.
3. Avila J, Lucas JJ, Perez M, Hernandez F (2004) Role of tau protein in both physiological and pathological conditions. Physiol Rev 84: 361–384.
4. Braak H, Braak E (1991) Neuropathological stageing of Alzheimer-related changes. Acta Neuropathol 82: 239–259.
5. Walsh DM, Lomakin A, Benedek GB, Condron MM, Teplow DB (1997) Amyloid beta-protein fibrillogenesis. Detection of a protofibrillar intermediate. J Biol Chem 272: 22364–22372.
6. Klein WL, Krafft GA, Finch CE (2001) Targeting small Abeta oligomers: the solution to an Alzheimer's disease conundrum? Trends Neurosci 24: 219–224.
7. LaFerla FM, Green KN, Oddo S (2007) Intracellular amyloid-beta in Alzheimer's disease. Nat Rev Neurosci 8: 499–509.
8. Lesne S, Koh MT, Kotilinek L, Kayed R, Glabe CG, et al. (2006) A specific amyloid-beta protein assembly in the brain impairs memory. Nature 440: 352–357.
9. Walsh DM, Klyubin I, Fadeeva JV, Cullen WK, Anwyl R, et al. (2002) Naturally secreted oligomers of amyloid beta protein potently inhibit hippocampal long-term potentiation in vivo. Nature 416: 535–539.
10. Cleary JP, Walsh DM, Hofmeister JJ, Shankar GM, Kuskowski MA, et al. (2005) Natural oligomers of the amyloid-beta protein specifically disrupt cognitive function. Nat Neurosci 8: 79–84.
11. Shankar GM, Bloodgood BL, Townsend M, Walsh DM, Selkoe DJ, et al. (2007) Natural oligomers of the Alzheimer amyloid-beta protein induce reversible synapse loss by modulating an NMDA-type glutamate receptor-dependent signaling pathway. J Neurosci 27: 2866–2875.
12. De Felice FG, Velasco PT, Lambert MP, Viola K, Fernandez SJ, et al. (2007) Abeta oligomers induce neuronal oxidative stress through an N-methyl-D-aspartate receptor-dependent mechanism that is blocked by the Alzheimer drug memantine. J Biol Chem 282: 11590–11601.
13. Renner M, Lacor PN, Velasco PT, Xu J, Contractor A, et al. (2010) Deleterious effects of amyloid beta oligomers acting as an extracellular scaffold for mGluR5. Neuron 66: 739–754.
14. Sepulveda FJ, Parodi J, Peoples RW, Opazo C, Aguayo LG (2010) Synaptotoxicity of Alzheimer beta amyloid can be explained by its membrane perforating property. PLoS One 5: e11820.
15. Klyubin I, Walsh DM, Lemere CA, Cullen WK, Shankar GM, et al. (2005) Amyloid beta protein immunotherapy neutralizes Abeta oligomers that disrupt synaptic plasticity in vivo. Nat Med 11: 556–561.
16. Hartman RE, Izumi Y, Bales KR, Paul SM, Wozniak DF, et al. (2005) Treatment with an amyloid-beta antibody ameliorates plaque load, learning deficits, and hippocampal long-term potentiation in a mouse model of Alzheimer's disease. J Neurosci 25: 6213–6220.
17. Walsh DM, Townsend M, Podlisny MB, Shankar GM, Fadeeva JV, et al. (2005) Certain inhibitors of synthetic amyloid beta-peptide (Abeta) fibrillogenesis block oligomerization of natural Abeta and thereby rescue long-term potentiation. J Neurosci 25: 2455–2462.
18. Morgan D, Diamond DM, Gottschall PE, Ugen KE, Dickey C, et al. (2000) A beta peptide vaccination prevents memory loss in an animal model of Alzheimer's disease. Nature 408: 982–985.
19. Blennow K, Hampel H, Weiner M, Zetterberg H (2010) Cerebrospinal fluid and plasma biomarkers in Alzheimer disease. Nat Rev Neurol 6: 131–144.
20. Flirski M, Sobow T (2005) Biochemical markers and risk factors of Alzheimer's disease. Curr Alzheimer Res 2: 47–64.
21. Mattsson N, Zetterberg H, Hansson O, Andreasen N, Parnetti L, et al. (2009) CSF biomarkers and incipient Alzheimer disease in patients with mild cognitive impairment. JAMA 302: 385–393.
22. Andreasen N, Minthon L, Vanmechelen E, Vanderstichele H, Davidsson P, et al. (1999) Cerebrospinal fluid tau and Abeta42 as predictors of development of Alzheimer's disease in patients with mild cognitive impairment. Neurosci Lett 273: 5–8.
23. Klunk WE, Engler H, Nordberg A, Wang Y, Blomqvist G, et al. (2004) Imaging brain amyloid in Alzheimer's disease with Pittsburgh Compound-B. Ann Neurol 55: 306–319.
24. Fagan AM, Mintun MA, Mach RH, Lee SY, Dence CS, et al. (2006) Inverse relation between in vivo amyloid imaging load and cerebrospinal fluid Abeta42 in humans. Ann Neurol 59: 512–519.
25. Forsberg A, Engler H, Almkvist O, Blomquist G, Hagman G, et al. (2008) PET imaging of amyloid deposition in patients with mild cognitive impairment. Neurobiol Aging 29: 1456–1465.
26. Funke SA, Birkmann E, Henke F, Gortz P, Lange-Asschenfeldt C, et al. (2007) Single particle detection of Abeta aggregates associated with Alzheimer's disease. Biochem Biophys Res Commun 364: 902–907.
27. Haes AJ, Chang L, Klein WL, Van Duyne RP (2005) Detection of a biomarker for Alzheimer's disease from synthetic and clinical samples using a nanoscale optical biosensor. J Am Chem Soc 127: 2264–2271.
28. Pitschke M, Prior R, Haupt M, Riesner D (1998) Detection of single amyloid beta-protein aggregates in the cerebrospinal fluid of Alzheimer's patients by fluorescence correlation spectroscopy. Nat Med 4: 832–834.
29. Georganopoulou DG, Chang L, Nam JM, Thaxton CS, Mufson EJ, et al. (2005) Nanoparticle-based detection in cerebral spinal fluid of a soluble pathogenic biomarker for Alzheimer's disease. Proc Natl Acad Sci U S A 102: 2273–2276.
30. Fukumoto H, Tokuda T, Kasai T, Ishigami N, Hidaka H, et al. (2010) High-molecular-weight beta-amyloid oligomers are elevated in cerebrospinal fluid of Alzheimer patients. FASEB J 24: 2716–2726.
31. Santos AN, Ewers M, Minthon L, Simm A, Silber RE, et al. (2012) Amyloid-beta oligomers in cerebrospinal fluid are associated with cognitive decline in patients with Alzheimer's disease. J Alzheimers Dis 29: 171–176.
32. Gao CM, Yam AY, Wang X, Magdangal E, Salisbury C, et al. (2010) Abeta40 oligomers identified as a potential biomarker for the diagnosis of Alzheimer's disease. PLoS One 5: e15725.
33. Bard F, Cannon C, Barbour R, Burke RL, Games D, et al. (2000) Peripherally administered antibodies against amyloid beta-peptide enter the central nervous system and reduce pathology in a mouse model of Alzheimer disease. Nat Med 6: 916–919.
34. Bard F, Barbour R, Cannon C, Carretto R, Fox M, et al. (2003) Epitope and isotype specificities of antibodies to beta -amyloid peptide for protection against Alzheimer's disease-like neuropathology. Proc Natl Acad Sci U S A 100: 2023–2028.
35. Folstein MF, Folstein SE, McHugh PR (1975) "Mini-mental state". A practical method for grading the cognitive state of patients for the clinician. J Psychiatr Res 12: 189–198.
36. McKhann G, Drachman D, Folstein M, Katzman R, Price D, et al. (1984) Clinical diagnosis of Alzheimer's disease: report of the NINCDS-ADRDA Work Group under the auspices of Department of Health and Human Services Task Force on Alzheimer's Disease. Neurology 34: 939–944.
37. Petersen RC (2004) Mild cognitive impairment as a diagnostic entity. J Intern Med 256: 183–194.
38. Horikoshi Y, Sakaguchi G, Becker AG, Gray AJ, Duff K, et al. (2004) Development of Abeta terminal end-specific antibodies and sensitive ELISA for Abeta variant. Biochem Biophys Res Commun 319: 733–737.
39. LeVine H 3rd (2004) Alzheimer's beta-peptide oligomer formation at physiologic concentrations. Anal Biochem 335: 81–90.
40. Ward RV, Jennings KH, Jepras R, Neville W, Owen DE, et al. (2000) Fractionation and characterization of oligomeric, protofibrillar and fibrillar forms of beta-amyloid peptide. Biochem J 348 Pt 1: 137–144.
41. El-Agnaf OM, Mahil DS, Patel BP, Austen BM (2000) Oligomerization and toxicity of beta-amyloid-42 implicated in Alzheimer's disease. Biochem Biophys Res Commun 273: 1003–1007.
42. Mustafiz T, Portelius E, Gustavsson MK, Holtta M, Zetterberg H, et al. (2011) Characterization of the brain beta-amyloid isoform pattern at different ages of Tg2576 mice. Neurodegener Dis 8: 352–363.
43. Barghorn S, Nimmrich V, Striebinger A, Krantz C, Keller P, et al. (2005) Globular amyloid beta-peptide oligomer - a homogenous and stable neuro-pathological protein in Alzheimer's disease. J Neurochem 95: 834–847.
44. Xia W, Yang T, Shankar G, Smith IM, Shen Y, et al. (2009) A specific enzyme-linked immunosorbent assay for measuring beta-amyloid protein oligomers in human plasma and brain tissue of patients with Alzheimer disease. Arch Neurol 66: 190–199.
45. Sehlin D, Sollvander S, Paulie S, Brundin R, Ingelsson M, et al. (2010) Interference from heterophilic antibodies in amyloid-beta oligomer ELISAs. J Alzheimers Dis 21: 1295–1301.

46. Terry RD, Masliah E, Salmon DP, Butters N, DeTeresa R, et al. (1991) Physical basis of cognitive alterations in Alzheimer's disease: synapse loss is the major correlate of cognitive impairment. Ann Neurol 30: 572–580.

47. Bjerke M, Portelius E, Minthon L, Wallin A, Anckarsater H, et al. (2010) Confounding factors influencing amyloid Beta concentration in cerebrospinal fluid. Int J Alzheimers Dis 2010.

48. Andreasen N, Hesse C, Davidsson P, Minthon L, Wallin A, et al. (1999) Cerebrospinal fluid beta-amyloid(1–42) in Alzheimer disease: differences between early- and late-onset Alzheimer disease and stability during the course of disease. Arch Neurol 56: 673–680.

49. Hansson O, Zetterberg H, Buchhave P, Londos E, Blennow K, et al. (2006) Association between CSF biomarkers and incipient Alzheimer's disease in patients with mild cognitive impairment: a follow-up study. Lancet Neurol 5: 228–234.

50. Olsson A, Vanderstichele H, Andreasen N, De Meyer G, Wallin A, et al. (2005) Simultaneous measurement of beta-amyloid(1–42), total tau, and phosphorylated tau (Thr181) in cerebrospinal fluid by the xMAP technology. Clin Chem 51: 336–345.

Aβ40 Oligomers Identified as a Potential Biomarker for the Diagnosis of Alzheimer's Disease

Carol Man Gao[1,9], Alice Y. Yam[1,9], Xuemei Wang[1], Erika Magdangal[1], Cleo Salisbury[1], David Peretz[1], Ronald N. Zuckermann[1,¤], Michael D. Connolly[1,¤], Oskar Hansson[3], Lennart Minthon[3], Henrik Zetterberg[2], Kaj Blennow[2], Joseph P. Fedynyshyn[1,*], Sophie Allauzen[1]

1 Research and Development, Novartis Vaccines and Diagnostics, Emeryville, California, United States of America, 2 Clinical Neurochemistry Laboratory, Department of Neuroscience and Physiology, Sahlgrenska University Hospital, Mölndal, Sweden, 3 Clinical Memory Research Unit, Department of Clinical Sciences Malmö, Lund University, Malmö, Sweden

Abstract

Alzheimer's Disease (AD) is the most prevalent form of dementia worldwide, yet the development of therapeutics has been hampered by the absence of suitable biomarkers to diagnose the disease in its early stages prior to the formation of amyloid plaques and the occurrence of irreversible neuronal damage. Since oligomeric Aβ species have been implicated in the pathophysiology of AD, we reasoned that they may correlate with the onset of disease. As such, we have developed a novel misfolded protein assay for the detection of soluble oligomers composed of Aβ x-40 and x-42 peptide (hereafter Aβ40 and Aβ42) from cerebrospinal fluid (CSF). Preliminary validation of this assay with 36 clinical samples demonstrated the presence of aggregated Aβ40 in the CSF of AD patients. Together with measurements of total Aβ42, diagnostic sensitivity and specificity greater than 95% and 90%, respectively, were achieved. Although larger sample populations will be needed to confirm this diagnostic sensitivity, our studies demonstrate a sensitive method of detecting circulating Aβ40 oligomers from AD CSF and suggest that these oligomers could be a powerful new biomarker for the early detection of AD.

Citation: Gao CM, Yam AY, Wang X, Magdangal E, Salisbury C, et al. (2010) Aβ40 Oligomers Identified as a Potential Biomarker for the Diagnosis of Alzheimer's Disease. PLoS ONE 5(12): e15725. doi:10.1371/journal.pone.0015725

Editor: Sergio T. Ferreira, Federal University of Rio de Janeiro, Brazil

Received August 2, 2010; **Accepted** November 21, 2010; **Published** December 30, 2010

Funding: This work was funded by Novartis Vaccines and Diagnostics. Several of the authors are or were employed by the funder and, as such, the funders played a role in the study design, data collection and analysis, decision to publish, and preparation of the manuscript.

Competing Interests: Several of the authors are employed by Novartis Vaccines and Diagnostics and thus may have a conflict of interest. In addition, the submitted work is included in a pending patent application on amyloid-beta aggregates as biomarkers for Alzheimer's Disease (patent #61/265,340, submitted by Novartis AG on Nov 30, 2009). This does not alter the authors' adherence to all the PLoS ONE policies on sharing data and materials.

* E-mail: joseph.fedynyshyn@novartis.com

¤ Current address: Lawrence Berkeley National Laboratory, Molecular Foundry, Berkeley, California, United States of America

9 These authors contributed equally to this work.

Introduction

Alzheimer's Disease (AD) is a neurodegenerative disorder characterized by progressive memory loss and cognitive dysfunction. It is the most prevalent form of dementia, estimated to affect 13 million people worldwide [1]. While the precise mechanism underlying the disease is not fully understood, the aggregation of amyloid beta (Aβ) appears to play an important role [2–4]. Aβ peptides of various lengths (typically 1–40 and 1–42) are cleavage products of the amyloid precursor protein that aggregate and form insoluble plaques in AD brains. Post mortem identification of these plaques together with neurofibrillary tangles and neuronal loss is currently the definitive and only fully accepted diagnostic confirmation of AD [5,6]. However, recent reports suggest that smaller, soluble Aβ oligomers are more likely to be the pathogenic agents of disease [3,4,7–10].

A growing number of in vitro generated oligomers of varied size and structure have been implicated in AD [4]. However, the actual identity of the oligomer participating in AD pathogenesis remains elusive. Its chemical composition is also poorly defined, although several lines of evidence suggest that AD-associated oligomers are primarily composed of Aβ42 [3]. For instance, one unifying feature of AD is the presence of Aβ42-containing plaques in the brain parenchyma [11,12]. This suggests that any soluble oligomers would also be composed of Aβ42. In addition, Aβ42 appears to be more amyloidogenic than Aβ40 and is found more frequently in plaques despite existing at much lower physiological concentrations [13]. Lastly, several presenilin mutations linked to familial forms of AD are known to increase production of Aβ42 cleavage products [14], further implicating this Aβ peptide in pathogenesis. Consequently, it is generally assumed that cytotoxic oligomers mediating AD are composed of Aβ42 peptides.

While the precise conformation of in vivo oligomers is unknown, several lines of evidence suggest that aggregated proteins share a number of structural properties. For instance, amyloid fibrils composed of different proteins have similar cross beta sheet structure, allowing binding and detection by a number of compounds such as Thioflavin T and Congo Red [15,16]. Smaller aggregated species such as oligomers and protofibrils also share structural properties recognized by conformation-sensitive antibodies [17,18]. Similarly, we have recently developed a series of peptides for the selective capture of aggregated prion protein (PrP) from plasma [19]. We now report the adaptation and integration of these peptides into a Misfolded Protein Assay (MPA) and the capture of aggregated Aβ from CSF. Given that soluble Aβ oligomers have been reported in the CSF of AD patients [10,20–22], we reasoned that the MPA could be utilized to detect oligomers found in vivo. Using this technology, we demonstrate for the first time the presence of Aβ40 oligomers in AD CSF. We propose that Aβ40 oligomers could be a novel biomarker for the early diagnosis of AD.

Methods

MPA capture of Aβ aggregates

Aggregate Specific Reagent 1 (ASR1) beads were generated by chemical conjugation of a thiolated ASR1 derivative to Dynal M270 carboxyl beads (Invitrogen Dynal AS, Oslo, Norway, 30 mg/mL) via maleimide chemistry (Figure 1). Control beads consisted of similarly conjugated glutathione molecules.

Aβ42 aggregates from AD brain homogenate (ADBH) were captured with 3 μl ASR1 beads for 1 hour at 37°C in 100 μl 80% plasma by spiking with 75 nl of 10% brain homogenate (Fig. 2C) or the indicated concentrations of Aβ aggregates (Fig. 2D) in capture buffer (50 mM Tris, 150 mM NaCl, 1% Tween-20, 1% Triton X-100 pH 7.5). 10% ADBH was estimated to contain ~1 pg/nL Aβ42 aggregates (data not shown). The beads were then washed with TBST (50 mM Tris, 150 mM NaCl, 0.05% Tween-20 pH 7.5), and bound proteins were eluted with 0.1 M NaOH at 80°C for 30 minutes and neutralized with 0.12 M NaH$_2$PO$_4$, 0.4% Tween-20. The eluted Aβ was subsequently detected by an Aβ42-specific ELISA, utilizing an Aβ x-42 specific capture antibody (12F4, Covance, Princeton, NJ) and HRP-conjugated 4G8 antibody (Covance) for detection. To test the conformational nature of ASR1 binding, ADBH was pretreated with 5.4 M guanidine thiocyanate for 30 minutes at room temperature prior to dilution into 80% plasma and MPA detection. AD and control brain samples were obtained from the tissue bank of the Swiss National Reference Centre of Prion Diseases (Zürich, Switzerland).

In vitro Aβ42 oligomers spiked into normal CSF and in vivo oligomers from clinical AD CSF were similarly detected by the MPA with a few modifications. 250 μl 80% human CSF in capture buffer was incubated with 30 μl ASR1 beads. ASR1 beads were subsequently washed with TBST and 1% Zwittergent 3-14 before Aβ42 and Aβ40 were eluted and detected in a multiplex format by MSD immunoassay (Meso Scale Discovery, Gaithersburg, Maryland) according to the manufacturer's instructions. In vitro Aβ42 oligomers are estimated to be 12mers and were prepared as described [23]. Normal pooled CSF for oligomer spiking experiments was purchased from Analytical Biological Services Inc. (Wilmington, DE).

Biochemical characterization of brain-derived aggregates

Solubility of brain-derived Aβ aggregates was assessed by differential centrifugation. 250 nl 10% ADBH diluted into 0.5x capture buffer was treated with or without 3 M guanidine thiocyanate for 10 minutes at 95°C and then centrifuged for 1.5 hour at 134,000 g at 4°C. Aβ42 in supernatant and pellet fractions were denatured with 3 M guanidine, diluted with TBST buffer, and detected by ELISA.

The size of brain-derived Aβ42 aggregates was estimated by separation of 75 μl of 10% ADBH on a Superdex200 10/300 GL column at a flow rate of 1 mL/min in TBS with 1 mM EDTA, 1% NP40. 1 mL fractions were collected and denatured with 0.1 N NaOH as stated above prior to ELISA detection.

ELISA

ELISA plates were coated with 2 μg/mL 12F4 antibody in coating buffer (0.1 M NaH$_2$PO$_4$, 1% NaCl, pH 6), washed with TBST, and blocked with 1% BSA, 3% sucrose in TBS for 1 hour at 37°C. 0.2 μg/mL HRP-conjugated 4G8 antibody in conjugate diluent (0.1% BSA, 0.01% casein in PBS) was diluted 1:1 with the sample and applied to the 12F4-coated plates for 1 hour at room temperature before detection by a chemiluminescent substrate (Pierce Supersignal ELISA Femto Substrate, Thermo Fisher Scientific, Rockford, IL).

Patients and CSF sampling

The AD group consisted of 26 patients consulting the memory disorder clinic at Malmö University Hospital, Sweden, mean age 71.8±7.3 years. All patients underwent physical, neurological and psychiatric examination, cognitive tests, careful clinical history and functional assessment. Patients diagnosed with AD had to meet the DSM-IIIR criteria of dementia [24] and the criteria of probable AD defined by NINCDS-ADRDA [25]. The AD patients were followed over time with repeated clinical evaluations, which increases the clinical diagnostic accuracy. The control group, in total 10 cases, mean age 69.4±9.7 years, was defined based on absence of memory complaints or any other cognitive symptoms, and no signs of active neurological or psychiatric disease. All patients and controls gave informed consent to participate in the study. The study was conducted according to the provisions of the Helsinki Declaration and was approved by the ethics committee of Lund University, Sweden. CSF was collected in polypropylene tubes, centrifuged, aliquoted, and stored at −80°C pending analyses.

Statistical analysis

Statistical comparison of two populations was performed using two-tailed t-test using GraphPad Prism for Windows, v 5.01 (GraphPad Software, San Diego, CA). Receiver operating

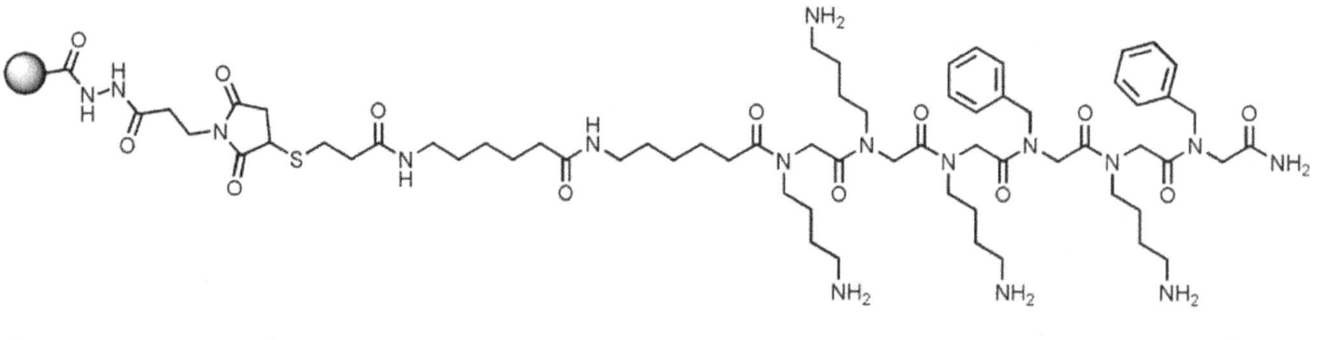

Figure 1. Aggregate Specific Reagent 1 (ASR1). Chemical structure of ASR1 peptoid conjugated to a solid surface.
doi:10.1371/journal.pone.0015725.g001

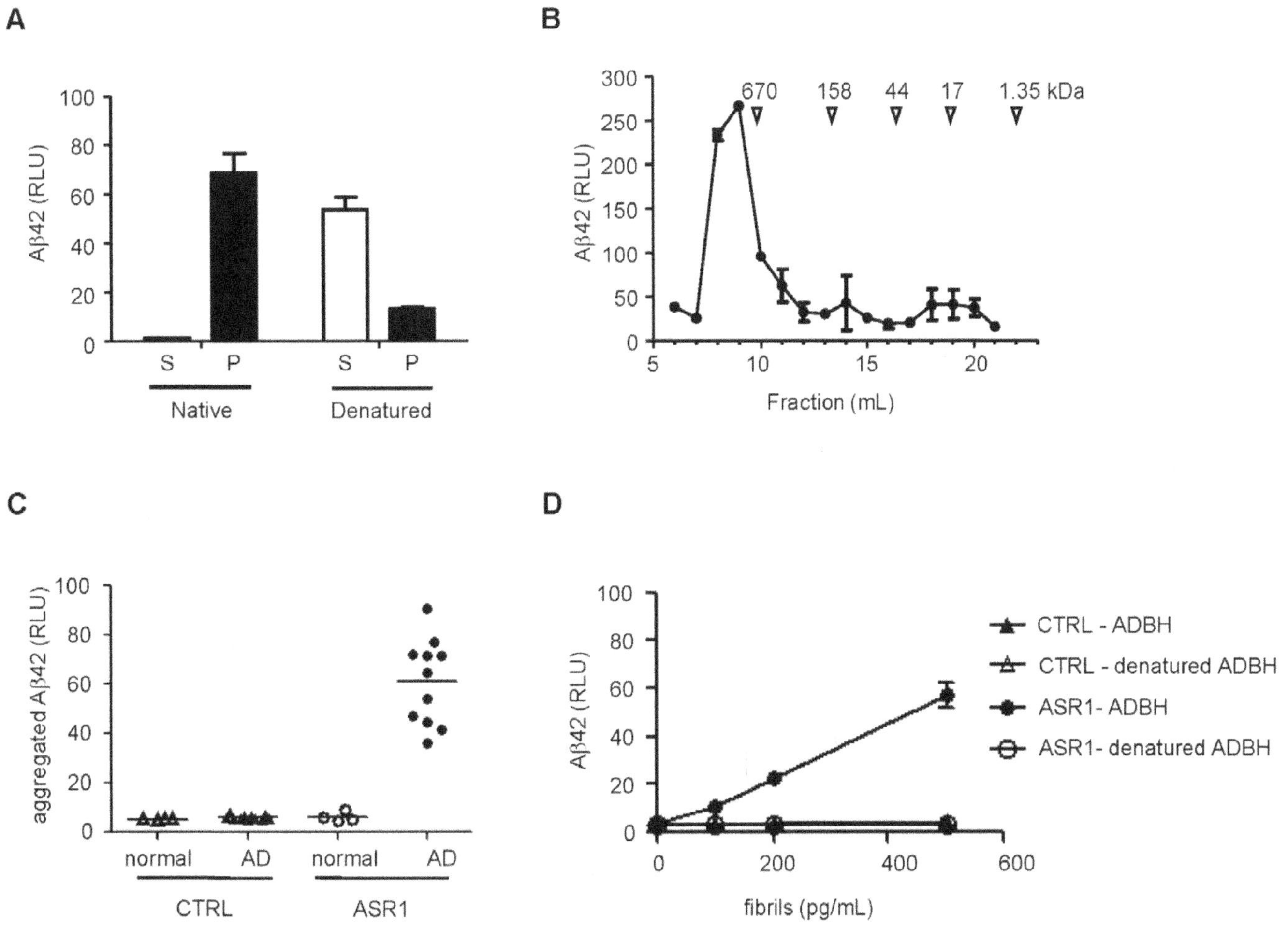

Figure 2. MPA detection of a conformational epitope in Aβ aggregates from AD brain homogenates (ADBH). *A.* ADBH was centrifuged at 134,000*g* for 1 hr, and denatured Aβ42 in the supernatant (S) and pellet (P) fractions was detected by ELISA. *B.* ADBH was fractionated by size exclusion chromatography and Aβ42 was detected by ELISA. *C.* 75 nl of normal (open symbols) or AD (closed symbols) brain homogenate was subjected to the MPA using control (triangles) or ASR1-coated (circles) beads. *D.* Aβ aggregates from an ADBH were examined by the MPA with (open symbols) or without (filled symbols) a pretreatment with 5.4 M guanidine thiocyanate using control (triangles) or ASR1-coated (circles) beads. Error bars represent the standard deviation of triplicate reactions.
doi:10.1371/journal.pone.0015725.g002

characteristic curves (ROC) were generated using R (R Foundation for Statistical Computing, Vienna, Austria).

Results

An aggregate-specific reagent captures Aβ aggregates from AD brain homogenate in a conformation-dependent manner

We have developed an Aggregate Specific Reagent (ASR1, Figure 1) that preferentially binds aggregated proteins over monomeric proteins. ASR1 is a peptoid, a peptidomimetic containing N-substituted glycines [26], which have been shown to be resistant to proteolytic digestion from enzymes commonly found in body fluids [27]. The ASR1 sequence is derived from a PrP peptide that has a strong ability to capture aggregated PrP in solution [19]. ASR1 can capture picomolar amounts of insoluble aggregated PrP from a solution containing an excess of normally folded PrP (Figure S1 and [19]).

As amyloid aggregates are characterized by similar cross-beta sheet structure, they share conformational epitopes that are recognized by amyloid-binding molecules such as Congo Red and thioflavin T [15,16] as well as conformation-specific antibodies [17,18]. We hypothesized that ASR1 might also

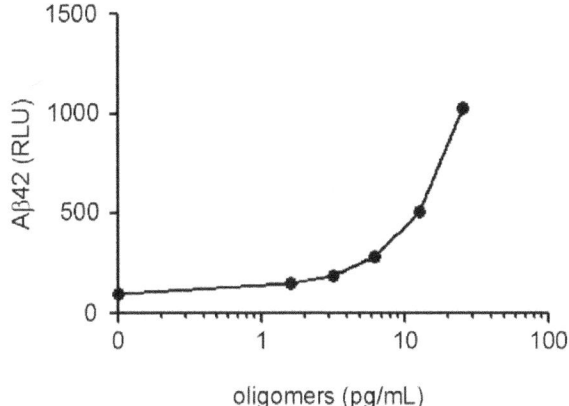

Figure 3. MPA detection of synthetic oligomers at subpicomolar levels. In vitro synthesized Aβ42 oligomers were diluted into normal CSF at the indicated concentrations and detected by the MPA. Error bars represent the standard deviation of triplicate reactions.
doi:10.1371/journal.pone.0015725.g003

recognize structural epitopes common to aggregated proteins rather than epitopes specific to PrP aggregates. As such, we asked if ASR1 could bind aggregates composed of Aβ. Like brain-derived PrP aggregates, aggregates from an AD brain homogenate (ADBH) were insoluble at 134,000 g (Figure 2A), suggesting that they were large. Fractionation by size exclusion chromatography demonstrated that these aggregates were larger than a 670 kDa molecular weight standard (Figure 2B).

To test if ASR1 could bind to Aβ aggregates, ASR1 beads were incubated with AD and normal brain homogenates, and then the bound Aβ42 was eluted, denatured, and then detected by an Aβ42-specific ELISA. This method, the MPA, could clearly distinguish between control and AD samples, while a parallel assay using a control bead could not (Figure 2C). Furthermore, ASR1 capture of Aβ42 was conformation-dependent since treatment of the aggregates with a chemical denaturant prior to the MPA abolished all binding (Figure 2D).

ASR1 captures soluble oligomers in CSF

We reasoned that ASR1 would be a powerful tool for early diagnosis of AD if, in addition to the large aggregates found in AD brain tissue, it could also capture the smaller oligomers implicated in AD pathogenesis. As such, we tested whether ASR1 could capture Aβ oligomers diluted into CSF. In vitro oligomers composed of ~12 Aβ42 monomers were prepared as described [23] and diluted at varying concentrations into normal CSF before being subjected to the MPA (Figure 3). Of note, the MPA could detect the oligomers with high sensitivity with a limit of detection of 5 pg/mL Aβ42 (corresponding to ~80 fM oligomer).

ASR1 detects Aβ40 oligomers in AD CSF

Because we achieved significant sensitivity at detecting in vitro oligomers spiked into normal CSF, we asked whether the MPA could detect endogenous oligomers reported to be present in AD

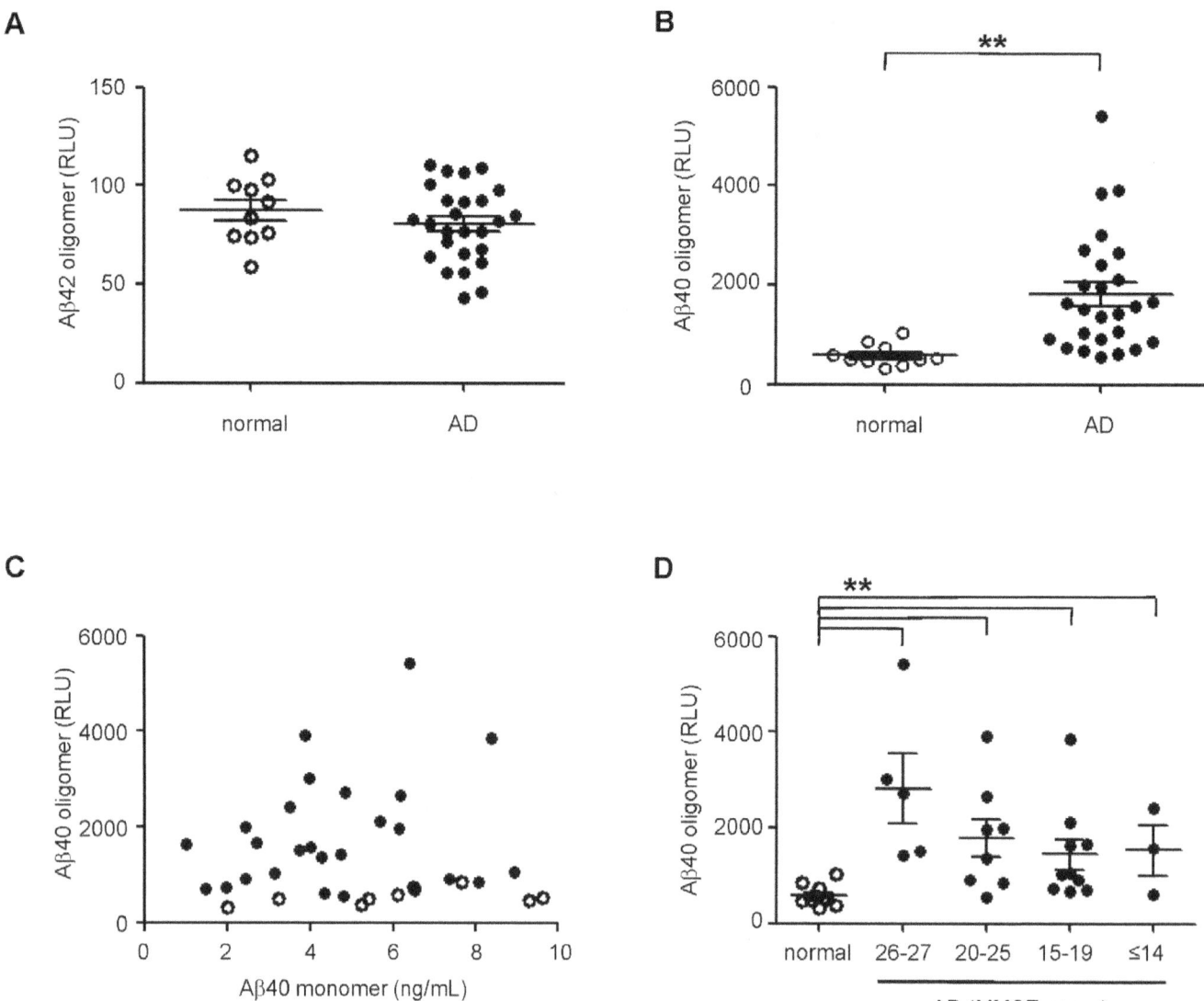

Figure 4. MPA detection of Aβ40 oligomers from AD CSF. Normal (open circles) and AD (closed circles) CSF were analyzed by the MPA. Oligomers containing Aβ42 *(A)* and Aβ40 *(B)* were captured by ASR1 beads followed by detection using a multiplex immunoassay. Significant differences between normal and AD population were calculated by t-test (Aβ42, $p = 0.31$; Aβ40, **$p < 0.01$). *C.* Lack of correlation between MPA-detected Aβ40 signal and the concentration of Aβ40 monomers in AD CSF ($R^2 = 0.037$). *D.* The distribution of Aβ40 oligomers by disease severity was examined by categorization of AD patients according to MMSE scores (**$p < 0.01$ between normal and all AD groups). The mean and standard error of the mean (SEM) are shown for all groups.
doi:10.1371/journal.pone.0015725.g004

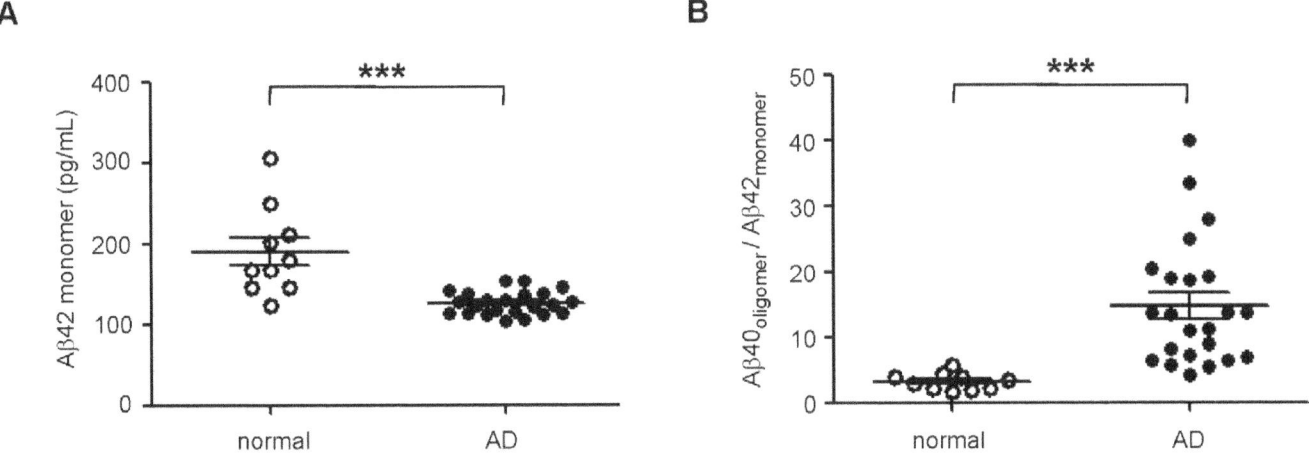

Figure 5. Synergistic combination of Aβ40 oligomer signal with monomeric Aβ42 concentration. *A.* The concentration of monomeric Aβ42 was measured in normal (open circles) and AD (closed circles) CSF (***$p<0.001$). *B.* The ratio of Aβ40 oligomers (RLU) and Aβ42 concentration (pg/mL) was calculated and plotted for both normal (open circles) and AD (closed circles) populations (***$p<0.001$). Three AD samples were not included in this analysis because of insufficient sample to measure Aβ42 concentrations. The mean and SEM are shown for all groups.
doi:10.1371/journal.pone.0015725.g005

CSF [20–22]. CSF from 26 clinically diagnosed AD patients at varying stages of disease and 10 aged-matched controls were examined by the MPA. As before, CSF was incubated with ASR1 beads and the captured Aβ was detected by a multiplex immunoassay specific for Aβ40 and Aβ42. Upon examination of captured Aβ42, we did not detect any difference between AD and control populations (Figure 4A). However, we observed surprisingly clear and significant differences in the Aβ40 signal between the two groups (Figure 4B). Importantly, Aβ40 signals from the MPA did not correlate with the concentration of total Aβ40 in the CSF (presumably this immunoassay format would bias the detection of total Aβ toward monomeric species, so they are indicated as such henceforth). This suggests that the Aβ40 signals were associated with specific MPA oligomeric capture and not nonspecific binding of Aβ40 monomers to the capture beads (Figure 4C). When we further categorized the AD samples into groups of increasing disease severity based on clinical Mini-Mental State Examination (MMSE) scores, we found that the Aβ40 oligomers were not only found in individuals with late-stage AD and low MMSE scores but also in patients with early stage AD and higher MMSE scores (Figure 4D). Therefore, using the MPA, we have identified Aβ40 oligomers as a potential biomarker that could diagnose AD in the early stages of disease.

Aβ40 oligomers are a novel biomarker for the diagnosis of AD

To validate our results against other investigated biomarkers for AD, we also measured the levels of monomeric Aβ42 in this set of samples. As expected, Aβ42 was significantly decreased in the CSF of AD patients relative to normal individuals (Figure 5A), consistent with previously published results [28]. Since low levels of monomeric Aβ42 and high levels of oligomeric Aβ40 are linked to AD, we combined the two biomarkers to strengthen their predictive value. The resulting ratio of oligomeric Aβ40 to monomeric Aβ42 indeed enhanced the differentiation of control and AD populations (Figure 5B). Additional ROC analysis demonstrated diagnostic sensitivity and specificity of 95% and 90%, respectively (Figure 6, Table 1). Positive and negative predictive value was estimated to be near 95% and 90%, respectively, whereas oligomeric Aβ40 and monomeric Aβ42 biomarkers alone had negative predictive values that were equal to or less than 75% (Table 1).

Discussion

AD is a growing epidemic that impacts nearly 50% of our elderly population greater than 85 years old [29]. However, the development of therapeutics to treat the disease has been hampered by the absence of suitable biomarkers to diagnose the disease. Currently, a clinical diagnosis of AD can only be confirmed with the identification of Aβ plaques in postmortem brain tissue [5,6]. Premortem clinical diagnosis is also problematic as it relies heavily on subjective reporting and observed cognitive decline that can occur over a period of years. Since the first clinical signs of cognitive dysfunction may appear after significant neuronal loss has occurred, there is a compelling need for biomarkers that can diagnose early AD.

Because Aβ oligomers are suggested to play a key role in AD pathogenesis [3,4,7–10] and because they have been detected in

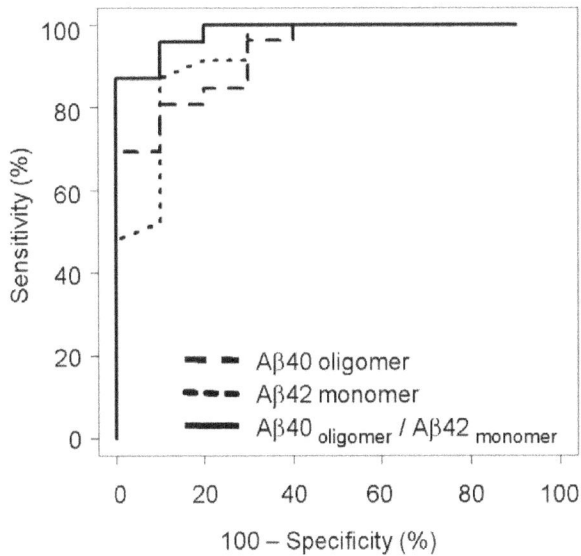

Figure 6. Receiver operating characteristic (ROC) curve. ROC analysis was performed to compare the diagnostic value of 3 biomarkers: oligomeric Aβ40 (– –), monomeric Aβ42 (- - -), and the ratio Aβ40oligomer/Aβ42monomer (——).
doi:10.1371/journal.pone.0015725.g006

67

Table 1. ROC analysis and diagnostic performance for Aβ40 oligomer, Aβ42 monomer, and Aβ40$_{oligomer}$/Aβ42$_{monomer}$ biomarkers.

Parameters	Aβ40 oligomer	Aβ42 monomer	Aβ40$_{oligomer}$/Aβ42$_{monomer}$
ROC AUC	0.93	0.93	0.98
Threshold value	850 RLU	150 pg/ml	4.3
Sensitivity (%)	81	87	96
Specificity (%)	90	90	90
Test accuracy (%)	83	88	94
Positive predictive value (%)	95	95	96
Negative predictive value (%)	64	75	90

doi:10.1371/journal.pone.0015725.t001

diagnostically relevant body fluids [10,20–22], we reasoned that Aβ oligomers could be a powerful AD biomarker predicting disease progression. However, the concentration of oligomers in CSF remains poorly defined and only a few studies estimate that they may exist at very low levels [21,22]. Furthermore, these studies did not distinguish between Aβ40 and Aβ42-containing oligomers since they utilized either antibodies recognizing oligomeric structure or oligomer-specific ELISAs that employed capture and detection antibodies recognizing the same amino-terminal epitopes. In this study, we report the development of a novel assay that specifically detected low concentrations of aggregated Aβ in a small population of AD CSF. Because AD is largely correlated with the accumulation of Aβ42 in the brain, we expected to identify oligomers composed of Aβ42. To our surprise, we found only an enrichment of Aβ40-containing oligomers in AD CSF. These oligomers were observed at multiple stages of AD, suggesting that they could be a biomarker for early diagnosis of AD.

Because Aβ42 oligomers are widely implicated in AD pathology, the correlation we observed of AD with Aβ40 but not Aβ42 oligomers was surprising. One explanation is that we detected oligomers associated with the vascular Aβ40 deposits that are seen in patients with cerebral amyloid angiopathy (CAA). CAA is a pathological feature of AD characterized by the cerebrovascular deposition of Aβ peptides with the major species being Aβ40 [30,31] and has been estimated to impact greater than 90% of AD cases [32,33]. Therefore, our findings might reflect an increase of oligomeric Aβ40 associated with these Aβ deposits.

Another possibility is that Aβ40 oligomers may be more soluble and reach CSF more readily than Aβ42 oligomers which may rapidly aggregate and deposit in the brain parenchyma. Consequently, high levels of Aβ40 oligomers in the CSF may be a surrogate marker of an amyloidogenic cascade in the brain.

A third explanation for our inability to identify Aβ42 oligomers may be the sensitivity of our detection system. While both Aβ40 and Aβ42 containing oligomers may be present in CSF and captured by ASR1 beads, the subsequent detection of the constituent monomers may be limited by the sensitivity of the immunoassay (Mesoscale detection limits for Aβ40 and Aβ42 are 5 and 8 pg/mL, respectively). Furthermore, the concentration of Aβ42 in CSF is approximately 10-fold lower than that of Aβ40, suggesting that any Aβ42-containing oligomers may exist at concentrations below our detection limit.

Although Aβ40 aggregates have been documented in AD, the biological relevance of Aβ40 oligomers in AD pathogenesis remains unclear. While nearly all cases of AD report Aβ42-containing plaques in the brain, approximately two thirds of them

also report Aβ40 deposits [11], and significant levels of Aβ40 have also been found in AD cortical brain tissue [34]. One interpretation of these results is that aggregation of the less soluble Aβ42 would precede and recruit subsequent aggregation of Aβ40, as has been previously suggested [12,35]. In support of this idea, purification of oligomers from AD brain tissues have isolated both Aβ40, Aβ42, and Aβ40/42 heterodimers [8,36]. The impact of Aβ40 oligomers on AD pathogenesis is unclear although some in vitro models suggest that Aβ42 oligomers are significantly more cytotoxic [37]. Nevertheless, preparations of soluble Aβ40 are sufficiently toxic to impact long term potentiation in cell culture systems and cognitive function when injected into mice [38].

Additional studies are clearly needed to understand the role of Aβ40 oligomers in AD pathogenesis. Since oligomeric Aβ is suggested to be a direct causative agent of AD, we believe they may be an ideal predictor of disease progression. Indeed, although the results do not reach significance, our data suggest that there could be an inverse correlation between oligomer concentration and disease severity (Figure 4D) similar to the decline that is observed in the Aβ42 levels of AD patients. Future studies will include larger patient populations and prospective CSF sampling to screen for incipient AD. Additionally, if Aβ oligomers are to become a relevant biomarker for AD, its predictive value must be measured in patients with mild cognitive impairment. Nevertheless, our results showing the detection of Aβ40 oligomers in CSF from patients in the initial stages of AD suggest that the MPA could be a sensitive assay for the early diagnosis of AD.

Supporting Information

Figure S1 Prion Protein (PrP) captured from plasma spiked with vCJD or normal brain homogenates. vCJD (closed circle) and normal (open circle) brain homogenates were spiked into normal human plasma at the indicated concentrations and subjected to the MPA. Captured prion protein was eluted and detected by a prion-specific ELISA. Materials and Methods: vCJD and normal 10% brain homogenates (w/v) ("Blue" and "Clear" samples, respectively, from National Institute for Biological Standards and Control, United Kingdom) were spiked into normal human plasma (SeraCare Life Sciences, West Bridgewater, MA), after which 200 μl of the solution was incubated with 50 μl of 5x capture buffer and 9 μl ASR1 beads for 1 hour at 37°C. The beads were washed and captured prion protein was subsequently eluted, denatured, and detected by sandwich ELISA [19]. The vCJD brain homogenate had an estimated 4 μg/mL of aggregated PrP.
(TIF)

Acknowledgments

We thank Ruixiao Lu and Ping Shi for helpful discussions on statistical analysis and assistance in generation of the ROC curve, and Dr. Adriano Aguzzi for generously providing samples.

Author Contributions

Conceived and designed the experiments: CMG AYY SA JPF DP. Performed the experiments: CMG EM AYY. Analyzed the data: CMG EM AYY JPF. Contributed reagents/materials/analysis tools: XW CS RNZ MDC OH LM HZ KB. Wrote the paper: AYY.

References

1. Ferri CP, Prince M, Brayne C, Brodaty H, Fratiglioni L, et al. (2005) Global prevalence of dementia: a Delphi consensus study. Lancet 366: 2112–2117.
2. Stefani M, Dobson CM (2003) Protein aggregation and aggregate toxicity: new insights into protein folding, misfolding diseases and biological evolution. J Mol Med 81: 678–699.
3. Haass C, Selkoe DJ (2007) Soluble protein oligomers in neurodegeneration: lessons from the Alzheimer's amyloid beta-peptide. Nat Rev Mol Cell Biol 8: 101–112.
4. Lansbury PT, Lashuel HA (2006) A century-old debate on protein aggregation and neurodegeneration enters the clinic. Nature 443: 774–779.
5. Caroli A, Frisoni GB (2009) Quantitative evaluation of Alzheimer's disease. Expert Rev Med Devices 6: 569–588.
6. Urbanelli L, Magini A, Ciccarone V, Trivelli F, Polidoro M, et al. (2009) New perspectives for the diagnosis of Alzheimer's disease. Recent Pat CNS Drug Discov 4: 160–181.
7. Lesne S, Koh MT, Kotilinek L, Kayed R, Glabe CG, et al. (2006) A specific amyloid-beta protein assembly in the brain impairs memory. Nature 440: 352–357.
8. Shankar GM, Li S, Mehta TH, Garcia-Munoz A, Shepardson NE, et al. (2008) Amyloid-beta protein dimers isolated directly from Alzheimer's brains impair synaptic plasticity and memory. Nat Med 14: 837–842.
9. Lambert MP, Viola KL, Chromy BA, Chang L, Morgan TE, et al. (2001) Vaccination with soluble Abeta oligomers generates toxicity-neutralizing antibodies. J Neurochem 79: 595–605.
10. Klyubin I, Betts V, Welzel AT, Blennow K, Zetterberg H, et al. (2008) Amyloid beta protein dimer-containing human CSF disrupts synaptic plasticity: prevention by systemic passive immunization. J Neurosci 28: 4231–4237.
11. Gravina SA, Ho L, Eckman CB, Long KE, Otvos L, Jr., et al. (1995) Amyloid beta protein (A beta) in Alzheimer's disease brain. Biochemical and immunocytochemical analysis with antibodies specific for forms ending at A beta 40 or A beta 42(43). J Biol Chem 270: 7013–7016.
12. Iwatsubo T, Odaka A, Suzuki N, Mizusawa H, Nukina N, et al. (1994) Visualization of A beta 42(43) and A beta 40 in senile plaques with end-specific A beta monoclonals: evidence that an initially deposited species is A beta 42(43). Neuron 13: 45–53.
13. Walsh DM, Selkoe DJ (2007) A beta oligomers - a decade of discovery. J Neurochem 101: 1172–1184.
14. Citron M, Westaway D, Xia W, Carlson G, Diehl T, et al. (1997) Mutant presenilins of Alzheimer's disease increase production of 42-residue amyloid beta-protein in both transfected cells and transgenic mice. Nat Med 3: 67–72.
15. Sawaya MR, Sambashivan S, Nelson R, Ivanova MI, Sievers SA, et al. (2007) Atomic structures of amyloid cross-beta spines reveal varied steric zippers. Nature 447: 453–457.
16. Leliveld SR, Korth C (2007) The use of conformation-specific ligands and assays to dissect the molecular mechanisms of neurodegenerative diseases. J Neurosci Res 85: 2285–2297.
17. Kayed R, Head E, Thompson JL, McIntire TM, Milton SC, et al. (2003) Common structure of soluble amyloid oligomers implies common mechanism of pathogenesis. Science 300: 486–489.
18. Kayed R, Head E, Sarsoza F, Saing T, Cotman CW, et al. (2007) Fibril specific, conformation dependent antibodies recognize a generic epitope common to amyloid fibrils and fibrillar oligomers that is absent in prefibrillar oligomers. Mol Neurodegener 2: 18.
19. Lau AL, Yam AY, Michelitsch MM, Wang X, Gao C, et al. (2007) Characterization of prion protein (PrP)-derived peptides that discriminate full-length PrPSc from PrPC. Proc Natl Acad Sci U S A 104: 11551–11556.
20. Pitschke M, Prior R, Haupt M, Riesner D (1998) Detection of single amyloid beta-protein aggregates in the cerebrospinal fluid of Alzheimer's patients by fluorescence correlation spectroscopy. Nat Med 4: 832–834.
21. Georganopoulou DG, Chang L, Nam JM, Thaxton CS, Mufson EJ, et al. (2005) Nanoparticle-based detection in cerebral spinal fluid of a soluble pathogenic biomarker for Alzheimer's disease. Proc Natl Acad Sci U S A 102: 2273–2276.
22. Fukumoto H, Tokuda T, Kasai T, Ishigami N, Hidaka H, et al. (2010) High-molecular-weight {beta}-amyloid oligomers are elevated in cerebrospinal fluid of Alzheimer patients. Faseb J.
23. Barghorn S, Nimmrich V, Striebinger A, Krantz C, Keller P, et al. (2005) Globular amyloid beta-peptide oligomer - a homogenous and stable neuropathological protein in Alzheimer's disease. J Neurochem 95: 834–847.
24. American Psychiatric Association Work Group to Revise DSM-III (1987) Diagnostic and statistical manual of mental disorders: DSM-III-R. Washington, DC: American Psychiatric Association. xxix, 567.
25. McKhann G, Drachman D, Folstein M, Katzman R, Price D, et al. (1984) Clinical diagnosis of Alzheimer's disease: report of the NINCDS-ADRDA Work Group under the auspices of Department of Health and Human Services Task Force on Alzheimer's Disease. Neurology 34: 939–944.
26. Nguyen JT, Porter M, Amoui M, Miller WT, Zuckermann RN, et al. (2000) Improving SH3 domain ligand selectivity using a non-natural scaffold. Chem Biol 7: 463–473.
27. Simon RJ, Kania RS, Zuckermann RN, Huebner VD, Jewell DA, et al. (1992) Peptoids: a modular approach to drug discovery. Proc Natl Acad Sci U S A 89: 9367–9371.
28. Blennow K, Hampel H, Weiner M, Zetterberg H (2010) Cerebrospinal fluid and plasma biomarkers in Alzheimer disease. Nat Rev Neurol 6: 131–144.
29. Hebert LE, Scherr PA, Bienias JL, Bennett DA, Evans DA (2003) Alzheimer disease in the US population: prevalence estimates using the 2000 census. Arch Neurol 60: 1119–1122.
30. Weller RO, Nicoll JA (2003) Cerebral amyloid angiopathy: pathogenesis and effects on the ageing and Alzheimer brain. Neurol Res 25: 611–616.
31. Haglund M, Kalaria R, Slade JY, Englund E (2006) Differential deposition of amyloid beta peptides in cerebral amyloid angiopathy associated with Alzheimer's disease and vascular dementia. Acta Neuropathol 111: 430–435.
32. Jellinger KA (2010) Prevalence and impact of cerebrovascular lesions in Alzheimer and lewy body diseases. Neurodegener Dis 7: 112–115.
33. Jellinger KA, Attems J (2005) Prevalence and pathogenic role of cerebrovascular lesions in Alzheimer disease. J Neurol Sci 229–230: 37–41.
34. Portelius E, Bogdanovic N, Gustavsson MK, Volkmann I, Brinkmalm G, et al. (2010) Mass spectrometric characterization of brain amyloid beta isoform signatures in familial and sporadic Alzheimer's disease. Acta Neuropathol.
35. Jarrett JT, Berger EP, Lansbury PT, Jr. (1993) The carboxy terminus of the beta amyloid protein is critical for the seeding of amyloid formation: implications for the pathogenesis of Alzheimer's disease. Biochemistry 32: 4693–4697.
36. Noguchi A, Matsumura S, Dezawa M, Tada M, Yanazawa M, et al. (2009) Isolation and characterization of patient-derived, toxic, high mass amyloid beta-protein (Abeta) assembly from Alzheimer disease brains. J Biol Chem 284: 32895–32905.
37. Hoshi M, Sato M, Matsumoto S, Noguchi A, Yasutake K, et al. (2003) Spherical aggregates of beta-amyloid (amylospheroid) show high neurotoxicity and activate tau protein kinase I/glycogen synthase kinase-3beta. Proc Natl Acad Sci U S A 100: 6370–6375.
38. Takeda S, Sato N, Niisato K, Takeuchi D, Kurinami H, et al. (2009) Validation of Abeta1-40 administration into mouse cerebroventricles as an animal model for Alzheimer disease. Brain Res 1280: 137–147.

Peptide Fingerprinting of Alzheimer's Disease in Cerebrospinal Fluid: Identification and Prospective Evaluation of New Synaptic Biomarkers

Holger Jahn[1]*[9], Stefan Wittke[2,3][9], Petra Zürbig[2], Thomas J. Raedler[1,4], Sönke Arlt[1], Markus Kellmann[5], William Mullen[6], Martin Eichenlaub[1], Harald Mischak[2,6], Klaus Wiedemann[1]

1 Department of Psychiatry, University Hospital Hamburg-Eppendorf, Hamburg, Germany, 2 Mosaiques Diagnostics GmbH, Hannover, Germany, 3 University of Applied Sciences, Bremerhaven, Germany, 4 Department of Psychiatry, Foothills Hospital, University of Calgary, Calgary, Canada, 5 Thermo Fisher Scientific GmbH, Bremen, Germany, 6 BHF Glasgow Cardiovascular Research Centre, University of Glasgow, Glasgow, United Kingdom

Abstract

Background: Today, dementias are diagnosed late in the course of disease. Future treatments have to start earlier in the disease process to avoid disability requiring new diagnostic tools. The objective of this study is to develop a new method for the differential diagnosis and identification of new biomarkers of Alzheimer's disease (AD) using capillary-electrophoresis coupled to mass-spectrometry (CE-MS) and to assess the potential of early diagnosis of AD.

Methods and Findings: Cerebrospinal fluid (CSF) of 159 out-patients of a memory-clinic at a University Hospital suffering from neurodegenerative disorders and 17 cognitively-healthy controls was used to create differential peptide pattern for dementias and prospective blinded-comparison of sensitivity and specificity for AD diagnosis against the Criterion standard in a naturalistic prospective sample of patients. Sensitivity and specificity of the new method compared to standard diagnostic procedures and identification of new putative biomarkers for AD was the main outcome measure. CE-MS was used to reliably detect 1104 low-molecular-weight peptides in CSF. Training-sets of patients with clinically secured sporadic Alzheimer's disease, frontotemporal dementia, and cognitively healthy controls allowed establishing discriminative biomarker pattern for diagnosis of AD. This pattern was already detectable in patients with mild cognitive impairment (MCI). The AD-pattern was tested in a prospective sample of patients (n = 100) and AD was diagnosed with a sensitivity of 87% and a specificity of 83%. Using CSF measurements of beta-amyloid1-42, total-tau, and phospho$_{181}$-tau, AD-diagnosis had a sensitivity of 88% and a specificity of 67% in the same sample. Sequence analysis of the discriminating biomarkers identified fragments of synaptic proteins like proSAAS, apolipoprotein J, neurosecretory protein VGF, phospholemman, and chromogranin A.

Conclusions: The method may allow early differential diagnosis of various dementias using specific peptide fingerprints and identification of incipient AD in patients suffering from MCI. Identified biomarkers facilitate face validity for the use in AD diagnosis.

Citation: Jahn H, Wittke S, Zürbig P, Raedler TJ, Arlt S, et al. (2011) Peptide Fingerprinting of Alzheimer's Disease in Cerebrospinal Fluid: Identification and Prospective Evaluation of New Synaptic Biomarkers. PLoS ONE 6(10): e26540. doi:10.1371/journal.pone.0026540

Editor: Koichi M. Iijima, Thomas Jefferson University, United States of America

Received April 19, 2011; Accepted September 28, 2011; Published October 26, 2011

Funding: This work was supported by grant No. 0313347 from the BioProfile Initiative and grant No. 01EW0909 to HJ by the German Federal Ministry of Education and Research in the frame of the ERA-NET NEURO project "ADtest: Role of proteases and their inhibitors in pathophysiology and diagnosis of Alzheimer Disease". The Memory Clinic of the Department of Psychiatry and Psychotherapy at the University Hospital Hamburg-Eppendorf is a member of the German National Dementia Competence Network. The funders had no role in study design, data collection and analysis, decision to publish, or preparation of the manuscript. HJ had full access to all of the data in the study and takes responsibility for the integrity of the data and the accuracy of the data analysis.

Competing Interests: PZ is an employee of Mosaiques Diagnostics GmbH. HM is founder and shareholder of Mosaiques Diagnostics GmbH. MK is an employee of Thermo Fisher Scientific GmbH. KW serves on the scientific advisory board of Mosaiques Diagnostics and Therapeutics AG. HJ, TJR, and SA are scientists at the Department of Psychiatry of the University of Hamburg and have nothing to declare. This does not alter the authors' adherence to all the PLoS ONE policies on sharing data and materials.

* E-mail: jahn@uke.uni-hamburg.de

[9] These authors contributed equally to this work.

Introduction

In an aging population dementias are a serious threat. Currently 30 million people worldwide suffer from Alzheimer's disease (AD) and the World Health organization projects that this number will triple over the next 20 years [1]. The cumulative incidence of AD has been estimated to rise from about 5% by age 70 to 50% by age 90 [2]. The clinical diagnosis of dementias is established late in the course of the disease process with poor sensitivity and specificity [3–5]. According to current diagnostic criteria, AD cannot be diagnosed before the disease has progressed so far that clinical dementia is present. The disease process, however, probably starts 20–30 years before first clinical signs emerge [6]. Hence we are in need of new diagnostic tools that are capable of detecting pre-clinical signs of neurodegenerative disorders. Recently different new analytical proteomic technologies like mass spectrometry coupled with protein separation or protein microarrays that can be applied on cerebrospinal fluid (CSF) have been developed to study proteins in neuroscience [7]. Due to the intimate relation between brain function and CSF composition, pathological brain-processes are more likely to be reflected in CSF than in other body-fluids (e.g. blood or urine). Since more than 70% of the CSF-proteins are isoforms of albumin, transferrin and immunoglobulines [8], and due to technical limitations only few studies have focused on the composition of proteins in CSF in the past [9]. Nonetheless an enormous wealth of information regarding pathological processes should be present in the less abundant CSF-proteins and the identification of changes in CSF composition at that level beside the current disease models would promote the understanding of the various dementias and their fundamental pathological processes. Such valid new biomarkers for AD could also serve as surrogate markers in detecting treatment effects while any earlier identification of AD patients is another goal to enable the development of treatments that stop or postpone the disease processes.

We report proteome analysis of CSF using capillary electrophoresis coupled to an electrospray ionisation time of flight mass spectrometer (CE-MS) and its potential use in the diagnosis of AD and other dementias. This approach allows the comprehensive analysis of low molecular weight peptides and protein fragments present in biological fluids in a single time-limited step. The method was already successfully applied to the examination of human urine for the differential diagnosis of renal diseases [10–13], the diagnosis of prostate or urothelial cancer [14–16], ureteropelvic junction obstruction [17], and rejection of renal transplants [18] demonstrating the broad application spectrum of this new technique that also allows the comparison of biomarker sequencing data by use of different mass spectrometer types [19]. In addition we already implemented the recommendations for studies in clinical proteomics that were recently formulated by experts in the field [20] to avoid pitfalls and circumvent methodological problems that became apparent in earlier studies in this fast developing field of science.

Methods

Ethics Statement

The study was approved by the ethics committee of the "Ärztekammer Hamburg, Germany" and all patients and/or their relatives gave written informed consent and all clinical investigations have been conducted according to the principles expressed in the Declaration of Helsinki. Furthermore, the University Hospital Hamburg-Eppendorf has carried out all investigations according to international Good Laboratory Practice (GLP) and Good Clinical Practice (GCP) standard.

Patient characteristics

Between April 2002 and December 2005 176 patients referred to the memory clinic of the University Hospital Hamburg-Eppendorf were recruited for this study. All patients underwent a diagnostic work-up and were diagnosed according to ICD-10 and the National Institute of Neurological and Communicative Disorders and the Stroke-Alzheimer's Disease and Related Disorders Association criteria (NINCDS-ADRDA) to identify patients with vascular dementia [21,22]. MCI diagnoses were made according to the criteria of Petersen [23] and FTD was diagnosed according to the Lund–Manchester criteria [24]. The structure of cognitive dysfunction was assessed with a neuropsychological test battery allowing the identification of MCI subtypes. Distinction of MCI and dementia was based on CDR rating (see **Table S3** for neuropsychological tests). Patients underwent lumbar puncture for diagnostic purposes. In a first step CSF of 17 control samples of cognitively healthy volunteers (these persons underwent a lumbar puncture in connection with a knee arthroscopy and agreed to obtain an additional cognitive testing apart from allowing to collect some CSF during peridural anaesthesia), 34 samples of patients with a clinical diagnosis of sporadic AD, 12 samples of patients with FTD and 13 samples of patients with schizophrenia (**Table 1**) was analyzed to establish disease specific peptide patterns. The clinical diagnoses of these training cases were supported by laboratory and image data from magnetic resonance imaging (MRI) and positron emission tomography (PET). The training set patients were selected to have no other major medical comorbidity. In a second step 100 patients (51 female, 49 male; mean age 65.3±12.3 years) (**Table S2**) with memory complaints were recruited for a prospective sample cohort, CSF was analysed to obtain a diagnosis and patients were clinically followed. These patients suffered from various dementias, MCI or memory complains of other causes. A few had further medical comorbidities like hypertension or diabetes type II or a history of insults or encephalitis.

Cerebrospinal fluid samples

Cerebrospinal fluid (CSF) was obtained by lumbar puncture in a sitting position according to standard procedures [25]. After collection of the 4 mL CSF for routine diagnosis, additional 5 ml of the CSF was sampled for this study into a polypropylene test tube. The CSF was centrifuged immediately after collection (1600 g, 4°C, 15 min), aliquoted into polypropylene test tubes (each aliquot, 750 µL), frozen within 30–40 min after the puncture and stored at −80°C until use. The CSF was at no time thawed/refrozen. After thawing, 700 µL of CSF were diluted with 700 µL buffer (pH 10.5; 2 M urea, 100 mmol/L NaCl, 0.0125% NH₃; Sigma-Aldrich, Taufkirchen, Germany) and ultracentrifugated using Centrisart ultrafiltration devices (cut off 20 kDa, Sartorius, Göttingen, Germany) at 4°C until 1.1 mL of filtrate was obtained.

Table 1. Demographic data of training sets.

Group	Number	Male	Female	Age [years±SD]	MMSE [mean±SD]
Controls	17	13	4	58.9±11,5	30.0±0.0
AD Training set	34	14	20	69.0±6.5	21.2±5.1
FTD Training set	12	4	8	65.6±7.9	22.4±2.5
Schizophrenia set	13	5	8	38.1±14.4	29.6±0.7

Baseline data of training sets for cognitively healthy controls and trainings sets for AD, FTD and schizophrenia. Given are numbers for gender, and the averages for age and the scores of the Mini Mental State Examination (MMSE).
doi:10.1371/journal.pone.0026540.t001

Subsequently the filtrate was applied onto a PD-10 desalting column (Amersham Bioscience, Uppsala, Sweden) equilibrated in 0.01% NH_4OH in HPLC-grade in water (Roth, Germany) to decrease matrix effects by removing urea, electrolytes, salts, and to enrich peptides present. Finally the eluate was lyophilized stored at 4°C and resuspended in 10 μL HPLC-grade water before CE-MS analysis.

Since blood contaminations may affect the proteome of CSF [26] we controlled our CSF samples for traces of haemoglobin and the presence of erythrocytes by microscopy of a centrifuged CSF sample. Using these two methods we can exclude any blood contamination of our CSF samples above 0.001% by that controlling a potential serious confounder of CSF biomarker studies with regard to proteins abundant in plasma.

Immunochemistry

The CSF levels of Aβ42, total tau, and phospho$_{181}$-tau were measured using commercial ELISAs (Innogenetics, Ghent, Belgium) according to the manufacturer's protocol. Cut-off values for AD suspicious biomarker concentrations were >540 pg/ml for total-tau, >61 pg/ml for phospho$_{181}$-tau and beta-amyloid1–42 values <240+1.18×total-tau pg/ml [4].

CE-MS

CE-MS analysis was performed as described using a P/ACE MDQ (Beckman Coulter, Fullerton, USA) system on-line coupled to a Micro-TOF MS (Bruker Daltonic, Bremen, Germany) [15–17].

Reproducibility and comparability

Analytical characteristics such as accuracy, mass accuracy, traceability and repeatability of the CE-MS application were recently described [15,27]. Thus, here we report about additional precision tests to underline the validity of the analytical data. Initially the sampling procedure was validated by fractionated extraction of six aliquots of CSF from one patient. **Figure S1** shows the protein contour plots of 4 different fractions. Classification of each fraction resulted in the same and correct classification as AD. We re-measured 10 samples twice and again all samples were classified correctly (**Table S4**). We were also able to re-puncture one patient with an AD pattern. The AD pattern was found again and stable after one year. Finally the reproducibility of the CE-MS approach is emphasized (**Figure S2**). Distinct lines (four to six) are visible in the peptide pattern due to the charge per peptide, which can be ascribed to the peptide structure (number of basic amino acids) and consequently allow the comparison of biomarker sequencing data even by use of different mass spectrometer types coupled with CE or liquid chromatography (LC) [19].

Data processing and cluster analysis

Mass spectral ion peaks representing identical molecules at different charge states were deconvoluted into single masses using MosaiquesVisu [27]. In addition the migration time and ion signal intensity (amplitude) were normalized using internal peptide standards [27,28]. The resulting peak list characterizes each peptide by its molecular mass (in Dalton), normalized CE-migration time (in minutes), and normalized signal intensity. All detected peptides were deposited, matched, and annotated in a Microsoft SQL database, allowing further analysis and comparison of multiple samples (patient groups) (**Table S5**). Peptides within different samples were considered identical if the mass deviation was less than 100 ppm and the migration time deviation was less than 1 min.

To define biomarker patterns we employed the following stringent quality control and selection criteria to avoid artefacts as well as to attain high levels in reproducibility and specificity: 1) the MS peaks list must contain 800–1400 peptides; 2) the normalized mean signal amplitude of each marker peptide must be >25 counts in one diagnostic group; 3) the frequency of occurrence (FOC) of each candidate biomarker must be >40% in one of the groups defined above; 4) the difference in the FOC between the two groups must be either >30% or, 5) if the difference in the FOC is less than 30%, the mean amplitude in one diagnostic group must be >1.4-fold higher compared to the other group and the FOC of the selected amplitude biomarker must be >70% in the diagnostic group with the higher mean amplitude.

Employing these criteria, a list of pre-defined peptides was obtained by the comparison of all available data sets (e.g. control vs. AD, FTD, schizophrenia patients, respectively) with MosaCluster software package [13]. The pre-defined set of peptides was further validated by randomly excluding 30% of available samples. This procedure was repeated 5 times to utilize markers (preliminary biomarker pattern) with consistently high discriminative value. Subsequently the preliminary biomarker patterns were refined by employing an unadjusted p-value limit of 0.01 and using one-out cross-validation to attain high sensitivity and specificity. This approach resulted in the definition of biomarker patterns consisting of 10–20 biomarkers.

Tandem sequencing

Tandem (MS/MS) sequencing was performed using Orbitrap instruments (Thermo Finnigan, Bremen, Germany). Orbitrap experiments were performed on a Dionex Ultimate 3000 nanoflow system connected to an LTQ Orbitrap hybrid mass spectrometer (Thermo Electron, Bremen, Germany) equipped with a nanoelectrospray ion source. Binding and chromatographic separation of the peptides took place on a fused silica nanocolumn (10 cm; 75-μm i.d.; C18, 5 μm; NanoSeparations, Nieuwkoop, Netherlands). The MS was operated in data-dependent mode to automatically switch between MS and MS/MS acquisition. Full scan MS spectra (from m/z 300–2000) were acquired in the Orbitrap with resolution $R = 60,000$ at m/z 400 (target value of 500,000 charges in the linear ion trap).

Statistical Analysis

To verify the diagnostic value of the potential biomarkers pre-selected by the criteria mentioned above, raw p-values (so called unadjusted p-values) were calculated using the natural logarithm transformed intensities and the Gaussian approximation to the t-distribution, both implemented as macros in the commercial statistical package SAS (SAS Institute, Cary, NC; www.sas.com). Estimates of sensitivity and specificity were calculated based on tabulating the number of correctly classified samples. The receiver operating characteristic (ROC) curve was obtained by plotting all sensitivity values (true positive fraction) on the y axis against their equivalent (1-specificity) values (false positive fraction) for all available thresholds on the x-axis (MedCalc Software, Mariakerke, Belgium, www.medcalc.be). The area under the ROC curve (AUC) was evaluated as it provides a single measure of overall accuracy that is not dependent upon a particular threshold. After the best suited biomarkers are selected disease specific biomarker patterns (model) were established and the internal sensitivity and specificity for the training set were determined by leave one-out cross-validation analysis as described [15].

Due to the difference of the mean age between the training sets for the control cohort and patients suffering on Alzheimer's disease we verified if the AD-pattern is related to age or not. For this purpose the control group was divided into two subgroups, whereas the first group consisted of controls aged 61 or younger (n = 10; mean age 54±12) and the second group of patients aged 63 or older (n = 7, mean age 65±4).

Adapting the AD-biomarker pattern to these two subgroups resulted in a misclassification rate of 43% after cross-validation. Hence the AD-biomarker pattern used in this study is not capable to discriminate between the two subgroups and therefore an age related inconsistency in the pattern is unlikely.

Results

CSF-samples were investigated using CE-MS with the aim to define a panel of disease-specific biomarkers that allow the identification and prospective diagnostic labelling of patients with various dementias, mild cognitive impairment (MCI) and their separation from healthy controls (for demographic data see **Table 1**).

Development of disease specific peptide patterns

In each sample we were able to tentatively identify >800 different peptides based on migration time and mass, with molecular weights ranging from 0.8 to 20 kDa. The data from the individual CE-MS analyses were compiled and specific biomarker patterns for AD, FTD and schizophrenia were developed with emphasis on a panel of biomarkers that should enable to detect AD-cases based solely on peptides in CSF.

Figure 1A shows the compiled data of 34 measurements of CSF from patients with sporadic Alzheimer's disease, while **Figure 1B** shows the data for the healthy controls from our training sets.

For the identification of AD specific peptides, analyses of these data with MosaCluster yielded 131 potentially biomarkers (**Table S1**), which fulfil the defined selection criteria (see Method section "Data processing and cluster analysis"). Given the number of cases and controls available, the pattern of 131 potential biomarkers was refined by statistical testing and employing an unadjusted p-value limit of 0.01, resulting in a preliminary diagnostic pattern of 35 potential biomarkers (**Table S1**, see bold marked peptides). Subsequently the preliminary pattern was iteratively refined by eliminating one potential biomarker and utilizing leave-one-out cross-validation for verification (while maintaining high sensitivity and specificity). Leave-one-out cross validation uses a single sample as the validation data and the remaining samples as the training data. Each sample is used once as the validation data, giving an indication of how well the training set will perform when it is applied on unknown samples. This approach yielded a final diagnostic pattern ("AD-pattern") based on 12 discriminatory peptides (**Figure 1C**). Utilizing support vector machines the AD-pattern allowed correct classification of 31/34 AD and 15/17 control samples, thus a sensitivity of 91% and specificity of 88%. The data including the AUC of the receiver operating characteristic (ROC) for these 12 biomarkers are shown in **Table 2** and **Figure 2**. The overall AUC for this biomarker pattern in the training set was calculated as 0.979 (95% CI: 0.893–0.997; p-value = 0.0001) pointing towards the potential of this multidimensional approach.

Subsequently this approach was also used to establish biomarker patterns for FTD (14 discriminatory peptides; data not shown) and schizophrenia (14 discriminatory peptides; data not shown). In the case that more than one disease specific pattern scores positive the use of differential diagnostic patterns is required for a final classification. Thus differential diagnostic patterns for AD versus

FTD and AD versus schizophrenia based on the disease specific biomarkers have also been established.

Blinded evaluation of prospectively collected samples

Using the defined patterns a blinded evaluation of additional prospective collected samples of 100 individuals followed. Whereas all non-AD samples in this study were used as disease controls, the blinded and prospective group consisted of samples from patients with multiple neurodegenerative disorders like MCI, vascular dementia, Parkinson's dementia, FTD, depression or other dementia syndromes. Given the need to differentiate against other forms of dementia and also other neuropsychological diseases, a hierarchical model for the classification of the blinded and prospectively collected samples was established. For this issue, in a first step the biomarker patterns for AD, FTD, and schizophrenia are applied onto the unknown sample for classification. If more than one disease-pattern scores positive differential diagnostic patterns are used for final classification. By this approach we circumvent the methodological problems of several investigations in proteomic research, which compare only two diagnostic groups [29,30].

Our method using the defined peptide pattern showed a sensitivity of 87% and a specificity of 83% for the diagnosis of AD of the prospective samples (**Table S2**). Using CSF measurements of beta-amyloid1–42, total-tau and phospho$_{181}$-tau, AD diagnosis had a sensitivity of 88% and a specificity of 67% in our clinical cohort. Interestingly, four patients diagnosed with primary progressive aphasia were classified as positive for both FTD and AD patterns.

Epidemiological studies have documented the accelerated rate of progression to dementia and AD in subjects with MCI. However, many MCI cases will never develop dementia [23]. To date there is no accepted clinical method to classify which MCI cases will progress to AD.

32 cases (17 male, 15 female; age: 66.1±6.6 years; MMSE: 27.8±1.9; values as mean ± SD) in the blinded set were originally diagnosed with MCI. After lumbar puncture the patients were clinically followed up for a mean of 57±7 months (mean ± SD; max 72, min 41 months). Twenty-one patients scored positive for the AD pattern, 11 patients scored negative for the AD pattern. The clinical outcome is shown in **Table 3**. In summary, the MCI cases with a positive AD pattern did clinically worse and showed a high conversion rate to AD. Furthermore, from 16 patients with a multi-domain or amnestic MCI, a diagnosis related to a higher risk of developing AD, 14 patients displayed a positive AD pattern in CSF. From the remaining 16 other MCI cases, only 7 patients showed a positive AD pattern. Using the Chi square test this difference is significant (p = 0.0255; p-value with continuity correction) pointing to an association of the former MCI subtypes with an AD pattern in CSF in our cohort.

Identification of biomarkers

In **Table 4** the identified peptide sequences out of the initial list of 131 potential AD biomarkers are shown: So far we identified 57 sequences deriving from 24 different protein precursors. We identified 2 fragments of amyloid beta A4 protein, 1 fragment of apolipoprotein E, 1 fragment of apolipoprotein J or clusterin, 6 fragments of amyloid-like protein 1 (APLP1), 1 fragment of amyloid-like protein 2 (APLP2), 1 fragment of collagen alpha 1(l) chain, 2 fragments of fibrinogen alpha chain, 1 fragment of complement C4-A, 1 fragment of son of sevenless homolog 2, 1 fragment of cystatin C, 1 fragment of cholecystokinin, 7 fragments of neurosecretory protein VGF, 7 fragments of proSAAS, 5 fragments of neuroendocrin protein 7B2, 7 fragments of

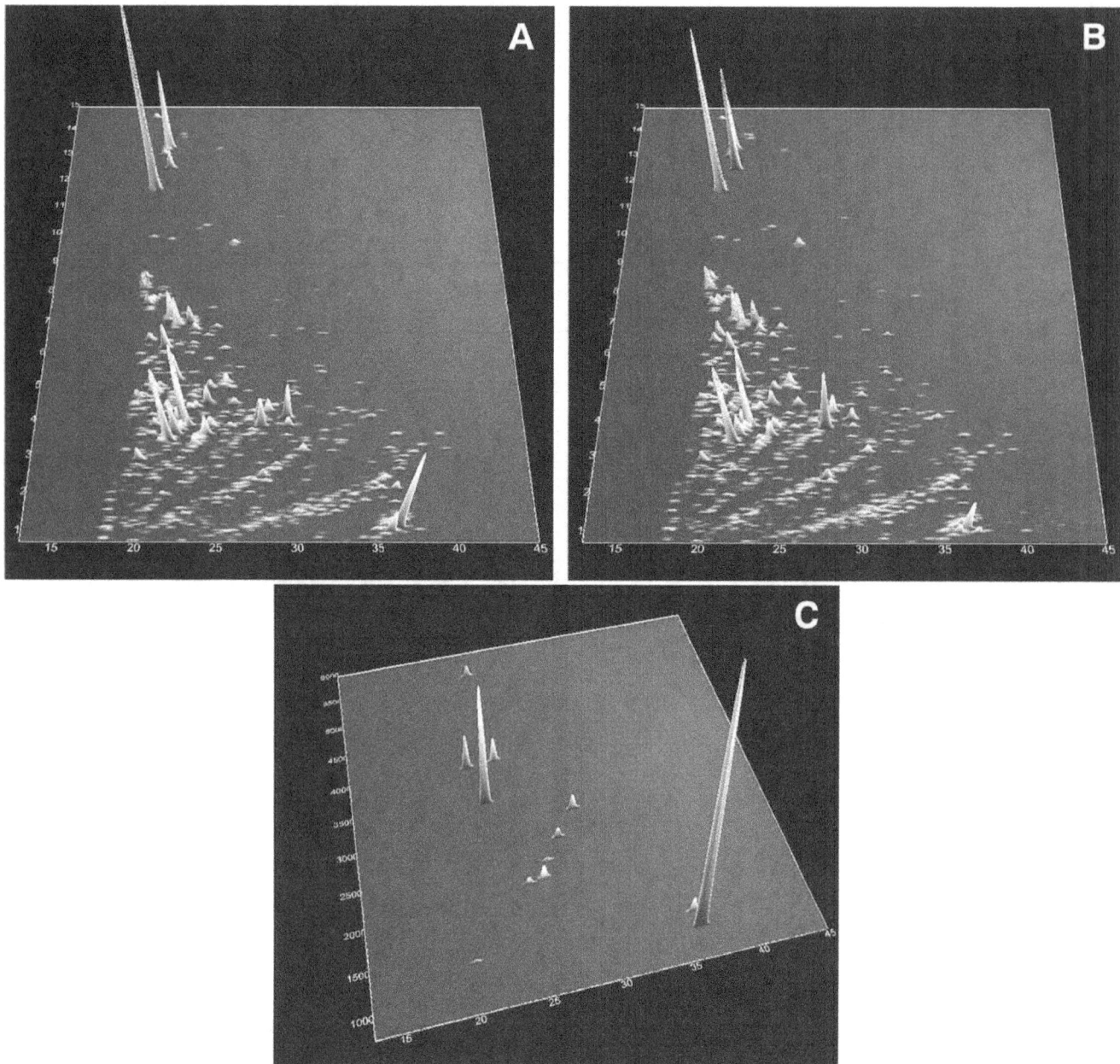

Figure 1. Contour-plots of the training set. A) Compiled 3-D protein contour plot from CSF samples of 34 patients with Alzheimer's disease. The normalized CE-migration time (in min) is plotted on the x-axis and the relative molecular mass (in kDa) on the y-axis. As a third dimension, the signal intensity is colour coded (blue lowest and white highest signal intensity). Each dot represents one peptide. **B**) Compiled 3-D protein contour plot for healthy controls (n = 17). **C**) Discriminative biomarker pattern for subjects suffering from Alzheimer's disease (n = 34). Depicted is a 3-D plot of 12 peptides that serve as specific biomarkers for AD brain damage. The normalized CE-migration time (in min) is plotted on the x-axis and the relative molecular mass (in Da) on the y-axis. As a third dimension, the signal intensity is colour coded.
doi:10.1371/journal.pone.0026540.g001

chromogranin A, 3 fragments of secretogranin I, and 1 fragment each of segretogranin II–III. We found 1 fragment of integral membrane protein 2B, 1 fragment of osteopontin, 2 fragments of testican-1, and 2 fragments of brevican core protein. Finally, we also identified 1 fragment of phospholemman (FXYD1) and FXYD6.

We have satisfactory mass spectra of all 12 AD biomarkers, which were used in the AD pattern (see **Figure S3**). However, we are not able to identify all peptides. The greater challenge of peptide identification in comparison to protein identification of classical proteomic studies is the missing availability of peptide mass fingerprint information. Sequencing is hindered by several obstacles associated with MS sequencing of naturally occurring

peptides (tryptic digests cannot be utilized because of a loss of connectivity to the original identification parameters [31]). Major obstacles are suboptimal use of proteomics search machines (like MASCOT or OMSSA) for naturally occurring peptides [32,33] as well as the chemical nature (e.g. post-translational modifications) of the peptides that prevents successful sequencing [19]. To date, sequences could be obtained from 5 of the final 12 best-of-selection of AD biomarkers with the ID 78842: AADHDVGSELPPEGVL-GALLRV, ProSAAS precursor [217–242]; ID 77519: SGELE-QEEERLSKEWEDS, chromogranin A [322–339], ID 86638: ESPKEHDPFTYDYQSLQIGGL, phospholemman (FXYD1) [21–41]; ID 102634: DQTVSDNELQEMSNQGSKYVN-KEIQNA, clusterin/apolipoprotein J [22–49]; and ID 110596:

Table 2. Peptide pattern identifying AD.

Peptide identification			Frequency by group [%]		Mean amplitude		
Protein ID	Mass [Da]	CE-time [min]	AD	Control	AD	Control	AUC
11229	1196.36	36.37	0.32	0.71	46658	49517	0.70
35146	1387.07	20.42	0.18	0.47	144	119	0.65
35998	1390.49	36.26	0.50	0.12	298	88	0.71
77519	**2179.03**	**25.31**	**0.76**	**0.35**	**85**	**32**	**0.83**
78842	**2214.22**	**26.48**	**0.85**	**0.29**	**149**	**83**	**0.84**
86638	**2423.19**	**27.03**	**0.62**	**0.18**	**48**	**47**	**0.72**
95324	2706.37	28.30	0.74	0.24	130	120	0.75
102634	**3068.46**	**30.03**	**0.76**	**0.29**	**185**	**84**	**0.81**
110596	**3401.73**	**23.48**	**1.00**	**1.00**	**2557**	**4518**	**0.82**
130889	4005.54	22.57	0.71	0.41	582	400	0.69
131863	4036.30	24.92	0.71	0.24	373	250	0.75
160599	5582.16	24.30	0.41	0	283	0	0.71

Shown are unique internal protein-IDs, mass, CE-migration time, observed frequency of occurrence, the corresponding mean amplitudes, and AUC values (as a biomarker quality measure) for the final peptide panel. Five peptides, which are marked in bold, are already identified (see **Table 4**).
doi:10.1371/journal.pone.0026540.t002

GRPEAQPPPLSSEHKEPVAGDAVPGPKDGSAPEV, neurosecretory protein VGF [26–59] (**Table 2**). Annotated mass spectra of these peptides are shown in **Figure S3**. Uniformly AD patients showed higher detection frequencies and amplitudes for most of these synaptic marker peptides in CSF that point toward alterations in vesicle maturation and transport in AD (**Table 4**). However, fragments of VGF, a peptide also found in synaptic vesicles, were detected with lower signal amplitude in AD patients.

A subset of the patient cohort (n = 61) could be screened for their apolipoprotein E (ApoE) allelic composition. About 50% carried an ApoE4 allele. The ApoE4 allele variant is a known risk factor for AD found in about 40–50% of all AD cases, while the ApoE4 allele frequency in a normal population is about 10% [34]. Although it is commonly not recommended as a screening test, a positive ApoE4 status predicts AD with a sensitivity of 80% when

clinical symptoms of a dementia are present [34]. The allelic status of 27 from 34 patients with clinical AD from our training set could be determined to investigate if the discriminative value of the AD-specific biomarkers changes in relationship to the ApoE4 status. 18 of 27 genotyped AD-patients were showing a positive ApoE4 status with at least one copy. The discriminative value of the 12 biomarkers in the final panel for AD (**Figure 2**) does not change significantly in view to a positive ApoE4 status. In contrast the N-terminal apolipoprotein E fragment ([19–32]; KVEQAVETEPE-PEL) originally included in the primary candidate list or the testican-1 fragments (**Table 4**) showed significantly better AUC values if patients carried the ApoE4 allele. We excluded affected biomarkers from the final list to avoid contamination with the already known risk factor due to the different allele frequencies in the diagnosis groups.

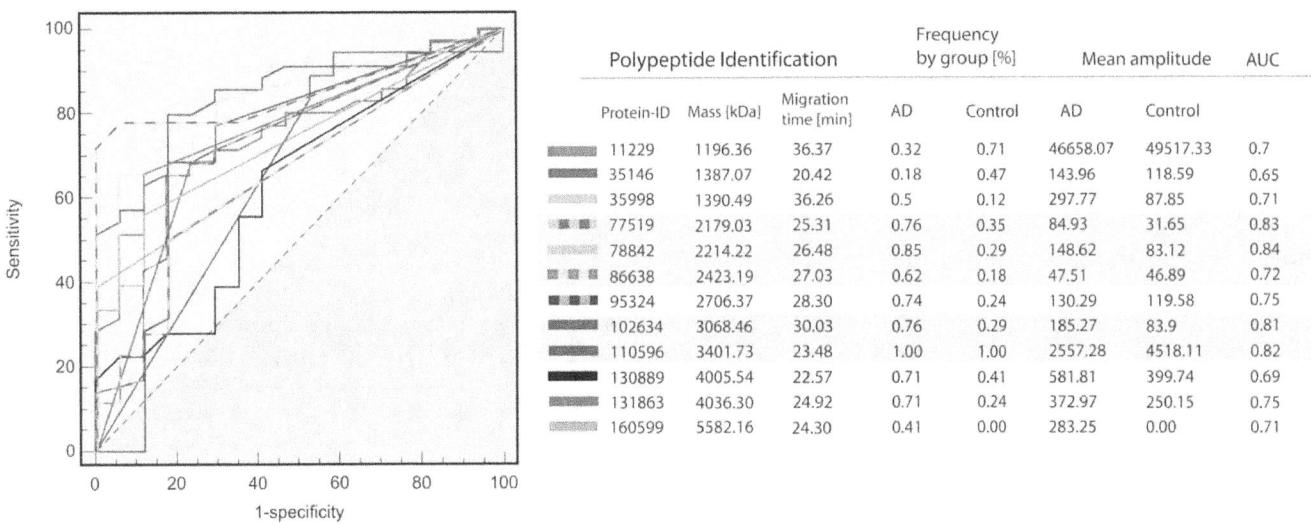

Figure 2. Peptide pattern identifying AD. Shown are the ROC analyses of all biomarkers. In the table unique internal protein-ID, mass, CE-migration time, observed frequency of occurrence, the corresponding mean amplitudes, and AUC values (as a biomarker quality measure) in the different groups for the final peptide panels. Five peptides, which are marked in yellow, are already identified (**Table 4**).
doi:10.1371/journal.pone.0026540.g002

Table 3. Clinical outcome of MCI cases by peptide pattern.

	Number	AD	OD	MCI	Remitter
Positve AD-Score	21	14	0	7	0
Negative AD-score	11	2	1	5	3

Clinical outcome of MCI cases (n = 32) followed up for a mean of 57 months. MCI cases with a positive score for the AD-pattern (n = 21) or a negative score for the AD-pattern (n = 11) according to our peptide panel. From 21 MCI patients originally identified as having a positive score for the AD pattern in CSF, only 7 patients are still clinically diagnosed with MCI, while 14 progressed into clinical AD. The other MCI group with negative score for the AD pattern showed a different outcome. Here only 2 patients progressed into AD so far, while 5 patients are still diagnosed with a stable MCI, one patient progressed into a vascular dementia (other dementia, OD), and 3 patients developed a complete remission of cognitive symptoms.
doi:10.1371/journal.pone.0026540.t003

Discussion

The urgent need of earlier and more precise diagnosis arises with the advent of first treatments [3]. Current treatments of AD may in some cases reduce disease progression, but certainly do not reverse the disease process. In addition, cholinesterase inhibitors or glutamate antagonists are currently applied to only a small fraction of patients [35].

The study focused on the analysis of proteins/peptides in CSF obtained from patients presenting to a memory clinic and suffering from various dementias. CE-MS does not require specific antibodies or specific knowledge about the peptides (e.g. solubility, binding or modifications) and yields a comprehensive display of the peptide populations present in CSF without being subject to selection-biases inherent to alternative proteomic methods like matrix-assisted techniques. The high sensitivity (detection limit in the low fmol to amol range) and reproducibility of the CE-MS technology enables the reliable analysis of >800 different peptides in CSF with molecular weights ranging from 0.8 kDa to about 20 kDa.

Disease specific peptide pattern

From the vast pool of peptides present in CSF, specific biomarkers and subsequent diagnostic models for AD and FTD could be established. The availability of proteome data from patient samples with clear clinical diagnoses enabled the definition of peptides that apparently allow the differentiation of dementias from healthy controls and the differentiation between dementias like AD and FTD in the blinded dataset with high sensitivity and specificity. The MCI data indicate that CE-MS can be utilized to identify incipient AD cases in MCI. Hence this approach may be used for stratification of patients in therapeutic intervention trials. Currently, clinical MCI trials of antidementiva are impaired due to low conversion rates and the inclusion of many patients that will not develop AD in the clinical course. In consequence many MCI trials fail or long term follow up of large patient cohorts are required to reach an acceptable statistical power, making such trials expensive and difficult in design [36].

As expected from earlier attempts to define biomarkers for AD [3,37,38], and as evident from the AUC values shown in **Table 2**, single biomarkers are often of limited diagnostic value. However, the classification model based on a combination of distinct and clearly defined single biomarkers shows a high discriminatory value that cannot be reached when using single biomarkers alone. Already our first attempt to use peptide patterns for diagnostic purposes in a prospective natural clinical sample yielded sensitivity

and specificity for AD diagnosis in the range that established methods like the measurement of T-tau, P-tau181, and beta-amyloid1–42 can reach only when combined. Fully developed, the new method should show its strength especially in the differential diagnosis of unclear cases. Having the potential to gather the information included in a multitude of peptides instead of detecting a single marker only, valuable and limited CSF samples can be analyzed more efficient and in-depth. This is in line with other studies, where e.g. levels of CSF beta-amyloid1–42 were lower in AD patients and levels of CSF tau were elevated in AD patients [39] and only the combination of these biomarkers allowed the detection and differentiation of AD from healthy controls with a sensitivity and specificity of greater than 80%. To date, the specificity to differentiate AD from other dementias especially in naturalistic samples, like in our prospective sample, is often considerably lower [3,4]. Similar approaches like the combination of classical AD markers were recently reported with the aim to identify incipient AD cases in patients suffering from MCI [38] or to predict cognitive decline in nondemented older adults [40]. In addition, Hansson et al. described that concentrations of T-tau, P-tau181, and beta-amyloid1–42 in CSF are associated with future development of AD in patients with MCI [41]. The application of CE-MS allowed the definition of a broader array of yet partially unknown biomarkers, which may have the potential of a more refined and earlier detection of the onset of AD. Interestingly our data also indicate an overlap in FTD and AD pathology especially in patients with primary progressive aphasia, which is line with recent observations made in brain biopsies [42]. This finding could have direct therapeutic impact. While there is currently no treatment option for FTD patients, the presence of AD pathology in this FTD subtype could justify the use of the available AD treatments.

A related approach using several unspecific blood plasma markers for inflammation and apoptosis processes in an ELISA array to identify AD claimed worldwide attention [43], but failed to work [44].

Identification of new AD-biomarkers using CE-MS

To date, we were able to sequence 279 from the 1104 reliable measured peptides and identified 57 peptides of the primary list of 131 potential AD-biomarkers (**Table 4**) present in cerebrospinal fluid of AD patients. The prevalence of sequences among these potential AD markers related to bioactive peptides derived from prohormones normally stored in neuronal dense-core vesicles is striking. In general, AD patients show higher detection frequencies and amplitudes for these synaptic marker peptides in CSF that could point toward alterations in vesicle maturation and transport in AD.

Cognitive decline in dementias is due to loss of synapses or synaptic functionality meaning loss of neurones, loss of synapses on still functioning neurones, or loss of function on still available synapses. Therefore biomarkers of synaptic function and/or damage or complementary changes in the brain, e.g. immunological responses or cellular stress may be especially suited as AD biomarkers with face validity [45]. Our method identified a set of AD biomarkers that are of synaptic origin: Long known suspects like chromogranin A [37] and some newer like neurosecretory protein VGF (VGF), clusterin (apolipoprotein J), ProSAAS, testican-1, and neuroendocrine protein 7B2. We also found fragments of proteins well known to be associated with AD like the amyloid beta peptides, one fragment of beta-amyloid1–42 and one fragment of a soluble form of APP, one fragment of APLP2 and apolipoprotein E [6,32]. Maybe most interestingly, we found 6 APLP1-derived 'A-beta-like peptide' species [46] among them

Table 4. Sequence analysis.

Pr ID	Mass [Da]	CE-time [min]	Sequence	Protein name	start	stop	calc. mass [Da]
2065	1013.43	25.18	FMSDTREE	Secretogranin-1	430	437	1013.4124
3251	1083.55	25.61	FENKFAVET	Integral membrane protein 2B	254	262	1083.5237
7029	1158.62	27.02	EDVGSNKGAIIG	Amyloid beta A4 protein	693	704	1158.5881
9404	1183.66	27.49	DPPAIPPRQPP	Son of sevenless homolog 2	1171	1181	1183.6350
9730	1186.56	27.21	HELDSASSEVN	Osteopontin	273	287	1186.5102
17258	1250.61	27.59	DHDVGSELPPEG	ProSAAS	223	234	1250.5415
19245	1265.63	27.22	SpGPDGKTGPpGPA	Collagen alpha-1(I) chain	546	559	1265.5888
24081	1300.67	29.70	DELAPAGTGVSRE	Amyloid-like protein 1	568	580	1300.6259
24573	1306.74	22.16	VSPAAGSSPGKPPR	Cystatin C	21	34	1306.6993
30960	1349.67	28.25	SGEGDFLAEGGGVR	Fibrinogen alpha chain	22	35	1349.6212
37415	1404.73	29.49	HDVGSELPPEGVLG	ProSAAS	224	237	1404.6885
41974	1448.69	29.41	EAVEEPSSKDVME	Chromogranin-A	119	131	1448.6341
44123	1475.77	30.05	HDVGSELPPEGVLGA	ProSAAS	224	238	1475.7256
45572	1499.74	29.89	LDDLQPWHSFGAD	Amyloid beta A4 protein	615	627	1499.6681
45788	1500.71	22.99	SVPHFSDEDKDPE	Neuroendocrine protein 7B2	200	212	1500.6369
47143	1519.76	31.87	DHDVGSELPPEGVLG	ProSAAS	223	237	1519.7155
48140	1535.74	30.00	ADSGEGDFLAEGGGVR	Fibrinogen alpha chain	20	35	1535.6852
49413	1552.61	30.78	VTEDDEDEDDDKE	Testican-1	420	432	1552.5537
51940	1596.83	30.32	KVEQAVETEPEPEL	Apolipoprotein E	19	32	1596.7883
53060	1614.84	31.54	DELAPAGTGVSREAVSG	Amyloid-like protein 1	568	584	1614.7849
58375	1727.92	32.13	DELAPAGTGVSREAVSGL	Amyloid-like protein 1	568	585	1727.8690
60472	1771.97	30.02	SVNPYLQGQRLDNVVA	Neuroendocrine protein 7B2	182	197	1771.9217
62126	1816.98	33.53	DHDVGSELPPEGVLGALL	ProSAAS	219	240	1816.9207
62500	1820.06	32.23	DVGSELPPEGVLGALLRV	ProSAAS	221	242	1820.0044
64448	1867.72	33.07	AVTEDDEDEDDDKEDE	Testican-1	419	434	1867.6603
64930	1873.00	21.26	ALHPEEDPEGRQGRLLG	Brevican core protein	879	895	1872.9442
66400	1900.07	24.19	SVNPYLQGQRLDNVVAK	Neuroendocrine protein 7B2	182	198	1900.0167
66858	1907.99	21.60	ADPAGSGLQRAEEAPRRQ	Cholecystokinin	26	43	1907.9562
67973	1927.02	21.00	VAKKSVPHFSDEDKDPE	Neuroendocrine protein 7B2	196	212	1926.9323
71613	2028.17	21.62	SVNPYLQGQRLDNVVAKK	Neuroendocrine protein 7B2	182	199	2028.1116
71707	2029.13	20.15	ALHPEEDPEGRQGRLLGR	Brevican core protein	879	896	2029.0453
72233	2041.99	32.56	ELSAERPLNEQIAEAEED	Secretogranin-3	35	52	2041.9440
74137	2085.12	33.75	DELAPAGTGVSREAVSGLLIM	Amyloid-like protein 1	568	588	2085.0776
75685	2128.97	26.03	EGQEEEEDNRDSSMKLSF	Chromogranin-A	359	376	2128.8855
77519	**2179.03**	**25.31**	**SGELEQEEERLSKEWEDS**	**Chromogranin-A**	**322**	**339**	**2178.9553**
78842	**2214.22**	**26.48**	**AADHDVGSELPPEGVLGALLRV**	**ProSAAS**	**217**	**242**	**2214.1644**
79150	2222.16	26.60	STKLHLPADDVVSIIEEVEE	Neurosecretory protein VGF	459	478	2222.1318
84897	2377.25	28.07	DDPDAPLQPVTPLQLFEGRRN	Complement C4-A	1429	1449	2377.2026
86638	**2423.19**	**27.03**	**ESPKEHDPFTYDYQSLQIGGL**	**Phospholemman**	**21**	**41**	**2423.1281**
86817	2428.11	27.16	SSQGGSLPSEEKGHPQEESEESN	Secretogranin-1	293	315	2428.0262
88199	2471.30	35.56	DELAPAGTGVSREAVSGLLIMGAGGGS	Amyloid-like protein 1	568	593	2471.2326
88418	2475.21	27.09	HSGFEDELSEVLENQSSQAELK	Chromogranin-A	97	118	2475.1401
90848	2549.29	27.66	VGGLEEERESVGPLREDFSLSSSA	Amyloid-like protein 2	671	694	2549.2244
91583	2584.37	35.60	DELAPAGTGVSREAVSGLLIMGAGGGSL	Amyloid-like protein 1	568	595	2584.3167
94378	2684.32	21.38	SAAEKEKEMDPFHYDYQTLRIGG	FXYD6	19	41	2684.2541
102634	**3068.46**	**30.03**	**DQTVSDNELQEMSNQGSKYVNKEIQNA**	**Clusterin**	**22**	**49**	**3068.3993**
104636	3173.68	22.95	GRPEAQPPPLSSEHKEPVAGDAVPGPKDGSAP	Neurosecretory protein VGF	26	57	3173.5742
108011	3302.68	23.31	GRPEAQPPPLSSEHKEPVAGDAVPGPKDGSAPE	Neurosecretory protein VGF	26	58	3302.6044

Table 4. Cont.

Pr ID	Mass [Da]	CE-time [min]	Sequence	Protein name	start	stop	calc. mass [Da]
110596	**3401.73**	**23.48**	**GRPEAQPPPLSSEHKEPVAGDAVPGPKDGSAPEV**	**Neurosecretory protein VGF**	**26**	**59**	**3401.6852**
115988	3595.77	23.89	PPGRPEAQPPPLSSEHKEPVAGDAVPGPKDGSAPEV	Neurosecretory protein VGF	24	59	3595.7907
116478	3614.82	22.01	GRPEAQPPPLSSEHKEPVAGDAVPGPKDGSAPEVRG	Neurosecretory protein VGF	26	61	3614.8077
119503	3685.86	22.21	GRPEAQPPPLSSEHKEPVAGDAVPGPKDGSAPEVRGA	Neurosecretory protein VGF	26	62	3685.8449
121774	3768.77	31.84	SGFEDELSEVLENQSSQAELKEAVEEPSSKDVME	Chromogranin-A	98	131	3768.7048
122653	3792.76	27.25	HSGFEDELSEVLENQSSQAELKEAVEEPSSKDVm	Chromogranin-A	97	130	3792.7160
126695	3921.82	27.74	HSGFEDELSEVLENQSSQAELKEAVEEPSSKDVmE	Chromogranin-A	97	131	3921.7586
139272	4319.85	23.64	DPADASEAHESSSRGEAGAPGEEDIQGPTKADTEKWAEGGGHS	Secretogranin-1	88	130	4319.8711
140319	4349.06	28.17	VPGQGSSEDDLQEEEQIEQAIKEHLNQGSSQETDKLAPVS	Secretogranin-2	527	566	4349.0419

Identified sequences of 57 out of the initial set of 131 putative AD biomarkers are listed. Shown are unique internal protein ID (Pr ID), molecular mass (in Dalton), CE-migration time (in minutes), sequence, originating protein name, and calculated mass (in Dalton). Peptides that are utilized in the final AD pattern are highlighted in bold letters.
doi:10.1371/journal.pone.0026540.t004

APL1β28, as putative AD biomarkers with our approach. This non-amyloidogenic peptide fragment is proposed to be a CSF surrogate marker of beta-amyloid production [47,48] and we also identify them as potential AD biomarkers using a different methodology.

So far we were able to identify 5 biomarkers of our diagnostic AD panel of 12 peptides used in this study:

A fragment of neurosecretory protein VGF was identified. For VGF a role in the regulation of energy balance is currently discussed and knockout mice are thin and hypermetabolic [49]. One may speculate whether there is a connection with the heavy weight losses observed in some AD patients. Furthermore, other proteomic approaches have also found decreased VGF as potential biomarker in CSF of AD patients [9].

Phospholemman (FXYD1) is a 72-residue protein, which is expressed in the CNS, e. g. in the choroid plexus and cerebellum. It is a homolog of the Na+/,K+-ATPase γ subunit (FXYD2), a small accessory protein that modulates ATPase activity. It forms ion channels selective for K+, Cl−, and taurine in lipid bilayers and colocalizes with the Na+/K+-ATPase and the Na+/Ca2+-exchanger, which may suggest a role in the regulation of cell volume [50,51]. Na+/K+-ATPase activity might be altered by amyloid in AD [52]. Interestingly, we also found a fragment of FXYD6 (Phosphohippolin).

Clusterin (also called apolipoprotein J) is a secreted glycoprotein. In the central nervous system, clusterin expression is elevated in neuropathological conditions such as AD, where it is found associated with amyloid-beta (Aβ) plaques. Clusterin also coprecipitates with Aβ from CSF, suggesting a physiological interaction with Aβ and can be found in Lewy Bodies [53]. A recent study using an ELISA found that clusterin is significantly increased in cerebrospinal fluid from Alzheimer patients, but concluded that due to individual overlap between the two groups cerebrospinal fluid clusterin measurement is not suitable as a biochemical marker in the diagnosis of AD [54]. With an AUC value of 0.81 derived from the ROC curve our findings suggest that maybe depending from the technique used clusterin fragments might be useful as AD marker. Two recent studies using 2D gel electrophoresis also found increased levels of clusterin in patients with AD [55,56]. A genome wide association study also identified clusterin as a risk gen for AD [57].

Chromogranin A, a prohormone that is a major ingredient of large dense core vesicles in neurones, is proteolytically processed into low molecular weight peptides in neurons prior to axonal transport and released into the synaptic cleft where they may act as neurotransmitters. Up-regulation of chromogranin A was reported in AD, it is found in beta-amyloid plaques in AD brain biopsies [58,59] and was proposed to be a marker for synaptic degeneration [37]. Chromogranins are soluble glycophosphoproteins capable of activating microglial cells and metabotropic glutamate receptors [60]. Chromogranin A might synergistically enhance with beta-amyloid peptides the microglial neurotoxic effect and diminish microglial phagocytic activity in senile plaques [61]. Chromogranin A was recently discovered to bind to mutant superoxid dismutase activity in amyotrophic lateral sclerosis increasing neurotoxicity [62]. Furthermore, chromogranin A fragments may be therefore stimulators of senile plaque development and neuronal toxicity and their concentration changes during AD-treatments could be used as surrogate markers. Compared to initial findings [37] chromogranin A fragments maybe contain more information about the disease process than the intact prohormone and may yield better AD biomarkers. Interestingly, beside 7 chromogranin A fragments, we also found fragments of secretogranin I–III.

Proprotein convertase subtilisin/kexin type 1 inhibitor (pro-SAAS) a recently discovered prohormone is found in synaptic vesicles [63]. N-terminal proSAAS fragments are found in the Tau inclusion bodies of Pick disease and other tauopathies [64,65]. ProSAAS is distributed abundantly in neuroendocrine tissues like pituitary and hypothalamus and other brain regions and is co-localised with prohormone convertase 1 (PC-1). The C-terminal fragments are potent inhibitors of PC-1 belonging to a family of calcium-dependent serin proteases, the major endoproteolytic processing enzymes of the secretory pathway which are responsible for the proteolytic cleavage of a wide variety of peptide precursors including proinsulin [63,66]. Endogenous binding and inhibiting proteins for PC-1 and PC-2 have been identified as proSAAS and neuroendocrine peptide 7B2, respectively. A recent study using the iTRAQ technique identified proSAAS and chromogranin A fragments as putative AD markers [67]. ProSAAS was also identified as potential AD marker in the study of Finehout and colleagues [55]. So far we identified 7 fragments of proSAAS to be putative AD biomarkers in our approach.

Most interestingly some of the identified potential AD markers like testican-1 and proSAAS are inhibitors of proteases or like neuroendocrine protein 7B2 are required for the function of prohormone convertases. Recent research has demonstrated the critical importance of such protease inhibitors and their neuro-proteases for the regulation of specific peptide neurotransmitters and for the production of toxic peptides in major neurodegenerative diseases like AD [68]. Several of the identified biomarkers are involved in vesicular transport and processing of synaptic neuropeptides. A disturbance in maturation and degradation processes of synaptic neuropeptides may be one reason for the cognitive malfunction and subsequent neuronal loss. One may speculate whether abnormal proteolysis caused by enhanced protease inhibitor activities due to the synaptic peptides identified in this study in AD patients might play a role in cognitive impairment and AD pathology well before tangle and plaque formation occur [69]. Hence, proteases like prohormone convertases could become new drug targets in the development of AD treatments. That we do not only identify new biomarkers but also established markers of AD like fragments of amyloid-beta peptides or currently discussed AD-markers like the APLP1 fragments points to the validity and high potential of our method. A limitation of our study is surely the lack of any neuropathological confirmation of our clinical diagnoses that could help to improve the specificity and sensitivity of our pure clinical approach. When fully developed and validated, this powerful new technique, CE-MS, may be especially suited to monitor drug effects on a synaptic level. To date the method already allows the early diagnosis of AD and differential diagnosis of other dementias showing promising practical advantages in respect to current diagnostic approaches like e. g. ELISAs and PET. New analytical proteomic technologies like ours are now becoming mature and can be applied to clinical problems in dementia research like diagnostic and therapeutic biomarker discovery as more and more studies prove [7,43,55,67].

Supporting Information

Figure S1   Reproducibility of the CE-MS measurements. Protein contour plots of 4 CSF-samples obtained by fractionated extraction of six aliquots of cerebrospinal fluid from one patient. The molecular mass (in kDa, logarithmic scale) on the y-axis is plotted against CE-migration time (in min) on the x-axis. (TIFF)

Figure S2   Comparability of the CE-MS measurements. (**A**) Contour plot of the entire cerebrospinal fluid proteome. The molecular mass (in kDa, logarithmic scale) on the y-axis is plotted against CE-migration time (in min) on the x-axis. The arrangement of the peptides in distinct lines is obvious. (**B**) Contour plot of 279 identified peptides. The lines already observed in (**A**) could be comprehended as a result of the number of positive charges z (at pH 2). (**C**) By means of several examples for determined peptide sequences the correlation between the effective netto-charge, molecular mass and the CE-migration time is demonstrated. Basic amino acids are colored in red. (TIFF)

Figure S3   Tandem mass spectra of the AD biomarkers. The mass spectra of all 12 AD biomarkers (see Protein ID) are shown in the following figures. Spectra of the identified peptides

are annotated with fragment assignments from the OMSSA (Open Mass Spectrometry Search Algorithm; http://pubchem.ncbi.nlm.nih.gov/omssa) searches. The corresponding sequence is displayed above each spectrum. Identified b-ions are marked in blue and y-ions in red color. (PDF)

Table S1   AD marker list. Initial set of 131 putative AD biomarkers present with high frequency in CSF of AD are listed. Shown are unique internal protein ID, molecular mass (in Dalton), CE-migration time (in minutes), observed frequency of occurrence and the corresponding mean amplitudes in AD and controls, and unadjusted p-values. Peptides that have an unadjusted p-value limit of 0.01 are highlighted in bold letters. (XLS)

Table S2   Prospective sample data. Patients (n = 100): Final diagnoses (clinical outcome) before unblinding: AD (52), still MCI (14), mixed dementia (6), vascular dementia (5), FTD (6), depression (6), schizophrenia (3), delusional disorder (1), encephalitis (2), Parkinson dementia (2), alcohol psychosis (1), amyotropic lateral sclerosis (1), Chorea Huntington (1). Scores: cut-off for AD>0, FTD>−0.1, schizophrenia>0.1. Row AD-MS and AD-IM contains the values for AD diagnosis for mass spectrometry and immunochemistry: tp, true positiv; tn, true negative, fp, false positive, fn, false negative for diagnosis AD. File further includes data for gender, age, diagnoses for the prospective patient sample, scores for peptide patterns and the values for the biomarker total tau, phospho$_{181}$-tau, and beta-amyloid1–42 if available. (XLS)

Table S3   Neuropsychological tests used to classify MCI according to Petersen et al. [70] and dementia cases. Mini-Mental State Examination (MMSE) [71], Clinical Dementia Rating (CDR) [72], CERAD test battery [73], WMS-R Logical Memory [74], Trail Making Test (TMT) [75], and Clock Drawing Test (CDT) [76]. (XLS)

Table S4   Precision data examples. Precision study for ten cerebrospinal fluid samples which are measured twice. (XLS)

Table S5   CE-MS raw data of the 176 samples used in the study. Only data that were actually utilized (that are present in at least 40% of the samples of one of the diagnostic groups, see section "Methods") are shown. The protein IDs of all peptides are given in the first column named "protein ID", the unique sample IDs constitute the first row. The MS data from each sample are reflected in one column. The number in each cell represents the normalized signal intensity of the mass spectrometric signal of each peptide detected in the sample. (XLS)

Author Contributions

Conceived and designed the experiments: HJ HM KW. Performed the experiments: HJ SW. Analyzed the data: HJ SW PZ. Contributed reagents/materials/analysis tools: HM MK HJ ME SA. Wrote the paper: HJ SW PZ. Enrolled patients: HJ TJR SA ME. Performed the sequence analysis: MK WM PZ. Performed statistical analysis: PZ HJ.

References

1. Wimo A, Jonsson L, Winblad B (2006) An estimate of the worldwide prevalence and direct costs of dementia in 2003. Dement Geriatr Cogn Disord 21: 175–181.

2. Hebert LE, Scherr PA, Beckett LA, Albert MS, Pilgrim DM, et al. (1995) Age-specific incidence of Alzheimer's disease in a community population. JAMA 273: 1354–1359.

3. Blennow K, de Leon MJ, Zetterberg H (2006) Alzheimer's disease. Lancet 368: 387–403.
4. Hulstaert F, Blennow K, Ivanoiu A, Schoonderwaldt HC, Riemenschneider M, et al. (1999) Improved discrimination of AD patients using beta-amyloid(1–42) and tau levels in CSF. Neurology 52: 1555–1562.
5. Mayeux R (1998) Evaluation and use of diagnostic tests in Alzheimer's disease. Neurobiol Aging 19: 139–143.
6. Davies L, Wolska B, Hilbich C, Multhaup G, Martins R, et al. (1988) A4 amyloid protein deposition and the diagnosis of Alzheimer's disease: prevalence in aged brains determined by immunocytochemistry compared with conventional neuropathologic techniques. Neurology 38: 1688–1693.
7. Choudhary J, Grant SG (2004) Proteomics in postgenomic neuroscience: the end of the beginning. Nat Neurosci 7: 440–445.
8. Bergquist J, Palmblad M, Wetterhall M, Hakansson P, Markides KE (2002) Peptide mapping of proteins in human body fluids using electrospray ionization Fourier transform ion cyclotron resonance mass spectrometry. Mass Spectrom Rev 21: 2–15.
9. Carrette O, Demalte I, Scherl A, Yalkinoglu O, Corthals G, et al. (2003) A panel of cerebrospinal fluid potential biomarkers for the diagnosis of Alzheimer's disease. Proteomics 3: 1486–1494.
10. Haubitz M, Wittke S, Weissinger EM, Walden M, Rupprecht HD, et al. (2005) Urine protein patterns can serve as diagnostic tools in patients with IgA nephropathy. Kidney Int 67: 2313–2320.
11. Haubitz M, Good DM, Woywodt A, Haller H, Rupprecht H, et al. (2009) Identification and validation of urinary biomarkers for differential diagnosis and dvaluation of therapeutic intervention in ANCA associated vasculitis. Mol Cell Proteomics 8: 2296–2307.
12. Rossing K, Mischak H, Dakna M, Zürbig P, Novak J, et al. (2008) Urinary proteomics in diabetes and CKD. J Am Soc Nephrol 19: 1283–1290.
13. Weissinger EM, Wittke S, Kaiser T, Haller H, Bartel S, et al. (2004) Proteomic patterns established with capillary electrophoresis and mass spectrometry for diagnostic purposes. Kidney Int 65: 2426–2434.
14. Schiffer E, Vlahou A, Petrolekas A, Stravodimos K, Tauber R, et al. (2009) Prediction of muscle-invasive bladder cancer using urinary proteomics. Clin Cancer Res 15: 4935–4943.
15. Theodorescu D, Wittke S, Ross MM, Walden M, Conaway M, et al. (2006) Discovery and validation of new protein biomarkers for urothelial cancer: a prospective analysis. Lancet Oncol 7: 230–240.
16. Theodorescu D, Schiffer E, Bauer HW, Douwes F, Eichhorn F, et al. (2008) Discovery and validation of urinary biomarkers for prostate cancer. Proteomics Clin Appl 2: 556–570.
17. Decramer S, Wittke S, Mischak H, Zürbig P, Walden M, et al. (2006) Predicting the clinical outcome of congenital unilateral ureteropelvic junction obstruction in newborn by urinary proteome analysis. Nat Med 12: 398–400.
18. Metzger J, Chatzikyrkou C, Broecker V, Schiffer E, Jäntsch L, et al. (2011) Diagnosis of subclinical and clinical acute T-cell mediated rejection in renal transplant patients by urinary proteome analysis. Proteomics Clin Appl;in press.
19. Zürbig P, Renfrow MB, Schiffer E, Novak J, Walden M, et al. (2006) Biomarker discovery by CE-MS enables sequence analysis via MS/MS with platform-independent separation. Electrophoresis 27: 2111–2125.
20. Mischak H, Apweiler R, Banks RE, Conaway M, Coon JJ, et al. (2007) Clinical Proteomics: a need to define the field and to begin to set adequate standards. Proteomics Clin Appl 1: 148–156.
21. WHO (2004) International Statistical Classification of diseases and Heathly Related Problems (The) ICD-10. WHO, Geneva.
22. McKhann G, Drachman D, Folstein M, Katzman R, Price D, et al. (1984) Clinical diagnosis of Alzheimer's disease: report of the NINCDS-ADRDA Work Group under the auspices of Department of Health and Human Services Task Force on Alzheimer's Disease. Neurology 34: 939–944.
23. Petersen RC (2004) Mild cognitive impairment as a diagnostic entity. J Intern Med 256: 183–194.
24. The Lund and Manchester Groups (1994) Clinical and neuropathological criteria for frontotemporal dementia. The Lund and Manchester Groups. J Neurol Neurosurg Psychiatry 57: 416–418.
25. Lewczuk P, Kornhuber J, Wiltfang J (2006) The German Competence Net Dementias: standard operating procedures for the neurochemical dementia diagnostics. J Neural Transm 113: 1075–1080.
26. You JS, Gelfanova V, Knierman MD, Witzmann FA, Wang M, et al. (2005) The impact of blood contamination on the proteome of cerebrospinal fluid. Proteomics 5: 290–296.
27. Good DM, Zürbig P, Argiles A, Bauer HW, Behrens G, et al. (2010) Naturally occurring human urinary peptides for use in diagnosis of chronic kidney disease. Mol Cell Proteomics 9: 2424–2437.
28. Jantos-Siwy J, Schiffer E, Brand K, Schumann G, Rossing K, et al. (2009) Quantitative Urinary Proteome Analysis for Biomarker Evaluation in Chronic Kidney Disease. J Proteome Res 8: 268–281.
29. Check E (2004) Proteomics and cancer: Running before we can walk. Nature 429: 496–497.
30. Petricoin EF, Ardekani AM, Hitt BA, Levine PJ, Fusaro VA, et al. (2002) Use of proteomic patterns in serum to identify ovarian cancer. Lancet 359: 572–577.
31. Chalmers MJ, Mackay CL, Hendrickson CL, Wittke S, Walden M, et al. (2005) Combined top-down and bottom-up mass spectrometric approach to characterization of biomarkers for renal disease. Anal Chem 77: 7163–7171.
32. Fliser D, Novak J, Thongboonkerd V, Argiles A, Jankowski V, et al. (2007) Advances in urinary proteome analysis and biomarker discovery. J Am Soc Nephrol 18: 1057–1071.
33. Mischak H, Julian BA, Novak J (2007) High-resolution proteome/peptidome analysis of peptides and low-molecular-weight proteins in urine. Proteomics Clin Appl 1: 792–804.
34. Mulder C, Scheltens P, Visser JJ, Van Kamp GJ, Schutgens RB (2000) Genetic and biochemical markers for Alzheimer's disease: recent developments. Ann Clin Biochem 37(Pt 5): 593–607.
35. Bullock R (2002) New drugs for Alzheimer's disease and other dementias. Br J Psychiatry 180: 135–139.
36. Jelic V, Kivipelto M, Winblad B (2006) Clinical trials in mild cognitive impairment: lessons for the future. J Neurol Neurosurg Psychiatry 77: 429–438.
37. Blennow K, Davidsson P, Wallin A, Ekman R (1995) Chromogranin A in cerebrospinal fluid: a biochemical marker for synaptic degeneration in Alzheimer's disease? Dementia 6: 306–311.
38. Borroni B, Di LM, Padovani A (2006) Predicting Alzheimer dementia in mild cognitive impairment patients. Are biomarkers useful? Eur J Pharmacol 545: 73–80.
39. Sunderland T, Linker G, Mirza N, Putnam KT, Friedman DL, et al. (2003) Decreased beta-amyloid1-42 and increased tau levels in cerebrospinal fluid of patients with Alzheimer disease. JAMA 289: 2094–2103.
40. Fagan AM, Roe CM, Xiong C, Mintun MA, Morris JC, et al. (2007) Cerebrospinal fluid tau/beta-amyloid(42) ratio as a prediction of cognitive decline in nondemented older adults. Arch Neurol 64: 343–349.
41. Hansson O, Zetterberg H, Buchhave P, Londos E, Blennow K, et al. (2006) Association between CSF biomarkers and incipient Alzheimer's disease in patients with mild cognitive impairment: a follow-up study. Lancet Neurol 5: 228–234.
42. Knibb JA, Xuereb JH, Patterson K, Hodges JR (2006) Clinical and pathological characterization of progressive aphasia. Ann Neurol 59: 156–165.
43. Ray S, Britschgi M, Herbert C, Takeda-Uchimura Y, Boxer A, et al. (2007) Classification and prediction of clinical Alzheimer's diagnosis based on plasma signaling proteins. Nat Med.
44. Soares HD, Chen Y, Sabbagh M, Roher A, Schrijvers E, et al. (2009) Identifying early markers of Alzheimer's disease using quantitative multiplex proteomic immunoassay panels. Ann N Y Acad Sci 1180: 56–67.
45. Wiltfang J, Lewczuk P, Riederer P, Grunblatt E, Hock C, et al. (2005) Consensus paper of the WFSBP Task Force on Biological Markers of Dementia: the role of CSF and blood analysis in the early and differential diagnosis of dementia. World J Biol Psychiatry 6: 69–84.
46. Bayer TA, Cappai R, Masters CL, Beyreuther K, Multhaup G (1999) It all sticks together–the APP-related family of proteins and Alzheimer's disease. Mol Psychiatry 4: 524–528.
47. Okochi M, Tagami S, Takeda M (2010) Analysis of APL1beta28, a surrogate marker for Alzheimer Abeta42, indicates altered precision of gamma-cleavage in the brains of Alzheimer disease patients. Neurodegener Dis 7: 42–45.
48. Yanagida K, Okochi M, Tagami S, Nakayama T, Kodama TS, et al. (2009) The 28-amino acid form of an APLP1-derived Abeta-like peptide is a surrogate marker for Abeta42 production in the central nervous system. EMBO Mol Med 1: 223–235.
49. Levi A, Ferri GL, Watson E, Possenti R, Salton SR (2004) Processing, distribution, and function of VGF, a neuronal and endocrine peptide precursor. Cell Mol Neurobiol 24: 517–533.
50. Feschenko MS, Donnet C, Wetzel RK, Asinovski NK, Jones LR, et al. (2003) Phospholemman, a single-span membrane protein, is an accessory protein of Na,K-ATPase in cerebellum and choroid plexus. J Neurosci 23: 2161–2169.
51. Geering K (2006) FXYD proteins: new regulators of Na-K-ATPase. Am J Physiol Renal Physiol 290: F241–F250.
52. Dickey CA, Gordon MN, Wilcock DM, Herber DL, Freeman MJ, et al. (2005) Dysregulation of Na+/K+ ATPase by amyloid in APP+PS1 transgenic mice. BMC Neurosci 6: 7.
53. Calero M, Rostagno A, Frangione B, Ghiso J (2005) Clusterin and Alzheimer's disease. Subcell Biochem 38: 273–298.
54. Nilselid AM, Davidsson P, Nagga K, Andreasen N, Fredman P, et al. (2006) Clusterin in cerebrospinal fluid: analysis of carbohydrates and quantification of native and glycosylated forms. Neurochem Int 48: 718–728.
55. Finehout EJ, Franck Z, Choe LH, Relkin N, Lee KH (2007) Cerebrospinal fluid proteomic biomarkers for Alzheimer's disease. Ann Neurol 61: 120–129.
56. Sihlbom C, Davidsson P, Sjogren M, Wahlund LO, Nilsson CL (2008) Structural and quantitative comparison of cerebrospinal fluid glycoproteins in Alzheimer's disease patients and healthy individuals. Neurochem Res 33: 1332–1340.
57. Harold D, Abraham R, Hollingworth P, Sims R, Gerrish A, et al. (2009) Genome-wide association study identifies variants at CLU and PICALM associated with Alzheimer's disease. Nat Genet 41: 1088–1093.
58. Munoz DG (1991) Chromogranin A-like immunoreactive neurites are major constituents of senile plaques. Lab Invest 64: 826–832.
59. Rangon CM, Haik S, Faucheux BA, Metz-Boutigue MH, Fierville F, et al. (2003) Different chromogranin immunoreactivity between prion and a-beta amyloid plaque. Neuroreport 14: 755–758.
60. Taylor DL, Diemel LT, Cuzner ML, Pocock JM (2002) Activation of group II metabotropic glutamate receptors underlies microglial reactivity and neurotox-

icity following stimulation with chromogranin A, a peptide up-regulated in Alzheimer's disease. J Neurochem 82: 1179–1191.

61. Twig G, Graf SA, Messerli MA, Smith PJ, Yoo SH, et al. (2005) Synergistic amplification of beta-amyloid- and interferon-gamma-induced microglial neurotoxic response by the senile plaque component chromogranin A. Am J Physiol Cell Physiol 288: C169–C175.

62. Urushitani M, Sik A, Sakurai T, Nukina N, Takahashi R, et al. (2006) Chromogranin-mediated secretion of mutant superoxide dismutase proteins linked to amyotrophic lateral sclerosis. Nat Neurosci 9: 108–118.

63. Fricker LD, McKinzie AA, Sun J, Curran E, Qian Y, et al. (2000) Identification and characterization of proSAAS, a granin-like neuroendocrine peptide precursor that inhibits prohormone processing. J Neurosci 20: 639–648.

64. Kikuchi K, Arawaka S, Koyama S, Kimura H, Ren CH, et al. (2003) An N-terminal fragment of ProSAAS (a granin-like neuroendocrine peptide precursor) is associated with tau inclusions in Pick's disease. Biochem Biophys Res Commun 308: 646–654.

65. Wada M, Ren CH, Koyama S, Arawaka S, Kawakatsu S, et al. (2004) A human granin-like neuroendocrine peptide precursor (proSAAS) immunoreactivity in tau inclusions of Alzheimer's disease and parkinsonism-dementia complex on Guam. Neurosci Lett 356: 49–52.

66. Mzhavia N, Qian Y, Feng Y, Che FY, Devi LA, et al. (2002) Processing of proSAAS in neuroendocrine cell lines. Biochem J 361: 67–76.

67. Abdi F, Quinn JF, Jankovic J, McIntosh M, Leverenz JB, et al. (2006) Detection of biomarkers with a multiplex quantitative proteomic platform in cerebrospinal fluid of patients with neurodegenerative disorders. J Alzheimers Dis 9: 293–348.

68. Hook VY (2006) Neuroproteases in peptide neurotransmission and neurode-generative diseases: applications to drug discovery research. BioDrugs 20: 105–119.

69. Kuki K, Maeda K, Takauchi S, Kakigi T, Maeda S, et al. (1996) Neurochemical and pathological alterations following infusion of leupeptin, a protease inhibitor, into the rat brain. Dementia 7: 233–238.

70. Petersen RC, Doody R, Kurz A, Mohs RC, Morris JC, et al. (2001) Current concepts in mild cognitive impairment. Arch Neurol 58: 1985–1992.

71. Folstein MF, Folstein SE, McHugh PR (1975) "Mini-mental state". A practical method for grading the cognitive state of patients for the clinician. J Psychiatr Res 12: 189–198.

72. Morris JC (1993) The Clinical Dementia Rating (CDR): current version and scoring rules. Neurology 43: 2412–2414.

73. Thalmann B, Monsch AU, Bernasconi F, Berres M, Schneitter M, et al. (1998) Die CERAD Neuropsychologische Testbatterie - Ein gemeinsames minimales Instrumentarium zur Demenzabklärung. Basel: Memory Clinic, Geriatrische Universitätsklinik Basel.

74. Härting C, Markowitsch HJ, Neufeld H, Calabrese P, Deisinger K (2000) Deutsche Adaptation der revidierten Fassung der Wechsler-Memory Scale (WMS-R). Göttingen: Verlag Hans Huber, Bern.

75. Reitan RM (1979) Trail Making Test (TMT). Göttingen: Hogrefe Verlag, Bern.

76. Shulman KI, Shedletsky R, Silver IL (1986) Challenge of time: Clock-drawing and cognitive function in the elderly. Int J Ger Psychiatr 1: 135–140.

Multiplexed Immunoassay Panel Identifies Novel CSF Biomarkers for Alzheimer's Disease Diagnosis and Prognosis

Rebecca Craig-Schapiro[1], Max Kuhn[7,8], Chengjie Xiong[2,3], Eve H. Pickering[7,8], Jingxia Liu[3], Thomas P. Misko[7,8], Richard J. Perrin[2,4,5], Kelly R. Bales[7,8], Holly Soares[7,8], Anne M. Fagan[1,2,6], David M. Holtzman[1,2,6]*

1 Department of Neurology, Washington University School of Medicine, St. Louis, Missouri, United States of America, 2 The Knight Alzheimer's Disease Research Center, Washington University School of Medicine, St. Louis, Missouri, United States of America, 3 Division of Biostatistics, Washington University School of Medicine, St. Louis, Missouri, United States of America, 4 Division of Neuropathology, Washington University School of Medicine, St. Louis, Missouri, United States of America, 5 Department of Pathology and Immunology, Washington University School of Medicine, St. Louis, Missouri, United States of America, 6 Hope Center for Neurological Disorders, Washington University School of Medicine, St. Louis, Missouri, United States of America, 7 Neuroscience Research Unit, Pfizer Global Research and Development, Groton, Connecticut, United States of America, 8 Neuroscience Research Unit, Pfizer Global Research and Development, St. Louis, Missouri, United States of America

Abstract

Background: Clinicopathological studies suggest that Alzheimer's disease (AD) pathology begins ~10–15 years before the resulting cognitive impairment draws medical attention. Biomarkers that can detect AD pathology in its early stages and predict dementia onset would, therefore, be invaluable for patient care and efficient clinical trial design. We utilized a targeted proteomics approach to discover novel cerebrospinal fluid (CSF) biomarkers that can augment the diagnostic and prognostic accuracy of current leading CSF biomarkers (Aβ42, tau, p-tau181).

Methods and Findings: Using a multiplexed Luminex platform, 190 analytes were measured in 333 CSF samples from cognitively normal (Clinical Dementia Rating [CDR] 0), very mildly demented (CDR 0.5), and mildly demented (CDR 1) individuals. Mean levels of 37 analytes (12 after Bonferroni correction) were found to differ between CDR 0 and CDR>0 groups. Receiver-operating characteristic curve analyses revealed that small combinations of a subset of these markers (cystatin C, VEGF, TRAIL-R3, PAI-1, PP, NT-proBNP, MMP-10, MIF, GRO-α, fibrinogen, FAS, eotaxin-3) enhanced the ability of the best-performing established CSF biomarker, the tau/Aβ42 ratio, to discriminate CDR>0 from CDR 0 individuals. Multiple machine learning algorithms likewise showed that the novel biomarker panels improved the diagnostic performance of the current leading biomarkers. Importantly, most of the markers that best discriminated CDR 0 from CDR>0 individuals in the more targeted ROC analyses were also identified as top predictors in the machine learning models, reconfirming their potential as biomarkers for early-stage AD. Cox proportional hazards models demonstrated that an optimal panel of markers for predicting risk of developing cognitive impairment (CDR 0 to CDR>0 conversion) consisted of calbindin, Aβ42, and age.

Conclusions/Significance: Using a targeted proteomic screen, we identified novel candidate biomarkers that complement the best current CSF biomarkers for distinguishing very mildly/mildly demented from cognitively normal individuals. Additionally, we identified a novel biomarker (calbindin) with significant prognostic potential.

Citation: Craig-Schapiro R, Kuhn M, Xiong C, Pickering EH, Liu J, et al. (2011) Multiplexed Immunoassay Panel Identifies Novel CSF Biomarkers for Alzheimer's Disease Diagnosis and Prognosis. PLoS ONE 6(4): e18850. doi:10.1371/journal.pone.0018850

Editor: Ashley I. Bush, Mental Health Research Institute of Victoria, Australia

Received November 28, 2010; **Accepted** March 21, 2011; **Published** April 19, 2011

Funding: This work was supported by a grant to Washington University from Pfizer. Max Kuhn, Eve H. Pickering, Thomas P. Misko, Kelly R. Bales and Holly Soares are employed by Pfizer Global Research and Development, Groton, CT, and St. Louis, MO and therefore, Pfizer Global played a role in study design, data collection and analysis, decision to publish, and preparation of the manuscript. This work was also supported by the National Institutes of Health grants P50 AG05681, P01 AG03991, P01 AG026276, P30 NS057105 and the Charles and Joanne Knight Alzheimer Research Initiative. This publication was made possible by Grant Number UL1 RR024992 from the National Center for Research Resources (NCRR), a component of the National Institutes of Health (NIH), and NIH Roadmap for Medical Research. Its contents are solely the responsibility of the authors and do not necessarily represent the official view of NCRR or NIH. In regard to the funders other than Pfizer, they had no role in study design, data collection and analysis, decision to publish, or preparation of the manuscript.

Competing Interests: The authors have read the journal's policy and have the following conflicts: Max Kuhn, Eve H. Pickering, Kelly R. Bales are paid employees of Pfizer. They have no other competing interests relevant to the data in this manuscript. Thomas P. Misko and Holly Soares were paid employees of Pfizer during the course of this study. They have no other competing interests relevant to the data in this manuscript. David M. Holtzman co-founded the company C2N Diagnostics and has ownership interests. He serves on the Scientific Advisory Boards of En Vivo and Satori. He has no other competing interests relevant to the data in this manuscript. This does not alter the authors' adherence to all the PLoS ONE policies on sharing data and materials. Rebecca Craig-Schapiro, Chengjie Xiong, Jingxia Liu, Richard J. Perrin, and Anne M. Fagan have no competing interests to declare.

* E-mail: holtzman@neuro.wustl.edu

Introduction

With the growing prevalence of Alzheimer's disease (AD), the ability to accurately and reliably diagnose AD in its earliest stages has become a public health priority. The concept of 'earliest stages,' however, warrants revision as it is increasingly clear there exists a 'preclinical' or 'presymptomatic' stage during which the pathological changes associated with AD, amyloid plaques, neurofibrillary tangles, and neuroinflammation, begin to appear without concomitant clinical features. This period has been estimated to be ~10–15 years in duration. Means to identify this preclinical phase of AD may facilitate medical intervention to prevent or slow neurodegeneration and the resulting cognitive impairment. Because clinical examination cannot detect preclinical disease and is less accurate with very mild stages of AD, there is a pressing need for biomarkers for AD. Furthermore, biomarkers may have significant utility in clinical trial design, providing greater diagnostic certainty for enrollment than is possible by clinical diagnosis alone, and allowing for the selective enrollment of individuals at greater risk of developing future cognitive impairment, ultimately resulting in trials of shorter duration, smaller size, and reduced cost.

The cerebrospinal fluid (CSF) is a logical source of potential AD biomarkers, as it reflects biochemical changes in the brain. Indeed, the fluid biomarkers thus far showing the greatest promise for use in AD diagnosis and prognosis are CSF amyloid-$\beta42$ (A$\beta42$), tau, and phosphorylated forms of tau (p-tau) [1]–[5]. Concentrations of CSF A$\beta42$ decrease in association with the deposition of A$\beta42$ into plaques within the brain [6]–[9]. This process occurs years prior to the clinical onset of AD and may mark the earliest phase of AD pathology. CSF A$\beta42$ levels remain low throughout the disease course [6], [10], [11]. In contrast, CSF tau and p-tau levels progressively increase with the advancing stages of AD, and in some individuals, begin to rise several years prior to diagnosis [7], [12], [13]. The ratios of tau or p-tau to A$\beta42$ have also proven useful for predicting clinical progression in individuals who have very mild dementia or mild cognitive impairment (MCI), and, importantly, for predicting future MCI and AD dementia among those who are cognitively normal [7], [14], [15]. Nevertheless, even for these analytes, there is substantial overlap between control and AD groups and a need for better prognostic ability [16]. Consequently, there remains a need for supplemental biomarkers to improve diagnosis and prognosis at different disease stages. Given the multifactorial nature of AD pathophysiology, it is likely that there will be other CSF biomarkers that will be useful in this regard. While proteomic screens have identified a number of other candidate AD biomarkers [17]–[26], few studies have utilized large, well-characterized cohorts or have looked for biomarkers in preclinical or very early stage disease.

In this study, a large number of CSF samples (N = 333) selected from well-characterized MCI/very early stage-AD and cognitively normal control cohorts were chosen for protein profiling using a commercially available panel that measures a variety of cytokines, chemokines, metabolic markers, growth factors, and other markers. Multiplex immunoassay platforms such as the one used here, Rules Based Medicine Discovery MAP 1.0 panel, allow for the simultaneous quantitation of many analytes, and by adhering to clinical laboratory improvement amendments (CLIA) standards, are amenable for clinical trial work. Using multiple statistical approaches, we have identified a set of novel biomarkers that may improve the ability of traditional AD biomarkers, A$\beta42$ and tau, to distinguish MCI/early-stage AD from cognitive normalcy and to predict the development of future cognitive impairment (i.e. detection of preclinical AD at increased risk of progression).

Methods

Ethics Statement

The study protocols were approved by the Human Studies Committees at all participating institutions, and written and verbal informed consent was obtained from participants at enrollment. All aspects of this study were conducted according to the principles expressed in the Declaration of Helsinki.

Participant Selection

Participants (N = 333) were community-dwelling volunteers enrolled in longitudinal studies of healthy aging and dementia at the Knight Alzheimer's Disease Research Center at Washington University (WU-ADRC). The study protocol was approved by the Human Studies Committee at Washington University, and written and verbal informed consent was obtained from participants at enrollment. At sample collection, participants were ≥60 years of age and in good general health, having no other neurological, psychiatric, or major medical diagnoses that could contribute importantly to dementia. Clinical diagnosis was evaluated based on criteria from the National Institute of Neurological and Communicative Diseases and Stroke-Alzheimer's Disease and Related Disorders Association (NINCDS-ADRDA) [27]. Cognitive status was rated with the clinical dementia rating scale (CDR); a CDR of 0 (N = 242) indicated no dementia, CDR 0.5 (N = 63) indicated very mild dementia, and CDR 1 (N = 28) indicated mild dementia [28]. Some of the CDR 0.5 study participants met the criteria for mild cognitive impairment (MCI) and some were more mildly impaired and were considered "pre-MCI" [29], [30]. A subset of participants (N = 179) in this cohort had also undergone positron emission tomography (PET) imaging with Pittsburgh Compound-B (PIB) for assessment of in vivo amyloid burden [32]. A mean cortical PIB binding potential value was obtained by averaging prefrontal cortex, precuneus, lateral temporal cortex, and gyrus rectus regions, as described previously [6], [31]. Apolipoprotein E (*APOE*) genotype was determined by the WU-ADRC Genetics Core. Twenty-five to 30 mL of CSF was collected by lumbar puncture (LP) at 8 AM following overnight fasting. Samples were inverted to avoid gradient effects, centrifuged briefly (2,000g, 5 minutes, 4°C) to remove any cellular elements, and aliquoted into polypropylene tubes for freezing and storage at −80°C [7].

Analyte Measurements

CSF A$\beta42$, total tau, and phospho-tau181 levels (henceforth referred to as 'traditional' biomarkers) were analyzed in duplicate by the WU-ADRC Biomarker Core by quantitative ELISA after a single freeze-thaw cycle according to the manufacturer's specifications (Innotest, Innogenetics, Ghent, Belgium).

CSF samples were also evaluated by Rules Based Medicine, Inc. (RBM) (Austin, TX) for levels of 190 analytes using the Human Discovery Multi-Analyte Profile (MAP) 1.0 panel and a Luminex 100 platform. This 190 analyte panel (from here on referred to as 'RBM analytes') was assembled by RBM to measure a range of cytokines, chemokines, growth factors, hormones, metabolic markers, and other proteins thought to be important in disease; a complete list of analytes is available at www.rulesbasedmedicine.com.

At RBM, the samples were thawed at room temperature (RT), vortexed, spun at 13,000g for 5 minutes for clarification, and 1.0 mL was removed into a master microtiter plate for MAP analysis. Using automated pipetting, an aliquot of each sample was introduced into one of the capture microsphere multiplexes of the Human DiscoveryMAP. The mixtures of sample and capture microspheres were thoroughly mixed and incubated at RT for 1 hour. Multiplexed cocktails of biotinylated reporter antibodies for each multiplex were then added robotically, and after thorough mixing, were incubated for an additional hour at RT. Multiplexes were developed using an excess of streptavidin-phycoerythrin solution which was thoroughly mixed into each multiplex and incubated for 1 hour at RT. The volume of each multiplexed reaction was reduced by vacuum filtration and then increased by dilution into matrix buffer for analysis. Analysis was performed in a Luminex 100 instrument and the resulting data stream was interpreted using proprietary data analysis software developed at RBM. For each multiplex, both calibrators and controls were included on each microtiter plate. Eight-point calibrators were run in the first and last column of each plate and 3-level quality controls were included in duplicate. Testing results were determined first for the high, medium and low controls for each multiplex to ensure proper assay performance. Unknown values for each of the analytes localized in a specific multiplex were determined using 4 and 5 parameter, weighted and non-weighted curve fitting algorithms included in the data analysis package.

Statistical Analysis

Statistical analyses were performed in SAS 9.2 (SAS Institute Inc, Cary, NC) for univariate analyses, ROC/AUC calculations, and Cox proportional hazards models, and in R version 2.10.1 for predictive modeling [packages/versions: caret (4.65), earth (2.4-0), kernlab (0.9–9), klaR (0.6–3), MASS (7.3–7), mda (0.4–1), nnet (7.3–1), pamr (1.44.0), pls (2.1–0), randomForest (4.5–34), spls (2.1–0)] [33]. Of the 190 RBM analytes, 65 had >10% of data missing or below the lower detection limit (LDL), and were therefore excluded from analysis, yielding 125 'measurable' analytes. Data below the LDL were imputed to LDL/2, and data more than five standard deviations beyond the mean were imputed using a nearest neighbor algorithm. Of the 125 measurable analytes, 24 analytes had at least one value below the LDL, imputed to LDL/2. For those 24 analytes, the percentage of data imputed ranged from < 1% (3 or fewer values) to 9.5% (33 values). There were a total of 82 outliers from 48 participants, with outliers in a maximum of 10 analytes for one participant, and in 2 – 9 analytes for the remaining participants. The distributions of analytes were tested for normality by Box-Cox analysis and, when appropriate, log10 transformed to approximate a normal distribution. Correlations between RBM analytes, traditional AD biomarkers, and demographic variables were evaluated using the Spearman rho correlation coefficient ($\alpha = 0.05$). Analysis of covariance (ANCOVA) using the General Linear Model (GLM) procedure in SAS was used to determine analytes that differed in concentration between AD and control groups while adjusting for the effects of age and gender. Bonferroni correction was used to adjust for multiple testing (128 RBM plus traditional analytes). For each analyte showing promise by univariate analysis, the area under the Receiver Operating Characteristic (ROC) curve (AUC) was calculated for discriminating CDR 0 versus CDR>0. The method of Xiong et al. [34] was implemented to determine the optimum linear combination of analytes and to calculate the confidence interval (CI) on the AUC and the sensitivity. A bootstrapping resampling technique was used to obtain robust estimates of expected future performance of the three marker panels in predicting CDR 0 versus CDR>0. Averages of performance measures (the 95% CI of the AUC, sensitivity at 80% specificity, and p-value) were taken over 100 iterations of the bootstrap.

Cox proportional hazard models assessed the ability of baseline biomarkers to predict conversion from cognitive normalcy (CDR

0) to very mild or mild dementia (CDR 0.5 and 1). Data from participants who did not convert during the follow-up were statistically censored at the date of last assessment. Biomarker measurements were treated as continuous variables and were converted to standard Z-scores. Baseline variables were considered for inclusion in multivariate models if they were associated with time to conversion in a univariate analysis (p<0.15). Variables were retained in multivariate proportional hazard models if p<0.05. AIC (Akaike Information Criterion), a measure of goodness of fit of an estimated statistical model, was used to compare different models, with a lower AIC indicating better model fit.

Several statistical machine learning techniques were utilized to predict CDR status as a function of baseline characteristics (e.g. age) and the candidate biomarkers. Rather than focusing on a specific model, a panel of predictive modeling techniques was applied to the data. Most of these models contain "tuning parameters" that cannot be directly estimated from the data; these values were chosen using resampling techniques. The models used were:

- Partial Least Squares (PLS) is a latent variable model that produces linear class boundaries and works well with correlated predictors [35]. Candidate values of the tuning parameter, the number of PLS components, ranged from 1 to 20.
- Sparse Partial Least Squares (SPLS) is a variant of PLS that incorporates feature selection in the model fitting [36]. The number of PLS components was varied in the same manner as the basic PLS model and the additional tuning parameter for regularization was varied from 0.1 to 0.9.
- Random Forests (RF) is a tree-based ensemble method [37]. The number of randomly selected variables at each split was varied over five values (generally 2 to the number of predictors in the model).
- Boosted Trees are another tree-based ensemble model [38]. The three tuning parameters are the depth of the tree (even values from 2 to 10 were evaluated), the number of boosting iterations (20 iterations to 2000 in 100 iteration increments) and the learning rate (fixed at 0.1).
- Support Vector Machine (SVM) are a kernel based method [39]. The radial basis function kernel was used. The kernel parameter was estimated analytically [40] and the five candidate values of the cost parameter ranged from 0.1 to 1,000 on the log10 scale.
- Nearest Shrunken Centroids (NCS) is a prototype model that incorporates feature selection [41]. The tuning parameter, the shrinkage threshold, was varied over 30 values (between 0.325 and 9.097 for the model using traditional biomarkers, and between 0.325 and 9.11 for the model using traditional and RBM markers.)
- Naïve Bayes (NB) is a simple classifier where each predictor variable contributes to the final class prediction independently [42]. The conditional distributions were computed using a simple Gaussian distribution or using a nonparametric density estimator.
- K-Nearest Neighbors (KNN) is a simple prototype based model [42]. Candidate values for the number of neighbors ranged from 5 to 15.
- Flexible Discriminant Analysis (FDA) is a partitioning based model that also incorporates feature selection [43]. The multivariate adaptive spline basis function was used. Ten

candidate values for the number of retained terms were evaluated.

To determine the values for the tuning parameters and to estimate performance, resampling methods were used. The entire data set was repeatedly split into training (80%) and test sets (20%). This process was repeated 200 times. Models were fit on the training sets and the associated held-out values were used to estimate performance (sensitivity, specificity, and the area under the ROC curve). The final estimates of performance were calculated by averaging the 200 sets of performance values from the resampling procedure.

Results

Levels of 37 markers are altered in MCI/very mild and mild AD CSF

To identify new candidate biomarkers for AD, multiplexed Luminex-based immunoassays were used to evaluate the levels of 190 analytes in the CSF of 242 cognitively normal participants (CDR 0), 63 participants with very mild dementia (CDR 0.5), and 28 participants with mild dementia (CDR 1) (participant characteristics at baseline assessment in Table 1). Since the number of CDR 1 participants was relatively smaller, and all CDR 0.5 and CDR 1 participants were clinically diagnosed as having AD, the CDR 0.5 and CDR 1 groups were combined in the statistical analyses. There were no statistically significant differences in age, gender, MCBP for PIB-PET, or $APOE$ genotype between the CDR 0.5 and CDR 1 groups. Of the 125 RBM analytes that were statistically assessed (Table S1), the mean concentrations of 37 CSF analytes were found to differ between cognitively normal (CDR 0) and very mildly/mildly demented (CDR 0.5 and 1) participants by analysis of covariance (ANCOVA) adjusting for age and gender ($p < 0.05$) (Table 2 and Table S2). Twelve of these 37 analytes remained significant after Bonferroni correction for multiple testing (n = 128, adjusted alpha = 0.0004). Additionally, participants with very mild/mild dementia exhibited the typical AD CSF biomarker profile characterized by significantly lower mean levels of CSF Aβ42 and higher mean levels of CSF tau and CSF p-tau181, as well as displaying higher mean cortical amyloid burden (MCBP assessed by PIB-PET

imaging) as has been seen previously (Tables 1 and 2) [6], [31], [32].

Correlation of RBM analytes with demographic features and other biomarker values

Because the CDR 0, 0.5, and 1 groups showed somewhat different distributions with regard to age at lumbar puncture and gender, levels of the 37 RBM analytes were evaluated for correlation with these variables. Many analytes were significantly associated with age or gender (Table 3). Additionally, seeking insight into the potential roles of the analytes in AD pathology, we evaluated their association with CSF Aβ42, tau, and p-tau181, and cortical amyloid burden measured by PIB-PET imaging. Many of the analytes correlated with CSF tau and CSF p-tau181 (31 and 30 analytes, respectively), while fewer correlated with CSF Aβ42 or cortical amyloid burden (8 and 5 analytes, respectively) (Table 3).

Diagnostic Utility of Candidate Biomarkers

To assess the potential of the analytes for identifying very mild/ mild dementia (combined CDR 0.5 and CDR 1), ROC curves and AUCs were calculated for each of the 37 RBM analytes and for traditional AD biomarkers Aβ42, tau, p-tau181 and the ratios tau/ Aβ42 and p-tau181/Aβ42 (Table 4 and Figure 1). Although none of the RBM analytes alone out-performed the traditional biomarkers, combining traditional biomarkers with RBM analytes improved upon the AUC of the traditional biomarkers in many cases; e.g., Aβ42: AUC = .7552, combinations ranging from .7553–.8201; tau/Aβ42: AUC = .8443, combinations ranging from .8444–.8819; p-tau181/Aβ42: AUC = .8065, combinations ranging from .8065–.8468 (Table 4 and Figure 1). For these '2-marker panels' of traditional biomarker plus RBM analyte, combinations with tau/Aβ42 consistently yielded the highest AUCs. To investigate whether combinations of three markers could yield a small panel with improved diagnostic accuracy, we utilized a targeted approach in which the four 2-marker panels with the highest AUCs (tau/Aβ42 + cystatin C, tau/Aβ42 + VEGF, tau/Aβ42 + KIM-1, tau/Aβ42 + PP) were combined with the 10 RBM analytes with the highest individual AUCs (indicated in Table 4). Because an independent validation cohort was not available for analysis, bootstrapping resampling with 100 iterations was performed to obtain relatively unbiased estimates of expected future performance of the '3-marker panels' in predicting CDR 0 versus CDR>0 (Table 5). A number of the 3-marker panels demonstrated significantly improved AUCs compared to the corresponding 2-marker panels, with the best achieving AUCs of ~.90 and sensitivities of ~84% at 80% specificity (Table 5).

Because AD is a complex, multifactorial disease and likely involves alterations in multiple biological pathways, it is possible that a larger panel of biomarkers encompassing various features of AD pathophysiology may be optimal for disease diagnosis. Thus, we utilized statistical machine learning algorithms, which are more amenable to potentially large numbers of analyte combinations and can identify highly complex nonlinear relationships, to discover whether groups of markers are capable of distinguishing very mildly/mildly demented (CDR 0.5 and 1 combined) from cognitively normal participants (CDR 0). A multi-pronged analytical approach including RF, PLS, SPLS, Boosted Tree, FDA, NB, NSC, LR, KNN, and SVM was used, as each approach has its own strengths and weaknesses. Models were fit with two sets of predictors: 1) traditional biomarkers, and 2) traditional biomarkers plus RBM analytes; additionally, age, gender, and ApoE genotype were included in all models. Model performance measures were based on cross-validation, in which the test set results were averaged from 200 splits of the data between training

Table 1. Demographic, clinical, and genotypic characteristics of the 333 study participants.

Characteristic	CDR 0	CDR 0.5	CDR 1
N	242	63	28
Gender (% Female)	65%	52%	50%
$APOE$ genotype, % ε4+	32%	54%	57%
Mean MMSE score (SD)	28.9 (1.3)	26.3 (2.8)	22.5 (4.0)
Mean age at LP (SD), yrs	71.6 (7.4)	74.6 (7.3)	76.8 (6.2)
Mean CSF Aβ42 (SD), pg/mL	607 (234)	436 (233)	355 (119)
Mean CSF tau (SD), pg/mL	315 (169)	547 (278)	557 (266)
Mean CSF p-tau181 (SD), pg/mL	56 (25)	85 (45)	78 (38)
Mean PIB MCBP (SD)	0.12 (0.24)	0.54 (0.34)	0.50 (0.50)

Abbreviations: CDR, Clinical Dementia Rating; *APOE*, apolipoprotein E; MMSE, Mini-Mental State Examination; LP, lumbar puncture; SD, standard deviation; CSF, cerebrospinal fluid; Aβ-42, amyloid-beta peptide 1-42; p-tau181, tau phosphorylated at threonine 181; PIB MCBP, Pittsburgh Compound B mean cortical PIB binding potential. MCBP data available for 179 study participants.
doi:10.1371/journal.pone.0018850.t001

Table 2. Analytes that differ in levels between cognitively normal (CDR 0) and very mildly/mildly demented (CDR 0.5 and 1) participants.

Marker	Adjusted mean CDR 0	Adjusted mean CDR>0	p	Raw mean CDR 0	Raw mean CDR>0
Aβ42 (pg/mL)*	607.45	418.85	<0.0001	606.90	411.18
Tau (pg/mL)*	315.59	533.60	<0.0001	314.80	549.96
p-tau181 (pg/mL)*	56.30	81.01	<0.0001	56.32	82.98
Growth-Regulated alpha protein (GRO-α) (pg/mL)*	18.27	22.09	<0.0001	18.30	22.44
Log Matrix Metalloproteinase-10 (MMP-10) (pg/mL)*	24.84	31.41	<0.0001	24.11	32.61
Log N-terminal pro-brain natriuretic peptide (NT-proBNP) (pg/mL)*	87.00	107.75	<0.0001	87.70	111.12
Log Plasminogen Activator Inhibitor 1 (PAI-1) (ng/mL)*	1.05	1.28	<0.0001	1.01	1.34
TNF-Related Apoptosis-Inducing Ligand Receptor 3 (TRAIL-R3) (ng/mL)*	0.55	0.63	<0.0001	0.55	0.65
Vascular Endothelial Growth Factor (VEGF) (pg/mL)*	441.57	378.30	<0.0001	437.83	386.01
Log Pancreatic Polypeptide (PP) (pg/mL)*	0.94	1.30	0.0001	0.88	1.41
Log FAS (ng/mL)*	0.57	0.65	0.0002	0.56	0.67
Log Macrophage Migration Inhibitory Factor (MIF) (ng/mL)*	0.15	0.17	0.0004	0.15	0.18
Interleukin-7 (IL-7) (pg/mL)	12.63	9.47	0.0006	12.23	9.68
Log Cystatin C (ng/mL)	5613.84	4750.89	0.0011	5551.50	4835.30
Thrombopoietin (ng/mL)	0.43	0.37	0.0016	0.42	0.37
Sortilin (ng/mL)	6.32	6.92	0.0019	6.33	6.96
Monocyte Chemotactic Protein 2 (MCP-2) (pg/mL)	4.03	4.61	0.0020	3.97	4.67
Log Fibrinogen (ug/mL)	0.63	0.78	0.0024	0.59	0.81
Log Creatine Kinase-MB (CKMB) (pg/mL)	26.55	20.97	0.0030	26.62	20.87
Cortisol (ng/mL)	11.21	12.65	0.0034	11.17	12.89
Thymus-Expressed Chemokine (TECK) (ng/mL)	6.38	6.85	0.0039	6.30	6.96
Eotaxin-3 (pg/mL)	56.78	62.09	0.0057	55.33	63.68
Interleukin-17E (IL-17E) (pg/mL)	8.63	7.75	0.0058	8.60	7.79
Kidney Injury Molecule-1 (KIM-1) (pg/mL)	78.97	83.46	0.0074	79.05	83.08
Log Heparin-binding epidermal growth factor-like growth factor (HB-EGF) (pg/mL)	24.98	28.77	0.0077	25.05	28.70
Log Osteopontin (ng/mL)	173.23	197.68	0.0078	174.15	202.31
Log α-1-Antitrypsin (ug/mL)	4.87	5.37	0.0102	4.73	5.49
Fatty Acid Synthase Ligand (FASL) (pg/mL)	4.85	5.40	0.0109	4.78	5.49
Log Insulin-like Growth Factor-Binding Protein 2 (IGFBP-2) (ng/mL)	199.58	212.16	0.0111	195.93	217.47
Log Interleukin-10 (IL-10) (pg/mL)	1.14	1.29	0.0131	1.12	1.29
Log Tumor necrosis factor-a receptor 2 (TNF RII) (ng/mL)	0.53	0.59	0.0141	0.52	0.62
Log Resistin (pg/mL)	26.28	30.76	0.0146	25.20	32.14
Log Fatty Acid Binding Protein (FABP) (ng/mL)	3.03	3.62	0.0209	2.93	3.81
Log Apolipoprotein D (ApoD) (ug/mL)	4.18	4.57	0.0318	4.02	4.65
Log Hepatocyte Growth Factor (HGF) (ng/mL)	1.18	1.28	0.0349	1.18	1.30
Log Insulin (uIU/mL)	0.22	0.19	0.0359	0.21	0.19
Log Hemofiltrate cysteine-cysteine chemokine (HCC-4) (pg/mL)	30.25	33.13	0.0418	28.98	33.87
Log Interferon gamma Induced Protein 10 (IP-10) (pg/mL)	299.63	341.86	0.0432	295.14	354.74
Log Gamma-Interferon-Induced Monokine (MIG) (pg/mL)	423.80	493.91	0.0452	400.16	572.75
Thrombomodulin (ng/mL)	0.17	0.18	0.0475	0.17	0.19

Analysis of covariance (ANCOVA) using the General Linear Model (GLM) procedure in SAS was used to determine analytes that differed in concentration (p<0.05) between CDR 0 and CDR>0 groups while adjusting for the effects of age and gender ("adjusted means").
*indicates analytes that were significant after Bonferroni correction based on the number of markers analyzed (128 markers, cutoff of 0.0004 for familywise p<0.05). For markers that were log transformed to approximate a normal distribution, the resulting Least Squares mean (or estimated marginal mean) was back-transformed to obtain the adjusted mean shown. Also provided are the raw mean concentrations for the CDR 0 and CDR>0 groups.
doi:10.1371/journal.pone.0018850.t002

(80%) and test (20%) (Table 6). Using either traditional biomarkers or traditional biomarkers with RBM analytes, no model clearly out-performed the others; however, the RBM analytes appeared to contribute additional specificity to the biomarker panels (traditional: sensitivity 80.6–91.4%, specificity 42.4–56.6%; traditional+ RBM: sensitivity 79.1–93.2%, specificity 59.6–77.6%). This

Table 3. Correlations of RBM analytes with age, gender, and other biomarker values.

Analyte	Gender	Age	Aβ42	Tau	p-tau181	tau/Aβ42	Cortical PIB
α1A	<0.001	0.255 (<0.0001)	0.031 (0.574)	0.117 (0.033)	0.105 (0.055)	0.048 (0.386)	-0.048 (0.525)
ApoD	<0.001	0.218 (<0.0001)	0.059 (0.280)	0.222 (<0.0001)	0.216 (<0.0001)	0.113 (0.039)	-0.103 (0.169)
Calbindin	0.001	0.196 (<0.001)	0.094 (0.088)	0.476 (<0.0001)	0.500 (<0.0001)	0.294 (<0.0001)	0.122 (0.104)
CKMB	0.524	-0.069 (0.211)	0.008 (0.877)	-0.200 (<0.001)	-0.186 (0.001)	-0.148 (0.007)	0.032 (0.673)
Cortisol	0.282	0.252 (<0.0001)	-0.051 (0.357)	0.187 (0.001)	0.189 (0.001)	0.159 (0.004)	0.012 (0.875)
Cystatin C	0.461	0.093 (0.089)	0.281 (<0.0001)	0.536 (<0.0001)	0.597 (<0.0001)	0.236 (<0.0001)	-0.041 (0.587)
Eotaxin-3	<0.001	0.317 (<0.0001)	0.058 (0.289)	0.367 (<0.0001)	0.342 (<0.0001)	0.217 (<0.0001)	0.003 (0.971)
FABP	0.031	0.296 (<0.0001)	0.012 (0.833)	0.727 (<0.0001)	0.725 (<0.0001)	0.505 (<0.0001)	0.159 (0.034)
FAS	<0.001	0.297 (<0.0001)	0.083 (0.132)	0.491 (<0.0001)	0.470 (<0.0001)	0.288 (<0.0001)	-0.074 (0.326)
FASL	0.165	0.192 (<0.001)	-0.060 (0.274)	0.189 (0.001)	0.200 (0.001)	0.129 (0.018)	-0.020 (0.795)
Fibrinogen	<0.001	0.284 (<0.0001)	-0.044 (0.422)	0.192 (<0.001)	0.178 (0.001)	0.145 (0.008)	0.034 (0.652)
GRO-α	0.178	0.279 (<0.0001)	-0.105 (0.056)	0.317 (<0.0001)	0.329 (<0.0001)	0.259 (<0.0001)	0.144 (0.054)
HB-EGF	0.975	0.017 (0.751)	0.079 (0.151)	0.348 (<0.0001)	0.359 (<0.0001)	0.202 (<0.001)	-0.024 (0.751)
HCC-4	<0.001	0.240 (<0.0001)	0.007 (0.895)	0.094 (0.088)	0.037 (0.504)	0.047 (0.388)	-0.095 (0.204)
HGF	0.918	0.222 (<0.0001)	0.088 (0.110)	0.619 (<0.0001)	0.639 (<0.0001)	0.386 (<0.0001)	0.004 (0.957)
IGFBP-2	<0.001	0.394 (<0.0001)	0.062 (0.262)	0.462 (<0.0001)	0.441 (<0.0001)	0.278 (<0.0001)	0.031 (0.685)
IL-17E	0.386	0.032 (0.563)	0.017 (0.760)	0.007 (0.899)	0.049 (0.371)	0.019 (0.725)	-0.101 (0.180)
IL-7	0.007	0-.002 (0.976)	0.147 (0.007)	-0.003 (0.961)	0.032 (0.557)	-0.091 (0.096)	-0.227 (0.002)
IL-10	<0.001	0.055 (0.313)	-0.026 (0.637)	0.070 (0.205)	0.075 (0.170)	0.053 (0.337)	-0.071 (0.342)
IP-10	0.327	0.236 (<0.0001)	0.023 (0.682)	0.249 (<0.0001)	0.282 (<0.0001)	0.147 (0.007)	-0.071 (0.344)
Insulin	<0.001	0.094 (0.088)	0.245 (<0.0001)	0.213 (<0.0001)	0.214 (<0.0001)	0.005 (0.921)	-0.190 (0.011)
KIM-1	0.636	0-.032 (0.561)	-0.057 (0.301)	-0.239 (<0.0001)	-0.331 (<0.0001)	-0.154 (0.005)	-0.060 (0.427)
MCP-2	0.013	0.146 (0.007)	-0.106 (0.053)	0.045 (0.408)	0.059 (0.282)	0.071 (0.199)	-0.011 (0.880)
MIF	0.239	0.330 (<0.0001)	-0.007 (0.901)	0.579 (<0.0001)	0.597 (<0.0001)	0.412 (<0.0001)	0.084 (0.264)
MIG	0.528	0.603 (<0.0001)	-0.017 (0.762)	0.282 (<0.0001)	0.289 (<0.0001)	0.207 (<0.001)	-0.053 (0.484)
MMP-10	0.002	0.325 (<0.0001)	-0.116 (0.034)	0.458 (<0.0001)	0.415 (<0.0001)	0.390 (<0.0001)	0.086 (0.252)
NT-proBNP	0.030	0.273 (<0.0001)	0.053 (0.338)	0.331 (<0.0001)	0.323 (<0.0001)	0.188 (0.001)	-0.007 (0.923)
Osteopontin	0.137	0.192 (<0.001)	0.030 (0.590)	0.680 (<0.0001)	0.701 (<0.0001)	0.466 (<0.0001)	0.162 (0.030)
PP	<.001	0.374 (<0.0001)	-0.072 (0.189)	0.226 (<0.0001)	0.179 (0.001)	0.192 (<0.001)	0.041 (0.586)
PAI-1	<.001	0.429 (<0.0001)	-0.064 (0.244)	0.334 (<0.0001)	0.327 (<0.0001)	0.266 (<0.0001)	-0.003 (0.973)
Resistin	<.001	0.355 (<0.0001)	0.072 (0.189)	0.255 (<0.0001)	0.198 (<0.0001)	0.120 (0.029)	-0.075 (0.320)
Sortilin	0.881	0.135 (0.014)	0.139 (0.011)	0.515 (<0.0001)	0.527 (<0.0001)	0.273 (<0.0001)	-0.003 (0.972)
TNF RII	0.205	0.426 (<0.0001)	0.059 (0.282)	0.678 (<0.0001)	0.702 (<0.0001)	0.442 (<0.0001)	0.002 (0.975)
TRAIL-R3	0.112	0.413 (<0.0001)	-0.011 (0.837)	0.509 (<0.0001)	0.476 (<0.0001)	0.356 (<0.0001)	0.008 (0.914)
Thrombomodulin	<.001	0.193 (<0.001)	0.109 (0.048)	0.215 (<0.0001)	0.205 (<0.001)	0.076 (0.168)	-0.063 (0.406)
Thrombopoietin	0.015	0.034 (0.531)	0.194 (<0.001)	-0.016 (0.768)	0.017 (0.758)	-0.130 (0.017)	-0.237 (0.001)
TECK	0.015	0.270 (<0.0001)	0.047 (0.389)	0.322 (<0.0001)	0.312 (<0.0001)	0.193 (<0.001)	0.001 (0.992)
VEGF	0.651	0.101 (0.065)	0.357 (<0.0001)	0.470 (<0.0001)	0.543 (<0.0001)	0.154 (0.005)	-0.059 (0.429)

Correlations were evaluated using the Spearman rho correlation coefficient ($\alpha = 0.05$); shown are the *r* and (p value). Gender differences were evaluated by Mann-Whitney test.
doi:10.1371/journal.pone.0018850.t003

improvement is further reflected in the Youden Index, a single statistic that captures the performance of a diagnostic test and is a function of sensitivity and specificity, which was higher on average for the models fitted with traditional plus RBM analytes (traditional: 0.230–0.438; traditional+RBM: 0.401–0.621). Additionally, models fitted with traditional plus RBM analytes yielded mostly higher AUCs (traditional: 0.680–0.827; traditional+RBM: 0.754–0.868). For the four models with a built-in importance statistic (i.e., Boosted Tree, NSC, RF, and PLS) there was considerable overlap in the top 15 predictors for each model

(Figure 2, Table 7). Importantly, nearly all of the markers found to best discriminate CDR 0 from CDR>0 participants in the more targeted ROC analyses (Table 5) were also identified as the top predictors in the machine learning models (Figure 2, Table 7), reconfirming the potential of these analytes as biomarkers for AD.

Prognostic Utility of Candidate Biomarkers

Identifying individuals with AD neuropathology while they are still in the preclinical phase will be critically important, as disease-modifying therapies currently in development are likely to be most

Table 4. ROC analyses.

AUC of Traditional Biomarkers			
log Aβ42	0.7552		
log tau	0.7830		
log p-tau181	0.7149		
log tau/Aβ42	0.8443		
log p-tau181/Aβ42	0.8065		

AUC of RBM Biomarkers: alone and in combination with traditional biomarkers			
	Marker	Marker+log tau/Aβ42	Marker+log p-tau181/Aβ42
log α1A	0.6296	0.8578	0.8234
log ApoD	0.6136	0.8489	0.8138
log CKMB	0.6106	0.8475	0.8118
Cortisol	0.6183	0.8510	0.8155
log Cystatin C	0.5965	0.8819 §	0.8468
Eotaxin-3	0.6448 §	0.8516	0.8202
log FABP	0.6163	0.8499	0.8080
log FAS	0.6689 §	0.8518	0.8209
FASL	0.6134	0.8479	0.8116
log Fibrinogen	0.6503 §	0.8564	0.8232
GRO-α	0.7024 §	0.8609	0.8305
log HB-EGF	0.5929	0.8445	0.8081
log HCC-4	0.6172	0.8596	0.8281
log HGF	0.5972	0.8458	0.8069
log IGF-BP2	0.6378	0.8462	0.8116
IL-7	0.6029	0.8508	0.8162
log IL-10	0.6075	0.8575	0.8215
IL-17E	0.5969	0.8487	0.8145
log Insulin	0.5406	0.8453	0.8077
log IP-10	0.5970	0.8460	0.8093
KIM-1	0.5894	0.8668 §	0.8343
MCP-2	0.6264	0.8554	0.8200
log MIF	0.6651 §	0.8455	0.8117
log MIG	0.6376	0.8544	0.8207
log MMP-10	0.6929 §	0.8518	0.8232
log NT-proBNP	0.6753 §	0.8562	0.8248
log Osteopontin	0.6050	0.8508	0.8100
log PP	0.6789 §	0.8644 §	0.8356
log PAI-1	0.6814 §	0.8587	0.8273
log Resistin	0.6218	0.8522	0.8211
Sortilin	0.6177	0.8444	0.8076
log TNF RII	0.6319	0.8447	0.8065
TRAIL-R3	0.6851 §	0.8523	0.8212
Thrombomodulin	0.6004	0.8503	0.8150
Thrombopoietin	0.5898	0.8465	0.8111
TECK	0.6371	0.8525	0.8190
VEGF	0.6146	0.8766 §	0.8441

To assess the ability of the markers to distinguish CDR>0 from CDR 0, ROC analyses were performed for each of the traditional biomarkers (Aβ42, tau, p-tau181 and the ratios tau/Aβ42 and p-tau181/Aβ42) and for the 37 RBM analytes with p<0.05 in the univariate analyses. Each traditional biomarker was then combined with each RBM analyte to identify '2-marker panels' with improved AUCs. Among the traditional biomarkers, the ratios tau/Aβ42 and p-tau181/Aβ42 demonstrated the highest AUCs; additionally, combining these ratios with the RBM analytes consistently yielded 2-marker panels with AUCs higher than combinations of the individual traditional biomarkers (Aβ42, tau, p-tau181) with the RBM analytes. Thus, only the most promising 2-marker panels (those with tau/Aβ42 and p-tau181/Aβ42) are shown here. To determine whether combinations of three markers could yield a small panel with improved diagnostic accuracy, the four 2-marker panels with the highest AUCs were combined with the 10 RBM analytes with the highest individual AUCs (indicated by §, results in Table 5).

doi:10.1371/journal.pone.0018850.t004

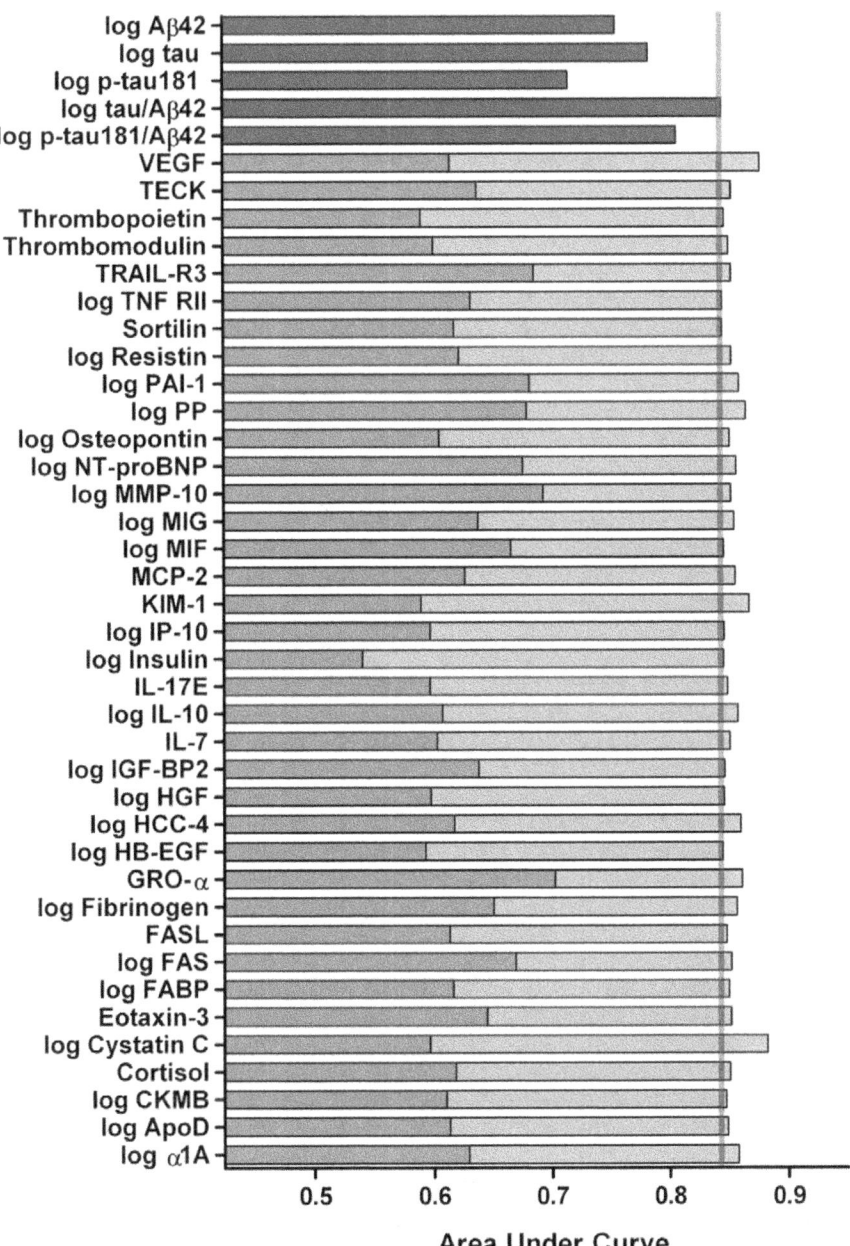

Figure 1. ROC analyses, graphical representation. ROC analyses assessed the ability of the traditional biomarkers (blue) and of the 37 RBM analytes with p<0.05 in the univariate analyses (red) to discriminate CDR>0 from CDR 0 individuals. Combining the best-performing of the traditional biomarkers, the tau/Aβ42 ratio, with RBM analytes improved upon the AUC of tau/Aβ42 in many cases (green). doi:10.1371/journal.pone.0018850.g001

effective early in the disease process before significant synaptic and neuronal loss has occurred. Thus, we used univariate and multivariate Cox proportional hazards models to evaluate the ability of the analytes to predict risk of developing cognitive impairment (conversion from CDR 0 to CDR>0). Of the 215 CDR 0 subjects with at least one follow-up annual clinical assessment, 29 received a CDR>0 at follow-up, and thus were classified as "converters." Analyte measurements were converted to standard Z-scores to allow for comparison of hazard ratios between the different analytes. Variables with p<0.15 in the univariate Cox analyses were considered for inclusion in the multivariate model; variables were retained in the final model if p<0.05. By univariate Cox analysis, calbindin (p = 0.0163), cortisol (p = 0.0688), HGF (p = 0.1364), MCP-2 (p = 0.0412), MIG (p = 0.0208), MIF (p = 0.0950), S100B (p = 0.1275), TNF

RII (p = 0.0645), TRAIL-R3 (p = 0.0833), Aβ42 (p = <0.0001), tau (p = 0.0071), and p-tau181 (p = 0.0087) were selected for further investigation by multivariate analysis. The final multivariate model consisted of calbindin (HR = 1.750, p = 0.0063), 1/Aβ42 (HR = 2.454, p<0.0001), and age at LP (HR = 1.096, p = 0.0002), with an overall HR of 4.704 (Table 8). Although calbindin and tau both had p<0.05 in the univariate analysis, the significant correlation between the two (r = 0.476, p<0.0001) prohibited inclusion of both variables in the multivariate model. Therefore, a second multivariate model consisted of tau (HR = 1.467, p = 0.0262), 1/Aβ42 (HR = 2.247, p<0.0001), and age at LP (HR = 1.098, p = 0.0003), with an overall HR of 3.619 (Table 8). However, the higher HR of calbindin than of tau, and the higher overall HR and lower AIC of the first model support it as the better model.

Table 5. ROC analyses of 3-marker panels.

Marker Panels	AUC	Stdev	95% CI	Sensitivity (at 80% specificity)	Stdev	95% CI	p-value	Stdev	95% CI
log tau/Aβ42 + log Cystatin C + TRAIL-R3	0.9014	0.0232	0.8969–0.9060	0.8367	0.0445	0.8280–0.8455	0.0299	0.0222	0.0255–0.0342
log tau/Aβ42 + log Cystatin C + log PAI-1	0.9063	0.0221	0.9020–0.9106	0.8470	0.0438	0.8384–0.8556	0.0283	0.0344	0.0215–0.0351
log tau/Aβ42 + log Cystatin C + log PP	0.9066	0.0203	0.9026–0.9106	0.8471	0.0400	0.8393–0.8550	0.0245	0.0319	0.0183–0.0307
log tau/Aβ42 + log Cystatin C + NT-proBNP	0.9041	0.0228	0.8996–0.9086	0.8422	0.0445	0.8335–0.8509	0.0287	0.0330	0.0223–0.0352
log tau/Aβ42 + log Cystatin C + log MMP-10	0.8987	0.0230	0.8942–0.9032	0.8317	0.0447	0.8230–0.8405	0.0647	0.0582	0.0533–0.0761
log tau/Aβ42 + log Cystatin C + log MIF	0.8964	0.0249	0.8915-0.9013	0.8272	0.0487	0.8177–0.8368	0.0699	0.0569	0.0588–0.0811
log tau/Aβ42 + log Cystatin C + GRO-α	0.9071	0.0218	0.9028–0.9113	0.8475	0.0412	0.8395–0.8556	0.0347	0.0410	0.0266–0.0427
log tau/Aβ42 + log Cystatin C + log Fibrinogen	0.9033	0.0219	0.8990–0.9075	0.8403	0.0429	0.8319–0.8487	0.0357	0.0502	0.0259–0.0455
log tau/Aβ42 + log Cystatin C + log FAS	0.9052	0.0220	0.9009–0.9095	0.8440	0.0425	0.8356–0.8523	0.0248	0.0248	0.0200–0.0297
log tau/Aβ42 + log Cystatin C + Eotaxin-3	0.9051	0.0219	0.9008–0.9094	0.8441	0.0427	0.8357–0.8524	0.0273	0.0350	0.0205–0.0342
log tau/Aβ42 + VEGF + TRAIL-R3	0.9004	0.0226	0.8960–0.9049	0.8347	0.0437	0.8262–0.8433	0.0208	0.0158	0.0177–0.0239
log tau/Aβ42 + VEGF + log PAI-1	0.9005	0.0225	0.8961–0.9049	0.8355	0.0445	0.8267–0.8442	0.0272	0.0320	0.0210–0.0335
log tau/Aβ42 + VEGF + log PP	0.9039	0.0215	0.8997–0.9081	0.8423	0.0422	0.8340–0.8506	0.0167	0.0250	0.0118–0.0216
log tau/Aβ42 + VEGF + NT-proBNP	0.9028	0.0224	0.8984–0.9072	0.8396	0.0439	0.8310–0.8482	0.0165	0.0207	0.0124–0.0205
log tau/Aβ42 + VEGF + log MMP-10	0.8947	0.0242	0.8900–0.8995	0.8241	0.0471	0.8149–0.8333	0.0534	0.0519	0.0432–0.0636
log tau/Aβ42 + VEGF + log MIF	0.8908	0.0261	0.8857–0.8959	0.8164	0.0506	0.8065–0.8264	0.0703	0.0570	0.0591–0.0815
log tau/Aβ42 + VEGF + GRO-α	0.9003	0.0238	0.8956–0.9049	0.8348	0.0452	0.8259–0.8436	0.0365	0.0371	0.0292–0.0437
log tau/Aβ42 + VEGF + log Fibrinogen	0.8988	0.0231	0.8943–0.9033	0.8317	0.0449	0.8229–0.8405	0.0327	0.0457	0.0237–0.0416
log tau/Aβ42 + VEGF + log FAS	0.9012	0.0232	0.8967–0.9058	0.8363	0.0445	0.8276–0.8451	0.0232	0.0248	0.0183–0.0281
log tau/Aβ42 + VEGF + Eotaxin-3	0.8991	0.0227	0.8947–0.9036	0.8325	0.0441	0.8239–0.8411	0.0293	0.0354	0.0224–0.0363
log tau/Aβ42 + KIM-1 + TRAIL-R3	0.8810	0.0256	0.8760–0.8860	0.7979	0.0486	0.7884–0.8075	0.1082	0.0747	0.0936–0.1229
log tau/Aβ42 + KIM-1 + log PAI-1	0.8866	0.0246	0.8818–0.8915	0.8087	0.0476	0.7993–0.8180	0.0614	0.0607	0.0495-0.0733
log tau/Aβ42 + KIM-1 + log PP	0.8905	0.0239	0.8858–0.8952	0.8162	0.0467	0.8070–0.8253	0.0357	0.0452	0.0269–0.0445
log tau/Aβ42 + KIM-1 + NT-proBNP	0.8821	0.0260	0.8770–0.8872	0.8001	0.0500	0.7903–0.8099	0.0926	0.0788	0.0772–0.1081
log tau/Aβ42 + KIM-1 + log MMP-10	0.8787	0.0270	0.8734–0.8840	0.7940	0.0511	0.7840–0.8040	0.1497	0.1015	0.1298–0.1696
log tau/Aβ42 + KIM-1 + log MIF	0.8775	0.0276	0.8721–0.8829	0.7918	0.0518	0.7816–0.8019	0.1478	0.0941	0.1294–0.1663
log tau/Aβ42 + KIM-1 + GRO-α	0.8897	0.0242	0.8850–0.8945	0.8153	0.0448	0.8065–0.8241	0.0513	0.0498	0.0416–0.0611
log tau/Aβ42 + KIM-1 + log Fibrinogen	0.8821	0.0267	0.8769–0.8874	0.8003	0.0507	0.7903–0.8102	0.0927	0.0809	0.0768–0.1085
log tau/Aβ42 + KIM-1 + log FAS	0.8806	0.0248	0.8757–0.8855	0.7973	0.0472	0.7881–0.8066	0.1157	0.0852	0.0990–0.1324
log tau/Aβ42 + KIM-1 + Eotaxin-3	0.8805	0.0264	0.8753–0.8857	0.7973	0.0498	0.7875-0.8071	0.1152	0.0943	0.0967–0.1337
log tau/Aβ42 + log PP + TRAIL-R3	0.8717	0.0249	0.8668–0.8766	0.7790	0.0488	0.7695–0.7886	0.2225	0.1023	0.2024–0.2425
log tau/Aβ42 + log PP + log PAI-1	0.8715	0.0250	0.8666–0.8764	0.7782	0.0498	0.7685–0.7880	0.2034	0.1052	0.1828–0.2240
log tau/Aβ42 + log PP + NT-proBNP	0.8723	0.0254	0.8674–0.8773	0.7806	0.0491	0.7710–0.7902	0.1705	0.1051	0.1499–0.1912
log tau/Aβ42 + log PP + log MMP-10	0.8702	0.0256	0.8652–0.8753	0.7761	0.0507	0.7662–0.7860	0.2394	0.1204	0.2158–0.2630
log tau/Aβ42 + log PP + log MIF	0.8685	0.0251	0.8635–0.8734	0.7723	0.0496	0.7625–0.7820	0.2909	0.1014	0.2711–0.3108
log tau/Aβ42 + log PP + GRO-α	0.8755	0.0250	0.8706–0.8804	0.7875	0.0472	0.7783–0.7968	0.1329	0.0908	0.1151–0.1507
log tau/Aβ42 + log PP + log Fibrinogen	0.8720	0.0255	0.8670–0.8769	0.7795	0.0498	0.7698–0.7893	0.1878	0.1160	0.1651–0.2106
log tau/Aβ42 + log PP + log FAS	0.8701	0.0244	0.8653–0.8749	0.7752	0.0487	0.7657–0.7847	0.2335	0.1091	0.2121–0.2548
log tau/Aβ42 + log PP + Eotaxin-3	0.8722	0.0245	0.8674–0.8770	0.7795	0.0487	0.7699–0.7890	0.1813	0.1087	0.1599–0.2026

AUC = area under the curve; Stdev = standard deviation; CI = confidence interval.
Receiver operating characteristic (ROC) analyses assessed the ability of three marker panels to discriminate CDR 0 from CDR>0 participants. Averages of performance measures were taken over 100 iterations of the bootstrap. "p-value" assesses the difference between the three marker panel and the corresponding two marker panel (e.g. log tau/Aβ42 + log Cystatin C + TRAIL-R3 vs. log tau/Aβ42 + log Cystatin C).
doi:10.1371/journal.pone.0018850.t005

Discussion

Biomarkers that can detect AD in its early stages and, importantly, predict future dementia will be invaluable for efficient clinical trial design and eventually patient care. This study identifies novel biomarkers that improve upon the ability of the best identified biomarkers to date to discriminate very mildly demented from cognitively normal participants, and identifies a novel biomarker with significant prognostic potential.

Using Luminex technology and a targeted multiplex panel, we identified 37 analytes (12 with Bonferroni correction) that are increased or decreased in the CSF of participants with early AD

Table 6. Performance measures of machine learning algorithms in discriminating cognitively normal (CDR 0) from very mildly/ mildly demented (CDR 0.5 and 1) participants.

Model	Traditional Biomarkers				Traditional + RBM Biomarkers			
	Sensitivity	Specificity	Youden Index	AUC	Sensitivity	Specificity	Youden Index	AUC
Boosted Tree	0.843	0.525	0.368	0.782	0.845	0.776	0.621	0.868
Flexible Discriminant Analysis	0.882	0.546	0.428	0.827	0.827	0.672	0.499	0.808
K-Nearest Neighbors	0.866	0.552	0.418	0.813	0.886	0.627	0.513	0.814
Logistic Regression	0.902	0.490	0.392	0.819	0.791	0.667	0.458	0.757
Naïve Bayes	0.898	0.492	0.390	0.799	0.802	0.599	0.401	0.754
Partial Least Squares	0.914	0.457	0.371	0.822	0.858	0.693	0.551	0.851
Sparse Partial Least Squares	0.914	0.457	0.371	0.822	0.858	0.694	0.552	0.851
Random Forests	0.872	0.566	0.438	0.810	0.932	0.596	0.528	0.866
Nearest Shrunken Centroids	0.882	0.527	0.409	0.805	0.833	0.643	0.476	0.802
Support Vector Machine	0.806	0.424	0.230	0.680	0.929	0.645	0.574	0.868

Ten statistical machine learning algorithms were used to determine groups of markers capable of distinguishing very mildly/mildly demented (CDR 0.5 and 1 combined) from cognitively normal participants (CDR 0). Models were fit with two sets of predictors: 1) traditional biomarkers, or 2) traditional biomarkers plus RBM analytes; additionally, age, gender, and ApoE4 allele status were included in all models. Model performance measures shown are based on cross-validation, in which the test set results were averaged from 200 splits of the data between training (80%) and test (20%).
doi:10.1371/journal.pone.0018850.t006

relative to cognitively normal controls. ROC analysis revealed that small combinations of a subset of these markers (cystatin C, VEGF, TRAIL-R3, PAI-1, PP, NT-proBNP, MMP-10, MIF, GRO-α, fibrinogen, FAS, and eotaxin-3) can enhance the ability of the best-performing of the traditional biomarkers, the tau/Aβ42 ratio, to discriminate CDR 0.5 and 1 from CDR 0 participants.

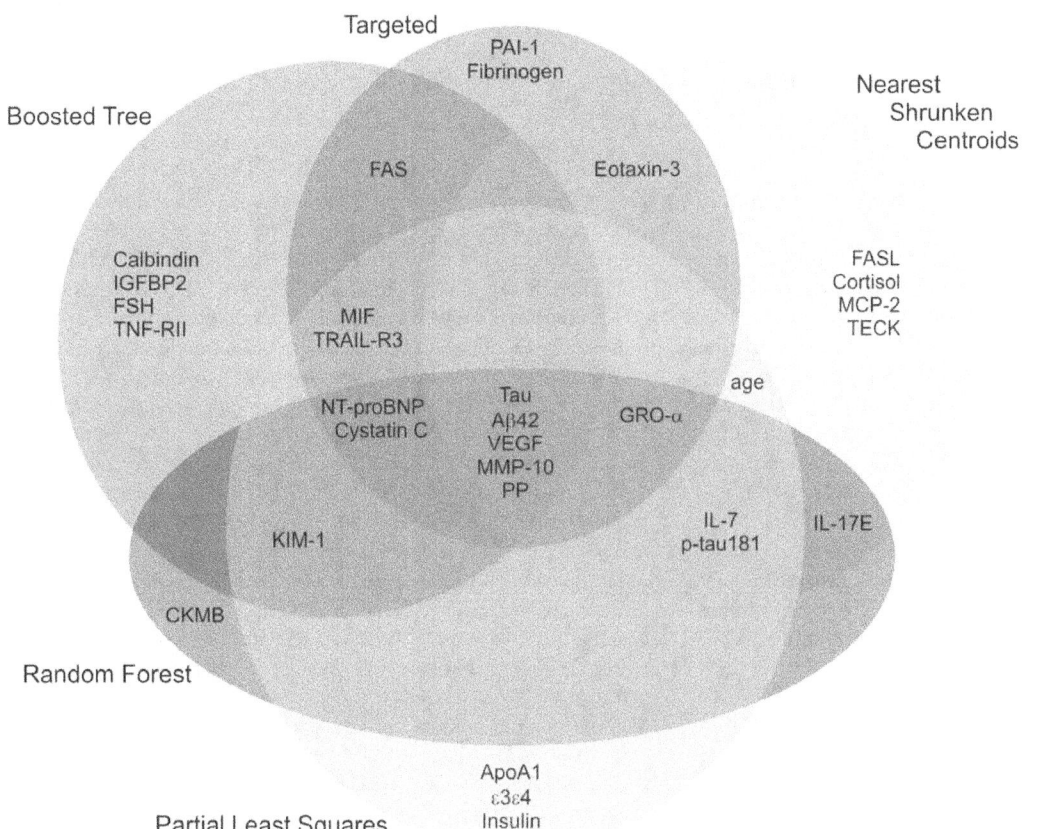

Figure 2. Venn diagram of the top 15 predictors for machine learning algorithms with a built-in importance measure. For the four models with a built-in importance statistic (i.e., Boosted Tree, Nearest Shrunken Centroids, Random Forests, and Partial Least Squares), there is considerable overlap in the top 15 predictors for each model. Additionally, nearly all of the markers found to best discriminate CDR 0 from CDR>0 participants in the more targeted ROC analyses (Table 5), as shown here ('Targeted'), were also identified as the top predictors in the machine learning models.
doi:10.1371/journal.pone.0018850.g002

Table 7. Top 15 predictors for machine learning algorithms with a built-in importance measure.

Predictor	Boosted Tree	Nearest Shrunken Centroids	Random Forests	Partial Least Squares
1	tau	Tau	Aβ42	Tau
2	Aβ42	Aβ42	tau	Aβ42
3	VEGF	p-tau181	MMP-10	VEGF
4	MMP-10	GRO-α	KIM-1	p-tau181
5	PP	VEGF	VEGF	GRO-α
6	KIM-1	Eotaxin-3	IL-7	PP
7	Cystatin C	Age	IL-17E	Cystatin C
8	Calbindin	PP	PP	NT-proBNP
9	NT-proBNP	Cortisol	NT-proBNP	MMP-10
10	MIF	MCP-2	TRAIL-R3	KIM-1
11	IGFBP-2	TECK	p-tau181	Apo A1
12	TRAIL-R3	MMP-10	Cystatin C	ε3ε4
13	FSH	IL-17E	MIF	IL-7
14	FAS	IL-7	GRO-α	Insulin
15	TNF RII	FASL	CKMB	Age

Ranking of the top 15 predictors for the four models with a built-in importance statistic demonstrates considerable overlap in the top predictors for each model. Furthermore, nearly all of the markers found to best discriminate CDR 0 from CDR>0 participants in the more targeted ROC analyses (Table 5) were also identified as the top predictors in the machine learning models, reconfirming their biomarker potential.
doi:10.1371/journal.pone.0018850.t007

Using alternative statistical strategies that are more amenable to the analysis of larger combinations of markers, multiple machine learning algorithms likewise showed that the novel biomarkers improved upon the diagnostic performance of the traditional biomarkers (Aβ42, tau, p-tau181). Importantly, nearly all of the markers found to best discriminate CDR 0 from CDR 0.5 and 1 participants in the more targeted ROC analyses were also identified as the top predictors in the machine learning models that contain a built-in importance statistic (10 of 12 markers). Thus, the potential of these analytes as biomarkers for AD is supported by alternative statistical approaches that yielded similar results. Further supporting these results is a recent report of the application of a smaller RBM Discovery MAP panel to a smaller cohort of AD, MCI, and control subjects [18]; this study identified a number of the same analytes as being differentially expressed in AD CSF as compared to control CSF and, although using different analytical approaches, included VEGF, TRAIL-R3, and eotaxin-3, in 'combined' models of novel and traditional biomarkers.

It is important to note that while the models used in our study suggest diagnostic value of the novel biomarkers, other combinations of these markers may be optimal; it will be of interest in future studies to validate the results of this discovery study in additional cohorts and to determine whether alternative combinations of these markers may demonstrate improved performance. The levels of at least 7 of the novel biomarkers have been evaluated in AD subjects in other studies: no change was observed in plasma PAI-1 levels [44]; in agreement with our findings, two studies have reported increased CSF MIF in AD and MCI subjects [45], [46]; also consistent with our findings, increased fibrinogen levels have been observed in AD and MCI CSF [47] and in AD plasma [48], and increased plasma levels have been associated with an increased risk of future dementia [49]; results have been mixed regarding CSF FAS levels in AD [50], [51]; AD plasma/serum VEGF levels have been reported to be unchanged [52], [53], decreased [54], and increased [55], while CSF levels have been reported to be

unchanged [56] or increased [57]; no change in CSF or serum levels of TNF RII in AD has been reported [58]; cystatin C findings have been inconsistent, with reports of serum/plasma levels unchanged [59], increased in AD [60] or in those who later develop AD [61], and decreased [62] or decreased levels associated with increased risk of future AD [63], while CSF levels have been reported to be unchanged [59], [64], decreased [65], or increased [21]. These inconsistent results may be due in part to the existence of a truncated form of cystatin C, which was found to be increased in AD CSF, while the full length protein was decreased [20], [21].

Furthermore, the potential involvement of each marker in AD pathophysiology necessitates investigation. The candidate biomarkers identified in the ROC and machine learning portions of this study belong to a wide variety of functional classes and pathways, including tissue remodeling and angiogenesis (MMP-10, VEGF), regulation of apoptosis (TRAIL-R3, FAS), neutrophil, eosinophil, and/or basophil chemotaxis (GRO-α, eotaxin-3), blood coagulation (Fibrinogen, PAI-1), intravascular volume homeostasis (NT-proBNP), and gastrointestinal and pancreatic secretions (PP). In addition, a number of molecules involved in inflammatory pathways were identified in the machine learning models (IL-7, IL-17E, TNF RII, MCP-2, FASL, MIF). The association of several of the candidate biomarkers with AD pathophysiology has already been probed, most notably for cystatin C, which appears to play a role in preventing Aβ oligomerization and amyloidogenesis [66–70], and to a lesser extent for PAI-1 [71–73], MIF [45], [74], fibrinogen [75], [76], FAS and FASL [77–80], VEGF [81–83], and TNF RII [84–86].

It will be important in future studies to assess each candidate biomarker's value in diagnosis in independent sample sets when combined with other existing biomarkers or imaging tools. The existing gold standard validated biomarkers include CSF tau, p-tau181, and amyloid imaging, which differ between control and AD populations and mark underlying AD pathology [4], [6], [31], [32]. Additionally, to follow up on these biomarker candidates, their ability to discriminate AD from other causes of dementia

Table 8. Cox proportional hazards models for predicting risk of developing cognitive impairment (conversion from CDR 0 to CDR>0).

	Marker	HR	95% CI	P	
A.	Marker	HR	95% CI	P	
	Log Calbindin	1.736	1.161–2.596	0.0072	
	Log 1/Aβ42	2.361	1.564–3.564	<0.0001	
	Age	1.094	1.043–1.147	0.0002	
	Gender	0.722	0.326–1.599	0.4216	
B.	Marker	HR	95% CI	P	
	Log Calbindin	1.752	1.176–2.609	0.0058	
	Log 1/Aβ42	2.485	1.655–3.731	<0.0001	
	Age	1.092	1.037–1.149	0.0008	
	ApoE4	0.847	0.355–2.025	0.7094	
C.	Marker	HR	95% CI	P	**Overall HR 4.704**
	Log Calbindin	1.750	1.172–2.613	0.0063	
	Log 1/Aβ42	2.454	1.637–3.679	<0.0001	
	Age	1.096	1.045–1.149	0.0002	
D.	Marker	HR	95% CI	P	
	Log Tau	1.462	1.039–2.057	0.0294	
	Log 1/Aβ42	2.221	1.477–3.339	0.0001	
	Age	1.096	1.041–1.154	0.0005	
	Gender	0.724	0.334–1.566	0.4113	
E.	Marker	HR	95% CI	P	**Overall HR 3.610**
	Log Tau	1.467	1.046–2.056	0.0262	
	Log 1/Aβ42	2.247	1.496–3.375	<0.0001	
	Age	1.098	1.043–1.156	0.0003	

Cox proportional hazards models were used to identify panels of biomarkers predictive of the risk of developing cognitive impairment (conversion from CDR 0 to CDR>0). Analyte measurements were converted to standard Z-scores to allow for comparison of hazard ratios between the different analytes. Variables with p<0.15 in the univariate Cox analyses were considered for inclusion in multivariate models; variables were retained in the final model if p<0.05. Because many of the analytes, including calbindin, demonstrated age and gender affects, both variables were entered into the multivariate models. However, as gender did not appear to contribute to the models (A, D), it was not included in the final panels (C, E). Similarly, apoE allelic status (E4+ vs. E4−) did not contribute to the models (B), and was not included in the final model (C). Although calbindin and tau both demonstrated p<0.05 in the univariate analyses, the significant correlation between the two (r = 0.476, p<0.0001) prohibited inclusion of both variables in the multivariate model. Therefore, a separate multivariate model that included tau was evaluated (D, E). The higher HR of calbindin than of tau, and the higher overall HR (4.704>3.610) and lower AIC (227.6<230.8) of the first model support it as the better model.
doi:10.1371/journal.pone.0018850.t008

needs to be examined; indeed, several of these markers have already shown promise for distinguishing AD from frontotemporal lobar degeneration (cystatin C [20], eotaxin-3 [18], and HGF [18]). Incorporation of such markers into a biomarker panel may improve diagnostic specificity. Beyond their clinical use, these markers may have great value in the design of and enrollment in trials of disease-modifying therapies. By enrolling only subjects with lower or higher values of a particular marker (or panels of markers) indicative of AD, and excluding potential subjects with intermediate or 'overlap' values, one might provide greater diagnostic certainty than is possible through clinical evaluation alone. This is especially relevant for the design and evaluation of primary prevention trials in cognitively normal cohorts. Enriching study populations for subjects displaying certain biomarker levels may result in studies of greater efficacy, translating to reduced cost and duration.

This study also suggests a novel biomarker, CSF calbindin, that can predict risk of future dementia in individuals who are still cognitively normal. Previous studies have shown that Aβ42, tau, YKL-40 (an astrocyte marker), and the ratios tau/Aβ42 and YKL-40/Aβ42 can predict subsequent cognitive decline in non-demented cohorts [7], [15], [87]. Using multivariate Cox proportional hazards models to determine the best combination of biomarkers for prognosis, we show here that a panel of markers consisting of calbindin, Aβ42, and age has predictive value comparable to, if not better than, a second panel consisting of tau, Aβ42, and age. Tissue culture studies have shown that increased expression of calbindin, a calcium binding protein present in central and peripheral nervous system neurons, correlates with increased resistance to cell death triggered by a variety of causes, including exposure to excitatory amino acids, ischemic injury, and Aβ [88–91]. Decreases in calbindin protein and mRNA levels [92] and number of calbindin-immunopositive neurons [93–95] have been observed in AD brains compared to controls. Further suggesting there may be a role for calbindin in AD pathophysiology is the large body of literature demonstrating that increased oxidative stress and altered calcium homeostasis appear to be interrelated mechanisms in AD pathogenesis. Interestingly, although not quite reaching statistical significance, we found that CSF calbindin levels trended higher in the very mildly/mildly demented group (p = .0660; CDR 0 = 145.9 ng/mL, CDR>0 = 157.4 ng/mL), suggesting that perhaps degenerating neurons release calbindin into the CSF. The immunohistochemical findings of a small study of 6 AD brains suggesting that calbindin-immunopositive neurons are relatively preserved in cases with moderate amyloid plaque and neurofibrillary content but are lost in more severe cases [94] prompts the question of whether CSF calbindin levels would be more significantly elevated in more severely demented individuals. Further studies are needed to confirm the prognostic potential of CSF calbindin, to determine if other complementary fluid or imaging biomarkers may improve upon its performance, and to more definitively elucidate its role in AD pathophysiology. As with the candidate diagnostic biomarkers, CSF calbindin may have value for clinical trial design by allowing for the selective enrollment of individuals who are at greater risk of developing cognitive impairment, resulting in clinical trials of shorter duration and reduced cost.

Supporting Information

Table S1 Means and standard deviations of the 125 RBM analytes and traditional biomarkers. The means and standard deviations of the 125 measurable RBM analytes and the traditional biomarkers are provided.
(DOC)

Table S2 ANCOVA: Age and gender interactions. As shown in Table 2, the mean concentrations of 37 CSF RBM analytes were found to differ between cognitively normal (CDR 0) and very mildly/mildly demented (CDR 0.5 and 1) participants by analysis of covariance (ANCOVA) adjusting for age and gender (p<0.05). ANCOVA showed that a number of these analytes demonstrated significant interactions with age or gender, as shown here.
(DOC)

Acknowledgments

We gratefully acknowledge the contributions of the volunteer participants, lumbar puncture physicians, and the Clinical, Psychometrics, Biomarker, Imaging and Biostatistics Cores of the Knight Alzheimer's Disease Research Center at Washington University.

Author Contributions

Conceived and designed the experiments: RC-S MK CX EHP TPM RJP KRB HS AMF DMH. Performed the experiments: RC-S MK CX TPM. Analyzed the data: RC-S MK CX EHP JL KRB HS DMH. Contributed reagents/materials/analysis tools: RC-S MK CX EHP TPM AMF DMH. Wrote the paper: RC-S MK TPM RJP HS DMH.

References

1. Craig-Schapiro R, Fagan AM, Holtzman DM (2009) Biomarkers of Alzheimer's disease. Neurobiol Dis 35: 128–140.
2. Hampel H, Burger K, Teipel SJ, Bokde AL, Zetterberg H, Blennow K (2008) Core candidate neurochemical and imaging biomarkers of Alzheimer's disease. Alzheimers Dement 4: 38–48.
3. Jack CR, Jr., Knopman DS, Jagust WJ, Shaw LM, Aisen PS, Weiner MW, et al. (2010) Hypothetical model of dynamic biomarkers of the Alzheimer's pathological cascade. Lancet Neurol 9: 119–128.
4. Perrin RJ, Fagan AM, Holtzman DM (2009) Multimodal techniques for diagnosis and prognosis of Alzheimer's disease. Nature 461: 916–922.
5. Blennow K, Hampel H (2003) CSF Markers for Incipient Alzheimer's Disease. Lancet Neurol 2: 605–613.
6. Fagan A, Mintun M, Mach R, Lee S-Y, Dence C, Shah A, et al. (2006) Inverse relation between in vivo amyloid imaging load and CSF Aβ42 in humans. Ann Neurol 59: 512–519.
7. Fagan A, Roe C, Xiong C, Mintun M, Morris J, Holtzman D (2007) Cerebrospinal fluid tau/Aβ42 ratio as a prediction of cognitive decline in nondemented older adults. Arch Neurol 64: 343–349.
8. Fagan AM, Mintun MA, Shah AR, Aldea P, Roe CM, Mach RH, et al. (2009) Cerebrospinal fluid tau and ptau(181) increase with cortical amyloid deposition in cognitively normal individuals: implications for future clinical trials of Alzheimer's disease. EMBO Mol Med 1: 371–380.
9. Jagust WJ, Landau SM, Shaw LM, Trojanowski JQ, Koeppe RA, Reiman EM, et al. (2009) Relationships between biomarkers in aging and dementia. Neurology 73: 1193–1199.
10. Andreasen N, Hess C, Davidsson P, Minthon L, Wallin A, Winblad B, et al. (1999) Cerebrospinal fluid β-amyloid(1-42) in Alzheimer's disease: Differences between early- and late-onset Alzheimer's disease and stability during the course of disease. Arch Neurol 56: 673–680.
11. Zetterberg H, Pedersen M, Lind K, Svensson M, Rolstad S, Eckerstrom C, et al. (2007) Intra-individual stability of CSF biomarkers for Alzheimer's disease over two years. J Alzheimers Dis 12: 255–260.
12. Andersson C, Blennow K, Almkvist O, Andreasen N, Engfeldt P, Johansson SE, et al. (2008) Increasing CSF phospho-tau levels during cognitive decline and progression to dementia. Neurobiol Aging 29: 1466–1473.
13. Buchhave P, Blennow K, Zetterberg H, Stomrud E, Londos E, Andreasen N, et al. (2009) Longitudinal study of CSF biomarkers in patients with Alzheimer's disease. PLoS One 4: e6294.
14. Hansson O, Zetterberg H, Buchhave P, Londos E, Blennow K, Minthon L (2006) Association Between CSF Biomarkers and Incipient Alzheimer's Disease in Patients with Mild Cognitive Impairment: A Follow-Up Study. Lancent Neurology 5: 228–234.
15. Li G, Sokal I, Quinn J, Leverenz J, Brodey M, Schellenberg G, et al. (2007) CSF tau/Aβ42 ratio for increased risk of mild cognitive impairment: A follow-up study. Neurology 69: 631–639.
16. Sunderland T, Linker G, Mirza N, Putnam K, Friedman D, Kimmel L, et al. (2003) Decreased β-amyloid1-42 and increased tau levels in cerebrospinal fluid of patients with Alzheimer's disease. JAMA 289: 2094–2103.
17. Zhang J, Goodlett DR, Quinn JF, Peskind E, Kaye JA, Zhou Y, et al. (2005) Quantitative proteomics of cerebrospinal fluid from patients with Alzheimer disease. J Alzheimers Dis 7: 125–133; discussion 173-180.
18. Hu WT, Chen-Plotkin A, Arnold SE, Grossman M, Clark CM, Shaw LM, et al. (2010) Novel CSF biomarkers for Alzheimer's disease and mild cognitive impairment. Acta Neuropathol 119: 669–678.
19. Simonsen A, McGuire J, Hansson O, Zetterberg H, Podust V, Davies H, et al. (2007) Novel panel of cerebrospinal fluid biomarkers for the prediction of progression to Alzheimer dementia in patients with mild cognitive impairment. Arch Neurol 64: 366–370.
20. Simonsen AH, McGuire J, Podust VN, Hagnelius NO, Nilsson TK, Kapaki E, et al. (2007) A novel panel of cerebrospinal fluid biomarkers for the differential diagnosis of Alzheimer's disease versus normal aging and frontotemporal dementia. Dement Geriatr Cogn Disord 24: 434–440.
21. Carrette O, Demalte I, Scherl A, Yalkinoglu O, Corthals G, Burkhard P, et al. (2003) A panel of cerebrospinal fluid potential biomarkers for the diagnosis of Alzheimer's disease. Proteomics 3: 1486–1494.
22. Davidsson P, Westman-Brinkmalm A, Nilsson C, Lindbjer M, Paulson L, Andreasen N, et al. (2002) Proteome analysis of cerebrospinal fluid proteins in Alzheimer patients. NeuroReport 13: 611–615.
23. Abdi F, Quinn J, Jankovic J, McIntosh M, Leverenz J, Peskind E, et al. (2006) Detection of biomarkers with a multiplex quantitative proteomic platform in cerebrospinal fluid of patients with neurodegenerative disorders. J Alzheimers Dis 9: 293–348.
24. Finehout EJ, Franck Z, Choe LH, Relkin N, Lee KH (2007) Cerebrospinal fluid proteomic biomarkers for Alzheimer's disease. Ann Neurol 61: 120–129.
25. Puchades M, Folkesson Hansson S, Nilsson C, Andreasen N, Blennow K, Davidsson P (2003) Proteomic studies of potential cerebrospinal fluid protein markers for Alzheimer's disease. Mol Brain Res 118: 140–146.
26. Hu Y, Hosseini A, Kauwe J, Gross J, Cairns N, Goate A, et al. (2007) Identification and validation of novel CSF biomarkers for early stages of Alzheimer's disease. Proteomics - Clin Appl 1: 1373–1384.
27. McKhann G, Drachman D, Folstein M, Katzman R, Price D, Stadlan E (1984) Clinical diagnosis of Alzheimer's disease: report of the NINCDS-ADRDA Work Group under the auspices of Department of Health and Human Services Task Force on Alzheimer's Disease. Neurology 34: 939–944.
28. Morris JC (1993) The Clinical Dementia Rating (CDR). Current version and scoring rules. Neurology 43: 2412–2414.
29. Storandt M, Grant E, Miller J, Morris J (2006) Longitudinal course and neuropathologic outcomes in original vs revised MCI and in pre-MCI. Neurology 67: 467–473.
30. Petersen R, Smith G, Waring S, Ivnik R, Tabgalos E, Kokmen E (1999) Mild cognitive impairment: Clinical characterization and outcome. Arch Neurol 56: 303–308.
31. Mintun M, LaRossa G, Sheline Y, Dence C, Lee S-Y, Mach R, et al. (2006) [11C]PIB in a nondemented population: Potential antecedent marker of Alzheimer disease. Neurology 67: 446–452.
32. Klunk W, Engler H, Nordberg A, Wang Y, Blomqvist G, Holt D, et al. (2004) Imaging brain amyloid in Alzheimer's disease with Pittsburgh Compound-B. Ann Neurol 55: 306–319.
33. Team RDC (2010) R: A language and environment for statistical computing. R Foundation for Statistical Computing.

34. Xiong C, McKeel D, Miller J, Morris J (2004) Combining correlated diagnostic tests---application to neuropathologic diagnosis of Alzheimer's disease. Medical Decision Making 24: 659–669.

35. Gerlach RW, Kowalski BR, Wold HOA (1979) Partial least-squares path modelling with latent variables. Analytica Chimica Acta 112: 417–421.

36. Chun H, Keleş S () Sparse partial least squares regression for simultaneous dimension reduction and variable selection. Journal of the Royal Statistical Society: Series B (Statistical Methodology) 72: 3–25.

37. Breiman L (2001) Random Forests. Mach Learn 45: 5–32.

38. Friedman JH (2001) Greedy Function Approximation: A Gradient Boosting Machine. The Annals of Statistics 29: 1189–1232.

39. Boser BE, Guyon IM, Vapnik VN (1992) A training algorithm for optimal margin classifiers. Proceedings of the fifth annual workshop on Computational learning theory. PittsburghPennsylvania, , United States: ACM.

40. Caputo B, Sim K, Furesjo F, Smola A (2001) Appearance-based object recognition using SVMs: which kernel should I use? Proceedings of Neural Information Processing Systems Workshop on Statistical methods for Computational Experiments In Visual Processing and Computer Vision. Whistler.

41. Tibshirani R, Hastie T, Narasimhan B, Chu G (2003) Class Prediction by Nearest Shrunken Centroids, with Applications to DNA Microarrays. Statistical Science 18: 104–117.

42. Hastie T, Tibshirani R, Friedman JH (2001) *The Elements of Statistical Learning*. New York: Springer-Verlag.

43. Hastie T, Tibshirani R, Buja A (1993) Flexible Discriminant Analysis by Optimal Scoring. Journal of the American Statistical Association 89: 1255–1270.

44. Ban Y, Watanabe T, Suguro T, Matsuyama TA, Iso Y, Sakai T, et al. (2009) Increased plasma urotensin-II and carotid atherosclerosis are associated with vascular dementia. J Atheroscler Thromb 16: 179–187.

45. Bacher M, Deuster O, Aljabari B, Egensperger R, Neff F, Jessen F, et al. (2010) The role of macrophage migration inhibitory factor in Alzheimer's disease. Mol Med 16: 116–121.

46. Popp J, Bacher M, Kolsch H, Noelker C, Deuster O, Dodel R, et al. (2009) Macrophage migration inhibitory factor in mild cognitive impairment and Alzheimer's disease. J Psychiatr Res 43: 749–753.

47. Lee JW, Namkoong H, Kim HK, Kim S, Hwang DW, Na HR, et al. (2007) Fibrinogen gamma-A chain precursor in CSF: a candidate biomarker for Alzheimer's disease. BMC Neurol 7: 14.

48. Chang CY, Liang HJ, Chow SY, Chen SM, Liu DZ (2007) Hemorheological mechanisms in Alzheimer's disease. Microcirculation 14: 627–634.

49. van Oijen M, Witteman JC, Hofman A, Koudstaal PJ, Breteler MM (2005) Fibrinogen is associated with an increased risk of Alzheimer disease and vascular dementia. Stroke 36: 2637–2641.

50. Tarkowski E, Wallin A, Regland B, Blennow K, Tarkowski A (2001) Local and systemic GM-CSF increase in Alzheimer's disease and vascular dementia. Acta Neurol Scand 103: 166–174.

51. Martinez M, Fernandez-Vivancos E, Frank A, De la Fuente M, Hernanz A (2000) Increased cerebrospinal fluid fas (Apo-1) levels in Alzheimer's disease. Relationship with IL-6 concentrations. Brain Res 869: 216–219.

52. Leyhe T, Hoffmann N, Stransky E, Laske C (2009) Increase of SCF plasma concentration during donepezil treatment of patients with early Alzheimer's disease. Int J Neuropsychopharmacol 12: 1319–1326.

53. Del Bo R, Scarlato M, Ghezzi S, Martinelli Boneschi F, Fenoglio C, Galbiati S, et al. (2005) Vascular endothelial growth factor gene variability is associated with increased risk for AD. Ann Neurol 57: 373–380.

54. Mateo I, Llorca J, Infante J, Rodriguez-Rodriguez E, Fernandez-Viadero C, Pena N, et al. (2007) Low serum VEGF levels are associated with Alzheimer's disease. Acta Neurol Scand 116: 56–58.

55. Chiappelli M, Borroni B, Archetti S, Calabrese E, Corsi MM, Franceschi M, et al. (2006) VEGF gene and phenotype relation with Alzheimer's disease and mild cognitive impairment. Rejuvenation Res 9: 485–493.

56. Blasko I, Lederer W, Oberbauer H, Walch T, Kemmler G, Hinterhuber H, et al. (2006) Measurement of thirteen biological markers in CSF of patients with Alzheimer's disease and other dementias. Dement Geriatr Cogn Disord 21: 9–15.

57. Tarkowski E, Issa R, Sjogren M, Wallin A, Blennow K, Tarkowski A, et al. (2002) Increased intrathecal levels of the angiogenic factors VEGF and TGF-beta in Alzheimer's disease and vascular dementia. Neurobiol Aging 23: 237–243.

58. Lanzrein AS, Johnston CM, Perry VH, Jobst KA, King EM, Smith AD (1998) Longitudinal study of inflammatory factors in serum, cerebrospinal fluid, and brain tissue in Alzheimer disease: interleukin-1beta, interleukin-6, interleukin-1 receptor antagonist, tumor necrosis factor-alpha, the soluble tumor necrosis factor receptors I and II, and alpha1-antichymotrypsin. Alzheimer Dis Assoc Disord 12: 215–227.

59. Kalman J, Marki-Zay J, Juhasz A, Santha A, Dux L, Janka Z (2000) Serum and cerebrospinal fluid cystatin C levels in vascular and Alzheimer's dementia. Acta Neurol Scand 101: 279–282.

60. Straface E, Matarrese P, Gambardella L, Vona R, Sgadari A, Silveri MC, et al. (2005) Oxidative imbalance and cathepsin D changes as peripheral blood biomarkers of Alzheimer disease: a pilot study. FEBS Lett 579: 2759–2766.

61. Lopez OL, Kuller LH, Mehta PD, Becker JT, Gach HM, Sweet RA, et al. (2008) Plasma amyloid levels and the risk of AD in normal subjects in the Cardiovascular Health Study. Neurology 70: 1664–1671.

62. Chuo LJ, Sheu WH, Pai MC, Kuo YM (2007) Genotype and plasma concentration of cystatin C in patients with late-onset Alzheimer disease. Dement Geriatr Cogn Disord 23: 251–257.

63. Sundelof J, Arnlov J, Ingelsson E, Sundstrom J, Basu S, Zethelius B, et al. (2008) Serum cystatin C and the risk of Alzheimer disease in elderly men. Neurology 71: 1072–1079.

64. Brettschneider J, Riepe MW, Petereit HF, Ludolph AC, Tumani H (2004) Meningeal derived cerebrospinal fluid proteins in different forms of dementia: is a meningopathy involved in normal pressure hydrocephalus? J Neurol Neurosurg Psychiatry 75: 1614–1616.

65. Hansson SF, Andreasson U, Wall M, Skoog I, Andreasen N, Wallin A, et al. (2009) Reduced levels of amyloid-beta-binding proteins in cerebrospinal fluid from Alzheimer's disease patients. J Alzheimers Dis 16: 389–397.

66. Kaeser SA, Herzig MC, Coomaraswamy J, Kilger E, Selenica ML, Winkler DT, et al. (2007) Cystatin C modulates cerebral beta-amyloidosis. Nat Genet 39: 1437–1439.

67. Selenica ML, Wang X, Ostergaard-Pedersen L, Westlind-Danielsson A, Grubb A (2007) Cystatin C reduces the in vitro formation of soluble Abeta1-42 oligomers and protofibrils. Scand J Clin Lab Invest 67: 179–190.

68. Sastre M, Calero M, Pawlik M, Mathews PM, Kumar A, Danilov V, et al. (2004) Binding of cystatin C to Alzheimer's amyloid beta inhibits in vitro amyloid fibril formation. Neurobiol Aging 25: 1033–1043.

69. Tizon B, Ribe EM, Mi W, Troy CM, Levy E (2010) Cystatin C protects neuronal cells from amyloid-beta-induced toxicity. J Alzheimers Dis 19: 885–894.

70. Mi W, Pawlik M, Sastre M, Jung SS, Radvinsky DS, Klein AM, et al. (2007) Cystatin C inhibits amyloid-beta deposition in Alzheimer's disease mouse models. Nat Genet 39: 1440–1442.

71. Fabbro S, Seeds NW (2009) Plasminogen activator activity is inhibited while neuroserpin is up-regulated in the Alzheimer disease brain. Journal of Neurochemistry 109: 303–315.

72. Melchor JP, Pawlak R, Strickland S (2003) The tissue plasminogen activator-plasminogen proteolytic cascade accelerates amyloid-beta (Abeta) degradation and inhibits Abeta-induced neurodegeneration. J Neurosci 23: 8867–8871.

73. Cacquevel M, Launay S, Castel H, Benchenane K, Cheenne S, Buee L, et al. (2007) Ageing and amyloid-beta peptide deposition contribute to an impaired brain tissue plasminogen activator activity by different mechanisms. Neurobiol Dis 27: 164–173.

74. Oyama R, Yamamoto H, Titani K (2000) Glutamine synthetase, hemoglobin alpha-chain, and macrophage migration inhibitory factor binding to amyloid beta-protein: their identification in rat brain by a novel affinity chromatography and in Alzheimer's disease brain by immunoprecipitation. Biochim Biophys Acta 1479: 91–102.

75. Cortes-Canteli M, Paul J, Norris EH, Bronstein R, Ahn HJ, Zamolodchikov D, et al. (2010) Fibrinogen and beta-amyloid association alters thrombosis and fibrinolysis: a possible contributing factor to Alzheimer's disease. Neuron 66: 695–709.

76. Paul J, Strickland S, Melchor JP (2007) Fibrin deposition accelerates neurovascular damage and neuroinflammation in mouse models of Alzheimer's disease. J Exp Med 204: 1999–2008.

77. Su JH, Anderson AJ, Cribbs DH, Tu C, Tong L, Kesslack P, et al. (2003) Fas and Fas ligand are associated with neuritic degeneration in the AD brain and participate in beta-amyloid-induced neuronal death. Neurobiol Dis 12: 182–193.

78. Erten-Lyons D, Jacobson A, Kramer P, Grupe A, Kaye J (2010) The FAS gene, brain volume, and disease progression in Alzheimer's disease. Alzheimers Dement 6: 118–124.

79. Ethell DW, Kinloch R, Green DR (2002) Metalloproteinase shedding of Fas ligand regulates beta-amyloid neurotoxicity. Curr Biol 12: 1595–1600.

80. Morishima Y, Gotoh Y, Zieg J, Barrett T, Takano H, Flavell R, et al. (2001) Beta-amyloid induces neuronal apoptosis via a mechanism that involves the c-Jun N-terminal kinase pathway and the induction of Fas ligand. J Neurosci 21: 7551–7560.

81. Burger S, Noack M, Kirazov LP, Kirazov EP, Naydenov CL, Kouznetsova E, et al. (2009) Vascular endothelial growth factor (VEGF) affects processing of amyloid precursor protein and beta-amyloidogenesis in brain slice cultures derived from transgenic Tg2576 mouse brain. Int J Dev Neurosci 27: 517–523.

82. Del Bo R, Ghezzi S, Scarpini E, Bresolin N, Comi GP (2009) VEGF genetic variability is associated with increased risk of developing Alzheimer's disease. J Neurol Sci 283: 66–68.

83. Patel NS, Mathura VS, Bachmeier C, Beaulieu-Abdelahad D, Laporte V, Weeks O, et al. (2010) Alzheimer's beta-amyloid peptide blocks vascular endothelial growth factor mediated signaling via direct interaction with VEGFR-2. J Neurochem 112: 66–76.

84. Cheng X, Yang L, He P, Li R, Shen Y (2010) Differential activation of tumor necrosis factor receptors distinguishes between brains from Alzheimer's disease and non-demented patients. J Alzheimers Dis 19: 621–630.

85. Patel JR, Brewer GJ (2008) Age-related differences in NFkappaB translocation and Bcl-2/Bax ratio caused by TNFalpha and Abeta42 promote survival in middle-age neurons and death in old neurons. Exp Neurol 213: 93–100.

86. Zhao M, Cribbs DH, Anderson AJ, Cummings BJ, Su JH, Wasserman AJ, et al. (2003) The induction of the TNFalpha death domain signaling pathway in Alzheimer's disease brain. Neurochem Res 28: 307–318.

87. Craig-Schapiro R, Perrin RJ, Roe CM, Xiong C, Carter D, et al. (2010) YKL-40: a novel prognostic fluid biomarker for preclinical Alzheimer's disease. Biol Psychiatry 68: 903–912.

88. Guo Q, Christakos S, Robinson N, Mattson MP (1998) Calbindin D28k blocks the proapoptotic actions of mutant presenilin 1: reduced oxidative stress and preserved mitochondrial function. Proc Natl Acad Sci U S A 95: 3227–3232.

89. Goodman JH, Wasterlain CG, Massarweh WF, Dean E, Sollas AL, Sloviter RS (1993) Calbindin-D28k immunoreactivity and selective vulnerability to ischemia in the dentate gyrus of the developing rat. Brain Res 606: 309–314.

90. Mattson MP, Rychlik B, Chu C, Christakos S (1991) Evidence for calcium-reducing and excito-protective roles for the calcium-binding protein calbindin-D28k in cultured hippocampal neurons. Neuron 6: 41–51.

91. Prehn JH, Bindokas VP, Jordan J, Galindo MF, Ghadge GD, Roos RP, et al. (1996) Protective effect of transforming growth factor-beta 1 on beta-amyloid neurotoxicity in rat hippocampal neurons. Mol Pharmacol 49: 319–328.

92. Iacopino AM, Christakos S (1990) Specific reduction of calcium-binding protein (28-kilodalton calbindin-D) gene expression in aging and neurodegenerative diseases. Proc Natl Acad Sci U S A 87: 4078–4082.

93. Lechner T, Adlassnig C, Humpel C, Kaufmann WA, Maier H, Reinstadler-Kramer K, et al. (2004) Chromogranin peptides in Alzheimer's disease. Exp Gerontol 39: 101–113.

94. Iritani S, Niizato K, Emson PC (2001) Relationship of calbindin D28K-immunoreactive cells and neuropathological changes in the hippocampal formation of Alzheimer's disease. Neuropathology 21: 162–167.

95. Greene JR, Radenahmad N, Wilcock GK, Neal JW, Pearson RC (2001) Accumulation of calbindin in cortical pyramidal cells with ageing; a putative protective mechanism which fails in Alzheimer's disease. Neuropathol Appl Neurobiol 27: 339–342.

Blood, plasma and serum biomarkers.

97

Diagnosis of Alzheimer's Disease Based on Disease-Specific Autoantibody Profiles in Human Sera

Eric Nagele[1,9], Min Han[2,3,9], Cassandra DeMarshall[2], Benjamin Belinka[1], Robert Nagele[3]*

1 Durin Technologies, Inc., New Brunswick, New Jersey, United States of America, 2 Graduate School of Biomedical Sciences, School of Osteopathic Medicine, University of Medicine and Dentistry of New Jersey, Stratford, New Jersey, United States of America, 3 New Jersey Institute for Successful Aging, School of Osteopathic Medicine, University of Medicine and Dentistry of New Jersey, Stratford, New Jersey, United States of America

Abstract

After decades of Alzheimer's disease (AD) research, the development of a definitive diagnostic test for this disease has remained elusive. The discovery of blood-borne biomarkers yielding an accurate and relatively non-invasive test has been a primary goal. Using human protein microarrays to characterize the differential expression of serum autoantibodies in AD and non-demented control (NDC) groups, we identified potential diagnostic biomarkers for AD. The differential significance of each biomarker was evaluated, resulting in the selection of only 10 autoantibody biomarkers that can effectively differentiate AD sera from NDC sera with a sensitivity of 96.0% and specificity of 92.5%. AD sera were also distinguishable from sera obtained from patients with Parkinson's disease and breast cancer with accuracies of 86% and 92%, respectively. Results demonstrate that serum autoantibodies can be used effectively as highly-specific and accurate biomarkers to diagnose AD throughout the course of the disease.

Citation: Nagele E, Han M, DeMarshall C, Belinka B, Nagele R (2011) Diagnosis of Alzheimer's Disease Based on Disease-Specific Autoantibody Profiles in Human Sera. PLoS ONE 6(8): e23112. doi:10.1371/journal.pone.0023112

Editor: Harish Pant, National Institutes of Health, United States of America

Received May 25, 2011; **Accepted** July 6, 2011; **Published** August 3, 2011

Funding: The authors gratefully acknowledge financial support from the Foundation Venture Capital Group, L.L.C, an affiliate of the New Jersey Health Foundation. The funders had no role in study design, data collection and analysis, decision to publish, or preparation of the manuscript.

Competing Interests: MH and CD have no competing interests. EPN is a paid consultant for Durin Technologies. BB is CEO of Durin Technologies and receives a salary from Durin. He also owns stock in Durin. RGN is Founder of Durin Technologies and has stock interest. This does not alter the authors' adherence to all the PLoS ONE policies on sharing data and materials.

* E-mail: nagelero@umdnj.edu

9 These authors contributed equally to this work.

Introduction

Alzheimer's disease (AD) is an increasingly prevalent and devastating neurodegenerative disease with tremendous social and economic costs, not only to the sufferers but also to caregivers and families. It is the most common cause of dementia worldwide, affecting over 5.4 million people in the United States alone, and has seen a rapidly growing incidence in the aging population [1]. Hallmarks of AD pathology include amyloid-β deposition in neurons, amyloid plaques, tau hyperphosphorylation, neurofibrillary tangles, synaptic loss, and progressive neurodegeneration [2–4]. The disease can span decades and is thought to progress unnoticed for 5–10 years before clear symptoms emerge and clinical detection is possible using conventional means [5,6].

Accurate diagnosis of AD has proven to be difficult to achieve. Current diagnostic practices include neuroimaging techniques, behavioral history assessments, and neuropsychiatric tests [7]. None of these methods by themselves or in combination provide for early detection or yield high accuracy. There has been a great deal of research emphasis on the search for blood-borne biomarkers indicative of AD pathology, but most attempts have found only limited success [7]. Other proposed tests have significant drawbacks in the form of patient discomfort or excessive cost. The Alzheimer's community is still in dire need of a diagnostic method that is accurate, relatively non-invasive, and inexpensive.

Our previous studies have shown that autoantibodies are surprisingly numerous in human sera regardless of age or disease

[8,9]. Suspecting that these autoantibodies may play a role in neurodegenerative diseases, we sought to determine if the presence of ongoing pathology causes changes in the spectrum of autoantibodies present in the serum. If so, then perhaps these changes could be used to identify specific autoantibodies that are useful as diagnostic indicators or biomarkers. Given the large number of autoantibodies present in human sera, we utilized high-throughput protein microarray technology to assess individual autoantibody expression profiles. We searched for disease group- and control group-specific variations in autoantibody expression patterns in an effort to identify potentially useful diagnostic biomarkers. Our results show that autoantibody expression profiles, determined using protein microarray technology, can be used to select a relatively small panel of useful autoantibody biomarkers that can detect the presence of specific diseases such as AD with great accuracy using only a small sample of blood.

Materials and Methods

Ethics Statement

Approval for the use of blood samples for this study was obtained from the UMDNJ-Stratford Institutional Review Board.

Patient Samples

Serum samples from 50 AD subjects and 40 non-demented controls (NDC) were obtained from *Analytical Biological Systems, Inc.* (Wilmington, DE). 30 breast cancer (BC) serum samples and 29

Parkinson's disease (PD) serum samples were obtained from *Asterand, Inc.* (Detroit, MI). To represent different disease stages reflecting disease severity, our AD serum pool contains samples with Mini-Mental State Examination (MMSE) scores ranging from 2–24. All samples were handled by standard procedures and stored at −80°C. Diagnosis of AD was based on a medical evaluation, neuropsychiatric testing, and on the National Institute of Neurological and Communicative Disorders and the Alzheimer's Disease and Related Disorders Association criteria. Demographic characteristics of the study population are shown in Table 1.

Human Protein Microarrays

To identify autoantibodies in human sera, we used *Invitrogen's* ProtoArray v5.0 Human Protein Microarrays (Cat. *No.* - PAH0525020, *Invitrogen*, Carlsbad, CA, USA), each containing 9,486 unique human protein antigens (www.invitrogen.com/protoarray). All proteins have been expressed as GST fusion proteins in insect cells, purified under native conditions, and spotted in duplicate onto nitrocellulose-coated glass slides. All arrays were probed and scanned according to the manufacturer's instructions using commercially prepared reagents. Briefly, microarray slides were blocked (Blocking Buffer, Cat. *No. PA055, Invitrogen*) and then incubated with serum samples, diluted 1:500 in washing buffer. After washing, the arrays were probed with anti-human IgG (H+L) conjugated to AlexaFluor 647 (Cat. *No.* A-21445, Invitrogen). Arrays were then washed, dried, and immediately scanned with a GenePix 4000B Fluorescence Scanner (*Molecular Devices*, Sunnyvale, CA, USA).

Dot Blot Analysis

One μl volumes of purified recombinant human FRMD8 (0.2 μg/μl) and PTCD2 (0.1 μg/μl) proteins (Cat. No. TP307879 and TP315253, OriGene Technologies, Inc., Rockville, MD, USA), were manually pipetted onto a nitrocellulose membrane. The proteins were blocked in a 5% non-fat milk PBS-Tween solution for one hour at room temperature (RT). The proteins were then probed with human serum samples diluted 1:2000 for one hour at RT. All sera were identical to those used to probe the human protein microarrays. The dot blots were probed with anti-human IgG (H+L) HRP conjugate antibody (Cat. No. 31410, Thermo Fisher Scientific Inc., Pittsburgh, PA, USA) for one hour at RT, incubated with ECL reagent (Cat. No. 34096, Thermo

Fisher Scientific Inc., Pittsburgh, PA, USA) for one minute, and then exposed to X-ray film at various intervals.

Data Analysis

The fluorescence data for each microarray was acquired by *Genepix Pro* analysis software after scanning, and then synced with Invitrogen's lot-specific *Genepix Array List* (GAL) files. The resulting *Genepix Results* (GPR) files were then imported into Invitrogen's *Prospector 5.2* for analysis. All data is MIAME compliant and have been deposited in NCBI's Gene Expression Omnibus and are accessible through GEO Series accession number GSE 29676. The "group characterization" and "two - group comparison" features in the *IRBP Toolbox* allowed for M-statistical analysis of autoantibody expression. Sorting detectable autoantibodies by difference of prevalence between AD and NDC groups in descending order, we selected the top 10 as our potential diagnostic biomarkers.

The selected biomarkers were re-verified as significant by *Predictive Analysis for Microarrays (PAM)* – an independent algorithm relying on nearest shrunken centroid analysis to identify proteins acting as significant class-differentiators. The predictive classification accuracy of the identified biomarkers was tested with *Random Forest (RF)* using the default settings, another significance algorithm run as an *R* package (v 2.12.1). In *RF*, partitioning trees are built by successively splitting the samples according to a measure of statistical impurity at a given node until terminal nodes are as homogenous as possible. Classification accuracy for a given set of diagnostic biomarkers is reported in a confusion matrix and misclassification as an Out-Of-Bag (OOB) error score.

Results

Protein Microarrays Reveal That Autoantibodies Are Numerous in Human Serum

To detect autoantibodies in sera, we probed protein microarrays with individual serum samples (n = 149) (Table 1). Results using the standard Chebyshev Inequality p-value threshold of 0.05 suggest an average of over one thousand different autoantibodies per serum sample; although the number varied widely from one individual to the next (n = 149, 1115±1096) (Table 2). This, along with our previous work showing the presence of abundant autoantibodies via western analysis [8,9], provides strong support for a large number of autoantibodies in human sera. It appears that this may be a generally unappreciated feature of the blood, with a function that remains to be elucidated.

Selection of Autoantibody Biomarkers for AD Diagnosis

A total of 90 human serum samples (50 AD and 40 NDC) were randomly assigned to either a Training or Testing Set composed of 25 AD and 20 NDC sera each; both containing equal proportions of earlier- and later-stage AD samples as well as older and younger controls. To identify potential diagnostic autoantibodies, we probed protein microarrays, each containing 9,486 antigens, with Training Set sera and analyzed the data as described in the methods section (Fig. 1). *Prospector* analysis software determined that 451 autoantibodies had a significantly higher prevalence in the AD group than in the NDC group (p<0.01). We selected the 10 biomarkers that demonstrated the largest difference in group prevalence between AD and NDC to serve as our diagnostic indicators (Table 3). As an independent verification of the 10 biomarkers selected, we also utilized *Predictive Analysis for Microarrays* (PAM) to re-evaluate our data [10]. *PAM* confirmed that the 10 biomarkers originally selected by *Prospector* were among the most significant classifiers of AD and NDC.

Table 1. Demographics of serum donors.

Group	n	Age		Sex	MMSE
		Mean	Range	(% male)	
Alzheimer's disease	50	78.5	61–97	40%	2–24
–Earlier-stage[1]	35	78.7	61–97	43%	15–24
–Later-stage[2]	15	78.0	65–94	33%	2–14
Non-demented Controls	40	40.4	19–86	82%	–
–Older Control	20	57.7	51–86	100%	–
–Younger Control	20	24.7	19–30	65%	–
Parkinson's disease	29	74.0	53–88	55%	–
Breast Cancer	30	46.7	32–54	0%	–

[1]Earlier-stage: AD patients with MMSE≥15.
[2]Later-stage: AD patients with MMSE<15.
doi:10.1371/journal.pone.0023112.t001

Table 2. Estimate of autoantibodies per sample group.

Sample Group	(n)	Median	σ	Range
All Samples	149	920	1096	0–6389
Alzheimer's disease	50	969.25	770	0–3311
–Earlier-stage	35	826.5	672	0–2805
–Later-stage	15	1321.5	865	110–3311
Non-demented controls	40	982	965	0–3585
–Older Controls	20	1066.25	896	32–2675
–Younger Controls	20	942.5	1050	0–3585
Parkinson's disease	29	539.5	762	0–2585
Breast Cancer	30	884.5	1723	5–6389

doi:10.1371/journal.pone.0023112.t002

Verification of Biomarkers via Training and Testing Set Analyses

To assess the Training and Testing set classification accuracies of the 10 selected biomarkers, we used *Random Forest* (*RF*) [11]. *RF* is a statistical algorithm which creates voting classes of decision-making trees to evaluate the significance of each marker and classify samples. Using our 10 biomarkers to "diagnose" the Training Set (n = 45; 25 AD and 20 NDC), *RF* had an overall accuracy of greater than 93% [Out-of-Bag (OOB) Error 6.67%, a positive predictive value (PPV) of 92.3%, and a negative predictive value (NPV) of 94.7%]. When the 10 biomarkers were used to classify the Testing Set sera (n = 45; 25 AD and 20 NDC), which played no part in the biomarker selection process, *RF* distinguished AD samples from NDCs with a similar accuracy (prediction error of 6.67%, PPV of 100.0%, and NPV of 87.0%).

Biomarker Performance in Different Sample Demographics

When the 10 autoantibody biomarkers were used to classify all AD and NDC samples combined (n = 90; 50 AD, 40 NDC) using

RF, they did so with a 96.0% sensitivity and 92.5% specificity. We also tested their performance in classifying samples from different demographics: earlier-stage AD, later-stage AD, older controls, and younger controls. The 10 biomarkers classified samples with over 90% accuracy in all subgroups tested (Table 4). AD samples were correctly differentiated from younger controls with high and consistent accuracy, a common-sense indication of biomarker credibility.

Distinction of AD From Other Diseases

One must be careful in the creation of a biomarker diagnostic to ensure disease specificity. Therefore, we sought to differentiate AD from other non-neurological and neurological diseases. We acquired 30 breast cancer serum samples and used our 10 selected diagnostic biomarkers to differentiate them from the 50 AD samples. *RF* reported an OOB Error of 7.5% (PPV and NPV of 90.7% and 96.2%, respectively). These results are similar to those of the AD versus NDC trials above and demonstrate no diagnostic bias toward general disease.

We next sought to determine if it is possible to differentiate between two closely related neurodegenerative diseases. For this, we selected Parkinson's disease (PD) because it shares much in common with Alzheimer's pathology [12,13]. There is also a significant overlap (22%~48%) at the pathological and clinical levels, making it difficult to clearly distinguish these two diseases by conventional means alone [14,15]. Again, we utilized *Prospector*, *PAM*, and *RF* to identify the most significant disease classifiers. We determined that by using only five diagnostic biomarkers (Table 5), it was possible to differentiate AD samples from PD samples with over 86% accuracy (sensitivity = 90.0%, specificity = 79.3%). To our knowledge, this is the highest efficiency ever achieved with blood biomarkers to distinguish these closely related neurodegenerative diseases [15,16].

Dot Blot Confirmation of Potential Biomarkers

To further validate the differential expression of autoantibodies detected with human protein microarrays, we carried out a comparative dot-blot analysis using commercially-obtained, puri-

Figure 1. Biomarker selection and Training / Testing Analysis. Before biomarker selection, our total sample pool was split into two randomized groups: the Training Set and Testing Set. *Prospector* and *PAM* statistical analyses were performed on the Training Set to identify the top 10 most significant autoantibody classifiers of AD and NDC. We then verified the diagnostic accuracy of these selected biomarkers by using *Random Forest* to predict sample classification in the Training Set, Testing Set, and then both sets combined.
doi:10.1371/journal.pone.0023112.g001

Table 3. Identity and significance of 10 ad vs. Ndc diagnostic biomarkers.

Database ID	Description	Prevalence in AD	Prevalence in Control	p
NM_024754.2	Pentatricopeptide repeat domain 2 (PTCD2)	94.23%	14.29%	8.03E-14
BC051695.1	FERM domain containing 8 (FRMD8)	73.08%	4.76%	4.06E-13
NM_018956.2	Chromosome 9 open reading frame 9 (C9orf9)	82.69%	14.29%	3.30E-09
NM_002305.2	Lectin, galactoside-binding, soluble, 1 (galectin 1) (LGALS1)	65.39%	9.52%	3.76E-08
NM_000939.1	Proopiomelanocortin (adrenocorticotropin/ beta-lipotropin/ alpha-melanocyte stimulating hormone/ beta-melanocyte stimulating hormone/ beta-endorphin) (POMC), transcript variant 2	65.39%	11.91%	1.18E-05
NM_003668.2	Mitogen-activated protein kinase-activated protein kinase 5 (MAPKAPK5), transcript variant 1	71.15%	11.91%	8.91E-09
BC033758.1	Centaurin, alpha 2 (CENTA2)	82.69%	23.81%	5.27E-08
NM_014280.1	DnaJ homolog subfamily C member 8	78.85%	11.91%	9.49E-12
NM_024668.2	Ankyrin repeat and KH domain containing 1 (ANKHD1), transcript variant 3	73.08%	14.29%	1.05E-06
NM_023937.1	Mitochondrial ribosomal protein L34 (MRPL34), nuclear gene encoding mitochondrial protein	73.08%	16.67%	3.15E-05

doi:10.1371/journal.pone.0023112.t003

fied native proteins. We selected two of the most potent differentiating antigens identified, PTCD2 and FRMD8, and sought to verify their reactivity. The two proteins were spotted onto nitrocellulose membrane and probed with identical sera to that used on the microarrays. Results from both AD and NDC sera show strong agreement in the relative intensities of the immunoreaction in protein microarrays and dot blots (Fig. 2). The majority of AD sera reacted intensely to purified PTCD2 and FRMD8 protein, while most control sera showed a weak or no reaction (Figs. 2b, 2d). Dot blot assays independently confirmed that anti-FRMD8 and anti-PTCD2 antibodies were more predominant in AD sera than in NDC sera, and so are potentially useful as diagnostic biomarkers. Continued efforts are needed to independently confirm the remaining biomarkers.

Discussion

The identification and development of blood-borne biomarkers for accurate diagnosis and early detection of AD has long been a central goal. In the present study, we used human protein microarrays to confirm our earlier discovery using western analysis that autoantibodies are unexpectedly numerous and perhaps universally present in human sera. We also demonstrated that the

presence of disease can cause characteristic alterations in serum autoantibody profiles such that specific autoantibodies and their cognate antigens can be used effectively as diagnostic biomarkers of ongoing disease. Lastly, we demonstrate that accurate detection and diagnosis of AD from a blood sample is possible with only a small subset of these autoantibody biomarkers.

Autoantibodies Are Numerous in Human Serum

The number of autoantibodies detected in sera using protein microarrays was found to be surprisingly high, averaging over one thousand per sample but displaying wide individual variations. Ascertaining the true number of autoantibodies in individual serum samples is difficult for several technical reasons. In addition, any determination of this number employing the protein microarrays used here will, of course, be an underestimate, since the available autoantigens represent only about one third of the estimated human proteome. Regardless of these limitations, it is clear that the number of autoantibodies in a single serum sample is much higher than previously thought. The function of such a large number of autoantibodies is unknown. We suspect that they have some hitherto unrecognized, but important, role that remains to be elucidated.

Table 4. Diagnostic accuracies of selected biomarkers.

	AD (n = 50) vs.					Earlier-stage AD (n = 35) vs.		Later-stage AD (n = 15) vs.	
	All NDC	Older Control	Younger Control	PD*	Breast Cancer	All NDC	Older Control	All NDC	Older Control
	n = 40	n = 20	n = 20	n = 29	n = 30	n = 40	n = 20	n = 40	n = 20
Sensitivity %	96.0	98.0	98.0	90.0	98.0	97.1	97.1	86.7	93.3
Specificity %	92.5	85.0	90.0	79.3	83.0	92.5	90.0	97.5	90
PPV%	94.1	94.2	96.1	88.2	90.7	91.9	94.4	92.9	87.5
NPV %	94.9	94.4	94.7	82.1	96.2	97.4	94.7	95.1	94.7

*The biomarkers used for this classification are those of Table 5; all others are the biomarkers identified in Table 3.
doi:10.1371/journal.pone.0023112.t004

Table 5. Identity and significance of five AD vs. PD diagnostic biomarkers.

Database ID	Description	Prevalence in AD	Prevalence in PD	p
BC051695.1	FERM domain containing 8 (FRMD8)	9.62%	45.16%	5.93E-04
NM_003177.3	Spleen tyrosine kinase (SYK)	19.23%	70.97%	1.35E-05
BC019015.2	Mediator complex subunit 29 (MED29)	9.62%	61.29%	1.61E-06
BC003551.1	Transglutaminase 2 (C polypeptide, protein-glutamine-gamma-glutamyltransferase) (TGM2)	13.46%	61.29%	9.67E-05
BC001755.1	Leiomodin-1	26.92%	70.97%	6.84E-05

doi:10.1371/journal.pone.0023112.t005

An AD diagnostic Based on Detection of Tell-tale Autoantibody Profiles

The present study demonstrates that AD can be linked to characteristic alterations in serum autoantibody expression profiles. These changes allow for the identification and selection of specific autoantibodies that can serve as diagnostic biomarkers. As exemplified above, with only 10 autoantibody diagnostic biomarkers, AD serum samples are readily distinguished from NDC sera with a sensitivity of 96.0% and a specificity of 92.5%. The fact that these serum autoantibody biomarkers show similar patterns of reactivity in dot blots spotted with purified, native proteins further confirms the validity of the immunoreactions on protein microarrays. We also tested the efficacy of our chosen biomarkers in differentiating multiple sample demographics of

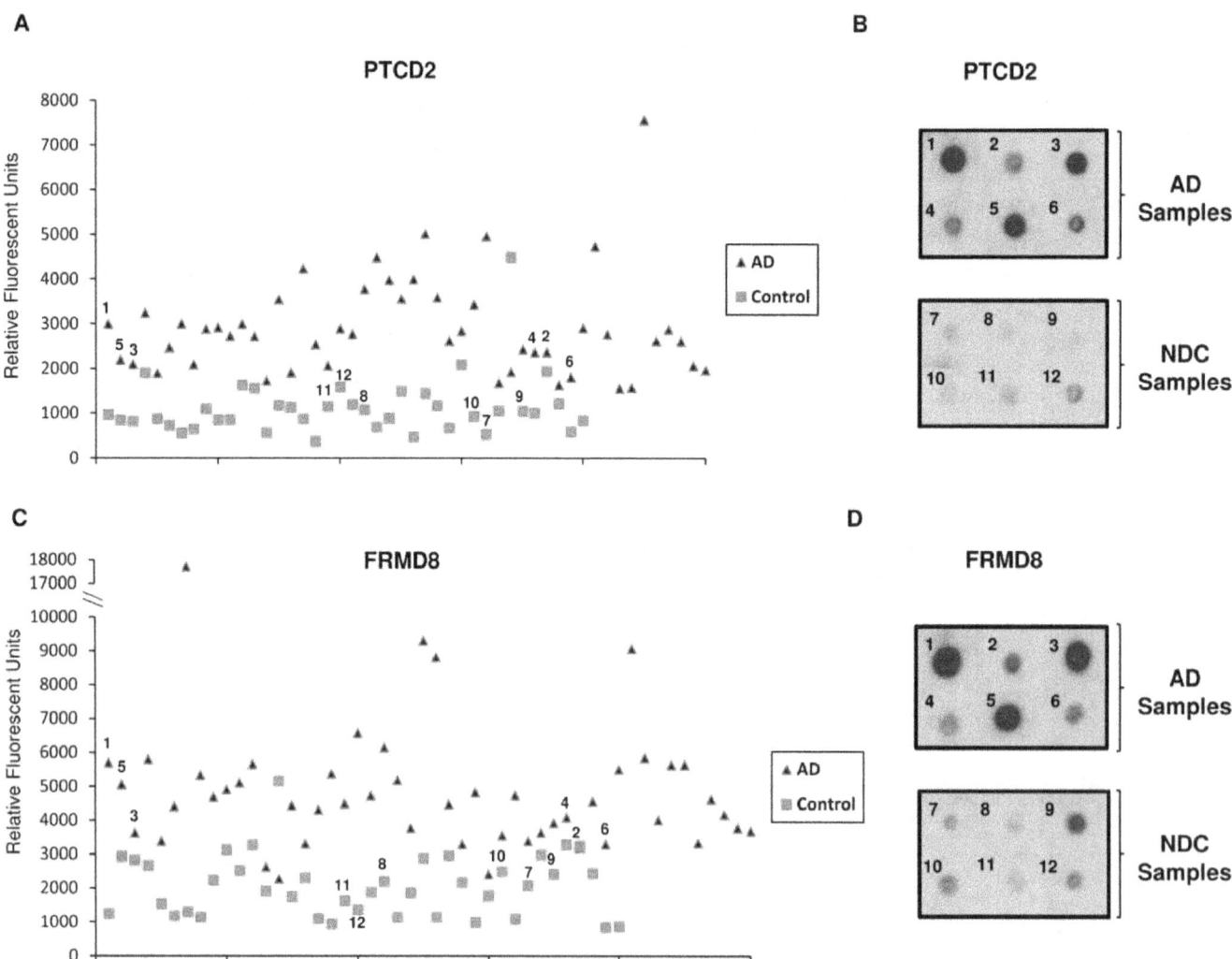

Figure 2. Differential Expression of PTCD2 and FRMD8 autoantibodies in AD and NDC sera. Microarray fluorescence values reflecting individual serum autoantibody titers demonstrate a difference in the expression of anti-PTCD2 and anti-FRMD8 in AD (n = 50) and NDC (n = 40) sera (a,c). This difference was confirmed in independent dot blots that assessed AD and NDC sera reactivity to purified PTCD2 and FRMD8 protein antigens (b,d).
doi:10.1371/journal.pone.0023112.g002

varying age and MMSE-score. We were able to distinguish AD patients from controls with over 90.0% accuracy in all subgroup comparisons. This successful classification of AD across the full range of available MMSE scores suggests that this approach is useful for AD diagnosis throughout the full course of the disease, and may also be useful for early detection, perhaps including patients with mild cognitive impairment and pre-symptomatic disease.

Future work involving more samples should extend our understanding of autoantibody expression and further optimize diagnostic success. Many of the samples used in this study were from living donors, and so their AD was diagnosed using standard clinical practices [17]. The highest accuracy claimed by these methods is roughly 90% [18–22] – thus, there is a possibility of inaccurate sample labeling. As our efforts continue with more samples and *post-mortem* validation of AD, the accuracies reported above should reflect a corresponding increase.

Multiplicity of the AD Diagnostic Panel

Aside from the discovery of so many autoantibodies being present in the blood, another unexpected finding was that many of these autoantibodies are differentially expressed in the AD and NDC groups, and so are potentially useful as diagnostic biomarkers. In fact, *Prospector* identified 199 differentiating autoantibodies with a p-value of less than 0.0001 and group prevalence differences of over 40%. Importantly, this evaluation of significance was duplicated by the other statistical algorithms used here, *PAM* and *RF*. Most autoantibodies considered significant in one program were repeatedly selected as significant diagnostic biomarkers by the other two programs. This finding suggests that many combinations of autoantibody biomarkers can be used to successfully distinguish AD sera from NDC sera with varying accuracies. Paradoxically, this multiplicity of diagnostic indicators often complicates bioinformatic analyses. The apparent inconsistency of biomarkers selected by algorithms like *RF* has been extensively discussed by others [23,24]. This has been blamed on many features of biological data, including number of variables and relative "closeness" of values. However, as reported above, we find that there are many relevant autoantibody biomarkers with diagnostic potential that make possible multiple "solutions" to a single diagnostic question. Thus, in this case, we contend that what often appears as inconsistency in this type of analysis might, in fact, simply be the selection of an equally viable set of biomarkers by the significance analysis programs.

Hypothesis Underlying the Generation of Diagnostic Autoantibodies

The underlying reason for the presence and abundance of autoantibodies in human sera, especially in younger and healthy individuals, is unknown. Although some autoantibodies may be vestiges of past diseases and reflect a history of immunological activity, it is clear that many are also present as a result of ongoing disease. We suggest that active diseases, resulting in cell damage and death, cause the production and release of antigenic cellular

products. In the case of AD, the somewhat selective early loss of pyramidal neurons provides a chronic, yet specific, source of such breakdown products. These products enter the cerebrospinal fluid, diffuse into the blood and lymph, with some presumably acting as antigens to elicit an immune response. We propose that this response leads to the production and appearance of a relatively large number of autoantibodies in the blood. Since many diseases exhibit damage to specific cell and tissue types, the biomarker discovery strategy described here could conceivably be applicable to the development of successful diagnostics for a wide variety of diseases.

Potential Benefits of Antigen Identification

One further advantage of using protein microarrays to detect disease-related autoantibodies in sera is that their antigen targets also become known. This knowledge may prove to have therapeutic implications, especially if it sheds new light on disease-relevant pathways. Such information could be used to develop therapies that combat pathology by targeting important members of these pathways. Currently, little is known about the functions of most of the antigens identified here as targets of the autoantibody biomarkers for AD. Many of them are explicit only at the genetic level as elucidated by efforts in creating comprehensive cDNA libraries [25]. As more is learned about the functions of autoantibodies in the sera and their targets, we anticipate that a better understanding of autoantibody profiles will eventually yield significant therapeutic benefits.

Conclusion

The development of a reliable and accurate blood test for AD will have profound clinical impact. The identification and use of a small panel of AD autoantibody biomarkers shown here has a diagnostic sensitivity of 96.0% and specificity of 92.5% using available samples. The relative non-invasiveness, low cost, and dynamism of protein microarrays make a diagnostic of this kind well-suited for incorporation into routine health care. We hope that with a diagnostic such as this, accessible early screening methods can be established so that patients will be better positioned to avail themselves of effective therapies as they arise.

Acknowledgments

The authors would like to thank Dr. Elizabetta Bini at the Rutgers School of Environmental and Biological Sciences for her technical help and generosity during the early phases of this work. The authors also thank Nimish Acharya for his constant help and encouragement.

Author Contributions

Conceived and designed the experiments: RGN EPN MH BB. Performed the experiments: EPN MH CD. Analyzed the data: RGN EPN MH CD. Contributed reagents/materials/analysis tools: RGN BB. Wrote the paper: RGN EPN MH CD.

References

1. Thies W, Bleiler L (2011) 2011 Alzheimer's disease facts and figures. Alzheimers Dement 7: 208–244.
2. Clifford PM, Zarrabi S, Siu G, Kinsler KJ, Kosciuk MC, et al. (2007) Abeta peptides can enter the brain through a defective blood-brain barrier and bind selectively to neurons. Brain Res 1142: 223–236.
3. Di Domenico F, Sultana R, Barone E, Perluigi M, Cini C, et al. (2011) Quantitative proteomics analysis of phosphorylated proteins in the hippocampus of Alzheimer's disease subjects. J Proteomics 74: 1091–1103.
4. Dickson DW (1997) Neuropathological diagnosis of Alzheimer's disease: a perspective from longitudinal clinicopathological studies. Neurobiol Aging 18: S21–26.
5. Morris JC (2005) Early-stage and preclinical Alzheimer disease. Alzheimer Dis Assoc Disord 19: 163–165.

6. Sperling RA, Aisen PS, Beckett LA, Bennett DA, Craft S, et al. (2011) Toward defining the preclinical stages of Alzheimer's disease: recommendations from the National Institute on Aging-Alzheimer's Association workgroups on diagnostic guidelines for Alzheimer's disease. Alzheimers Dement 7: 280–292.
7. McKhann GM, Knopman DS, Chertkow H, Hyman BT, Jack CR, Jr., et al. (2011) The diagnosis of dementia due to Alzheimer's disease: recommendations from the National Institute on Aging-Alzheimer's Association workgroups on diagnostic guidelines for Alzheimer's disease. Alzheimers Dement 7: 263–269.
8. Levin EC, Acharya NK, Han M, Zavareh SB, Sedeyn JC, et al. (2010) Brain-reactive autoantibodies are nearly ubiquitous in human sera and may be linked to pathology in the context of blood-brain barrier breakdown. Brain Res 1345: 221–232.

9. Nagele RG, Clifford PM, Siu G, Levin EC, Acharya NK, et al. (2011) Brain-reactive autoantibodies prevalent in human sera increase intraneuronal amyloid-beta1-42 deposition. J Alzheimers Dis;In press.

10. Tibshirani R, Hastie T, Narasimhan B, Chu G (2002) Diagnosis of multiple cancer types by shrunken centroids of gene expression. Proc Natl Acad Sci U S A 99: 6567–6572.

11. Breiman L (2001) Random Forests. Machine Learning 45: 5–32.

12. Haggerty T, Credle J, Rodriguez O, Wills J, Oaks AW, et al. (2011) Hyperphosphorylated Tau in an alpha-synuclein-overexpressing transgenic model of Parkinson's disease. Eur J Neurosci 33: 1598–1610.

13. Cheng F, Vivacqua G, Yu S (2010) The role of alpha-synuclein in neurotransmission and synaptic plasticity. J Chem Neuroanat: In press.

14. Aarsland D, Kurz MW (2010) The epidemiology of dementia associated with Parkinson's disease. Brain Pathol 20: 633–639.

15. Strobel G (2009) The spectrum series: grappling with the overlap between Alzheimer's and Parkinson's diseases. 9th International Conference on Alzheimer's and Parkinson's Diseases, 11–15 March 2009, Prague,Czech Republic. J Alzheimers Dis 18: 625–640.

16. DeKosky ST, Marek K (2003) Looking backward to move forward: early detection of neurodegenerative disorders. Science 302: 830–834.

17. McKhann G, Drachman D, Folstein M, Katzman R, Price D, et al. (1984) Clinical diagnosis of Alzheimer's disease: report of the NINCDS-ADRDA Work Group under the auspices of Department of Health and Human Services Task Force on Alzheimer's Disease. Neurology 34: 939–944.

18. Lopponen M, Raiha I, Isoaho R, Vahlberg T, Kivela SL (2003) Diagnosing cognitive impairment and dementia in primary health care – a more active approach is needed. Age Ageing 32: 606–612.

19. Ranginwala NA, Hynan LS, Weiner MF, White CL, 3rd (2008) Clinical criteria for the diagnosis of Alzheimer disease: still good after all these years. Am J Geriatr Psychiatry 16: 384–388.

20. Mayeux R, Saunders AM, Shea S, Mirra S, Evans D, et al. (1998) Utility of the apolipoprotein E genotype in the diagnosis of Alzheimer's disease. Alzheimer's Disease Centers Consortium on Apolipoprotein E and Alzheimer's Disease. N Engl J Med 338: 506–511.

21. Jobst KA, Barnetson LP, Shepstone BJ (1998) Accurate prediction of histologically confirmed Alzheimer's disease and the differential diagnosis of dementia: the use of NINCDS-ADRDA and DSM-III-R criteria, SPECT, X-ray CT, and Apo E4 in medial temporal lobe dementias. Int Psychogeriatr 10: 271–302.

22. Aretouli E, Brandt J (2010) Episodic memory in dementia: Characteristics of new learning that differentiate Alzheimer's, Huntington's, and Parkinson's diseases. Arch Clin Neuropsychol 25: 396–409.

23. Diaz-Uriarte R, Alvarez de Andres S (2006) Gene selection and classification of microarray data using random forest. BMC bioinformatics 7: 3.

24. Lubomirski M, D'Andrea MR, Belkowski SM, Cabrera J, Dixon JM, et al. (2007) A consolidated approach to analyzing data from high-throughput protein microarrays with an application to immune response profiling in humans. J Comput Biol 14: 350–359.

25. Gerhard DS, Wagner L, Feingold EA, Shenmen CM, Grouse LH, et al. (2004) The status, quality, and expansion of the NIH full-length cDNA project: the Mammalian Gene Collection (MGC). Genome Res 14: 2121–2127.

A Blood-Based Screening Tool for Alzheimer's Disease That Spans Serum and Plasma: Findings from TARC and ADNI

Sid E. O'Bryant[1][*][9], Guanghua Xiao[2][9], Robert Barber[3], Ryan Huebinger[4], Kirk Wilhelmsen[5], Melissa Edwards[6], Neill Graff-Radford[7], Rachelle Doody[8], Ramon Diaz-Arrastia[9], for the Texas Alzheimer's Research & Care Consortium[¤a], for the Alzheimer's Disease Neuroimaging Initiative[¤b]

1 Department of Neurology, F. Marie Hall Institute for Rural and Community Health, Garrison Institute on Aging, Texas Tech University Health Sciences Center, Lubbock, Texas, United States of America, 2 Department of Clinical Sciences, University of Texas Southwestern Medical Center, Dallas, Texas, United States of America, 3 Department of Pharmacology and Neuroscience, Institute for Aging and Alzheimer's Disease Research, University of North Texas Health Science Center, Fort Worth, Texas, United States of America, 4 Department of Surgery, University of Texas Southwestern Medical Center, Dallas, Texas, United States of America, 5 Department of Genetics, University of North Carolina School of Medicine, Chapel Hill, North Carolina, United States of America, 6 Department of Psychology, Texas Tech University, Lubbock, Texas, United States of America, 7 Department of Neurology, Mayo Clinic, Jacksonville, Florida, United States of America, 8 Department of Neurology, Alzheimer's Disease and Memory Disorders Center, Baylor College of Medicine, Houston, Texas, United States of America, 9 Center for Neuroscience and Regenerative Medicine, Uniformed Services University of the Health Sciences, Rockville, Maryland, United States of America

Abstract

Context: There is no rapid and cost effective tool that can be implemented as a front-line screening tool for Alzheimer's disease (AD) at the population level.

Objective: To generate and cross-validate a blood-based screener for AD that yields acceptable accuracy across both serum and plasma.

Design, Setting, Participants: Analysis of serum biomarker proteins were conducted on 197 Alzheimer's disease (AD) participants and 199 control participants from the Texas Alzheimer's Research Consortium (TARC) with further analysis conducted on plasma proteins from 112 AD and 52 control participants from the Alzheimer's Disease Neuroimaging Initiative (ADNI). The full algorithm was derived from a biomarker risk score, clinical lab (glucose, triglycerides, total cholesterol, homocysteine), and demographic (age, gender, education, *APOE*E4* status) data.

Major Outcome Measures: Alzheimer's disease.

Results: 11 proteins met our criteria and were utilized for the biomarker risk score. The random forest (RF) biomarker risk score from the TARC serum samples (training set) yielded adequate accuracy in the ADNI plasma sample (training set) (AUC = 0.70, sensitivity (SN) = 0.54 and specificity (SP) = 0.78), which was below that obtained from ADNI cerebral spinal fluid (CSF) analyses (t-tau/Aβ ratio AUC = 0.92). However, the full algorithm yielded excellent accuracy (AUC = 0.88, SN = 0.75, and SP = 0.91). The likelihood ratio of having AD based on a positive test finding (LR+) = 7.03 (SE = 1.17; 95% CI = 4.49–14.47), the likelihood ratio of not having AD based on the algorithm (LR−) = 3.55 (SE = 1.15; 2.22–5.71), and the odds ratio of AD were calculated in the ADNI cohort (OR) = 28.70 (1.55; 95% CI = 11.86–69.47).

Conclusions: It is possible to create a blood-based screening algorithm that works across both serum and plasma that provides a comparable screening accuracy to that obtained from CSF analyses.

Citation: O'Bryant SE, Xiao G, Barber R, Huebinger R, Wilhelmsen K, et al. (2011) A Blood-Based Screening Tool for Alzheimer's Disease That Spans Serum and Plasma: Findings from TARC and ADNI. PLoS ONE 6(12): e28092. doi:10.1371/journal.pone.0028092

Editor: Ashley I. Bush, Mental Health Research Institute of Victoria, Australia

Received August 26, 2011; **Accepted** November 1, 2011; **Published** December 7, 2011

Funding: This study was made possible by the Texas Alzheimer's Research Consortium funded by the state of Texas through the Texas Council on Alzheimer's Disease and Related Disorders. Investigators at the UTSW acknowledge NIH, NIA grant P30AG12300. The investigations at Baylor's Alzheimer's Disease and Memory Disorders Center were supported by the Cynthia and George Mitchell Foundation. Investigators at Texas Tech University Health Sciences Center were supported by The CH Foundation. ADNI. Data collection and sharing for this project was funded by the Alzheimer's Disease Neuroimaging Initiative (ADNI) (National Institutes of Health Grant U01 AG024904). ADNI is funded by the National Institute on Aging, the National Institute of Biomedical Imaging and Bioengineering, and through generous contributions from the following: Abbott, AstraZeneca AB, Bayer Schering Pharma AG, Bristol-Myers Squibb, Eisai Global Clinical Development, Elan Corporation, Genentech, GE Healthcare, GlaxoSmithKline, Innogenetics, Johnson and Johnson, Eli Lilly and Co., Medpace, Inc., Merck and Co., Inc., Novartis AG, Pfizer Inc, F. Hoffman-La Roche, Schering-Plough, Synarc, Inc., as well as non-profit partners the Alzheimer's Association and Alzheimer's Drug Discovery Foundation, with participation from the U.S. Food and Drug Administration. Private sector contributions to ADNI are facilitated by the Foundation for the National Institutes of Health (www.fnih.org). The grantee organization is the Northern California Institute for Research and Education, and the study is coordinated by the Alzheimer's Disease Cooperative Study at the University of California San Diego. ADNI data are disseminated by the Laboratory for Neuro Imaging at the University of California Los Angeles. This research was also supported by NIH grants P30 AG010129, K01 AG030514, and the Dana Foundation. The funders had no role in study design, data collection and analysis, decision to publish, or preparation of the manuscript.

Competing Interests: The authors have the following competing interest: In the TARC, a patent has been submitted on this blood-based screener. There are no other products in development or marketed products to declare. This does not alter the authors' adherence to all PLoS ONE policies on sharing data and materials, as detailed online in the guide for authors. ADNI has received funding from the following commercial sources: Abbott, AstraZeneca AB, Bayer Schering Pharma AG, Bristol-Myers Squibb, Eisai Global Clinical Development, Elan Corporation, Genentech, GE Healthcare, GlaxoSmithKline, Innogenetics, Johnson and Johnson, Eli Lilly and Co., Medpace, Inc., Merck and Co., Inc., Novartis AG, Pfizer Inc, F. Hoffman-La Roche, Schering-Plough, Synarc, Inc. This does not alter the authors' adherence to all PLoS ONE policies on sharing data and materials, as detailed online in the guide for authors. ADNI data is freely available to any interested scientists.

* E-mail: Sid.Obryant@ttuhsc.edu

❥ These authors contributed equally to this work.

¤a For a full list of the investigators from the Texas Alzheimer's Research Consortium please see the Acknowledgments section
¤b For more information about the Alzheimer's Disease Neuroimaging Initiative please see the Acknowledgments section

Introduction

Alzheimer's disease (AD) is a devastating disease affecting millions of people worldwide. While a Food and Drug Administration (FDA) working group recently provided preliminary approval for a beta amyloid (Aβ) neuroimaging technique as a biological marker (Amyvid©, Elli Lilly), no blood-based biomarker screening tool has received approval to date. However, blood-based biomarkers present significant advantages over neuroimaging modalities. For example, blood-based screenings offer a cost effective method of screening candidates for therapeutic trials [1], provide a rapid, cost-effective means of screening for AD at the population level [2,3,4,5], and provide an optimal starting point for a multi-stage assessment process that can be followed-up by clinical modalities (i.e. medical exam, neuropsychological testing, standard neuroimaging, clinical blood-work), specialized neuroimaging (i.e. Aβ imaging, fMRI, volumetric MRI analyses), and/or CSF (i.e. t-tau, $A\beta_{1-42}$, and/or t-tau/$A\beta_{1-42}$ ratio score) analyses [4] for screen positive cases. The 2009 U.S. Census estimates suggested that there were nearly 40 million Americans age 65 and above with an additional 34 million reaching 65 within 10 years; there are many more world-wide. Given their cost and limited availability, available imaging, clinical, and CSF modalities are not reasonable first-line approaches for screening all elders at risk of having AD or that have concerns about having the disease. The purpose of this study was to generate and cross-validate a blood-based screener for AD that can be incorporated into the existing medical infrastructure with additional assessments (e.g. clinical, imaging, CSF analysis) to confirm those who screen positive.

In the last several years, there have been significant advancements in the search for blood-based biomarkers for Alzheimer's disease (AD). In 2007, Ray and colleagues [6] analyzed a panel of plasma-based proteins among samples from 259 controls, AD and mild cognitive impairment (MCI) cases and generated a biomarker algorithm that accurately identified 89% of those with and without the disease; however, this work has not been replicated [7]. Buerger and colleagues [8] examined blood-based microcirculation markers as possible diagnostic markers for AD (AD n = 94, controls n = 53). These authors found that a ratio score of pro-atrial natriuretic peptide (MR-proANP) to C-terminal endothelin-1 precursor fragment (CT-proET-1)(MR-proANP/CT-proET-1 ratio) from plasma yielded a sensitivity of 0.81 and specificity of 0.82 in discriminating probable AD from healthy controls. More recently, we created a biomarker risk score from serum proteins (AD n = 197, controls n = 203) that yielded a 91% overall accuracy [2]. Our approach took the algorithm a step further by combining both demographic (i.e. age, gender, education, and *APOE*E4* status) and clinical lab values (i.e. cholesterol, triglycerides, high density lipoproteins, low density lipoproteins, lipoprotein-associated phospholipase, homocysteine, and C-peptide) into the algorithm, which improved the overall accuracy to 95% [5]. Analyzing samples from 22 AD cases, 22 controls, and 12 non-AD disease comparison subjects, Reddy and colleagues [9] took a novel approach by examining serum IgG antibodies as potential biomarkers of AD

status obtaining impressive results (AUC = 0.99); however, the sample size was very small (n = 15 AD cases in test set) limiting the generalizability of the findings at this point. Together, these studies suggest that a blood-based screening tool for AD is on the horizon.

Although this work is promising, there is little consistency as to what biological fluid is used for biomarker assays (i.e. serum versus plasma), which may explain many inconsistent findings found in the literature. While some assays must be conducted in one medium or another, there are numerous studies linking a variety of blood-based markers to AD from both mediums. Mayeux and colleagues [10] analyzed *plasma* amyloid β (Aβ) peptides $A\beta_{1-40}$ and $A\beta_{1-42}$ on 530 participants and found that $A\beta_{1-42}$ (but not $A\beta_{1-40}$) levels were higher among baseline AD cases as well as those who developed AD over a three-year period as compared to those who did not. Luis et al. [11] analyzed *serum* $A\beta_{1-40}$ and $A\beta_{1-42}$ levels among a sample of 87 AD and MCI cases as well as controls. In that study, serum $A\beta_{1-40}$ levels did not differ between groups whereas serum $A\beta_{1-42}$ levels where highest among MCI cases (versus AD cases and controls) and controls and AD levels were intermediate between those of the MCI cases and controls. The *serum* $A\beta_{1-42/1-40}$ ratio was also highest among the MCI group. In a sample of 40 AD cases and controls, Laske et al. [12] found that *serum* brain derived neurotrophic factor (BDNF) levels varied according to AD severity, suggesting BDNF as a potential biomarker for AD, though we failed to cross-validate these findings in a sample of 198 AD cases and controls from the Texas Alzheimer's Research Consortium (TARC) cohort [13]. In a follow-up study of 399 AD cases and controls, *elevated* serum BDNF was found to be specifically related to poorer memory performance among AD cases [14] whereas Komulainen and colleagues [15] found that *lower plasma* BDNF levels were significantly related to poorer scores on tests of language and memory among women in a population based sample of aging men and women (n = 1389).

To date, we are aware of no prior work that has explicitly sought to find blood-based biomarkers of AD across both serum and plasma and with no previous attempts at identifying blood-based screening tools utilizing markers across blood fractions. Additionally, no previously created blood-based tools have been cross-validated in independent cohorts. The current study was designed to (1) identify blood-based proteins that were highly correlated across both serum and plasma that also were significantly related to AD status, and (2) generate a screening algorithm for AD utilizing those markers from serum in the TARC cohort and validate that algorithm in the Alzheimer's Disease Neuroimaging Initiative (ADNI) plasma-samples. We hypothesized that, as with our prior work, we would be able to generate a screening algorithm that accurately identified AD across cohorts.

Methods

Participants

Texas Alzheimer's Research Consortium (TARC). Serum protein data were analyzed from 396 participants (197 AD subjects, 199 controls) from the TARC longitudinal cohort. In addition, plasma protein data were analyzed on a matched sample of 40 AD cases from the TARC. Blood samples for comparison of plasma and serum proteins were drawn concurrently from the same individuals. The methodology of the TARC project has been described in detail elsewhere [2,16]. Briefly, each participant undergoes a standardized annual examination at the respective sites, which includes a medical evaluation, neuropsychological testing, interview, and blood draw for storage of samples in the TARC biobank. Diagnosis of AD was based on NINCDS-ADRDA criteria [17] utilizing consensus review. Institution Review Board approval was obtained for this study with each participant (or caregiver) providing written informed consent. The Institution Review Board (IRB) at Texas Tech University Health Sciences Center, Baylor College of Medicine, University of North Texas Health Science Center, the University of Texas Southwestern Medical Center, and the University of Texas Health Science Center - San Antonio approved this research.

Alzheimer's Disease Neuroimaging Initiative (ADNI). Data used in the preparation of this article were obtained from the ADNI database (adni.loni.ucla.edu). The ADNI was launched in 2003 by the National Institute on Aging (NIA), the National Institute of Biomedical Imaging and Bioengineering (NIBIB), the Food and Drug Administration (FDA), private pharmaceutical companies and non-profit organizations, as a $60 million, 5-year public-private partnership. The primary goal of ADNI has been to test whether serial magnetic resonance imaging (MRI), positron emission tomography (PET), other biological markers, and clinical and neuropsychological assessment can be combined to measure the progression of mild cognitive impairment (MCI) and early Alzheimer's disease (AD). The Principal Investigator of this initiative is Michael W. Weiner, MD, VA Medical Center and University of California – San Francisco. ADNI is the result of efforts of many co-investigators from a broad range of academic institutions and private corporations, and subjects have been recruited from over 50 sites across the U.S. and Canada. For up-to-date information, see www.adni-info.org. Data from 170 participants from ADNI (58 controls and 112 AD cases) for whom plasma-based protein results were available were utilized in this study.

Blood Assays. In TARC, non-fasting samples were collected whereas ADNI utilized a fasting blood collection procedure. Serum blood samples were collected in serum-separating tubes during clinical evaluations, allowed to clot at room temperature for 30 minutes, centrifuged, aliquoted, and stored in polypropylene tubes at −80°C. In both TARC and ADNI, plasma samples were collected in lavender-top tubes and gently mixed 10–12 times. Next tubes were centrifuged at room temperature and plasma extracted and frozen until assay. In both studies, serum and plasma samples were sent to Rules Based Medicine (RBM, www.rulesbasedmedicine.com, Austin, TX) for assay on the RBM multiplexed immunoassay human Multi-Analyte Profile (human-MAP). Individual proteins were quantified with immunoassays on colored microspheres. Information regarding the least detectable dose (LDD), inter-run coefficient of variation, dynamic range, overall spiked standard recovery, and cross-reactivity with other humanMAP analytes can be readily obtained from RBM. Clinical lab data. Homocysteine, hemoglobin A1c, c-peptide, and lipoprotein-associated phospholipase A2 (Lp-PLA2) was provided by the Ballantyne laboratory at Baylor College of Medicine. Sample collection and storage was as described above. Lipids were measured using a AU400e automated chemistry analyzer (Olympus America; Center Valley, PA), serum total homocysteine (tHcy) by recombinant enzymatic cycling assay (Roche Hitachi

911), c-peptide by enzyme-linked immunosorbent assay (ELISA), HbA1c measurement by turbidimetric inhibition immunoassay (TINIA) for hemolyzed whole blood and Lp-PLA2 levels by diaDexus PLAC® test (diaDexus, Inc, San Francisco, CA). Clinical lab data from ADNI was conducted using kits provided by Covance. ADNI CSF Biomarkers. Our blood-based algorithm was compared to the diagnostic accuracy of the total tau (t-tau) to beta amyloid ($A\beta_{1-42}$) ratio (t-tau/$A\beta_{1-42}$) previously completed as part of the ADNI protocol. The CSF methods for ADNI have been described in detail elsewhere [18]. Lumbar punctures were conducted with a median of one day after baseline clinical visit. Once CSF was transferred into polypropylene tubes it was frozen and shipped to the ADNI Biomarker Core laboratory at the University of Pennsylvania Medical Center where biomarker assays were conducted [18].

Statistical Analyses. Analyses were performed using R (V 2.10) statistical software [19]. Biomarker data were transformed using Box-Cox [20] transformation so that the distribution of each protein is approximately normal. Analyses took place in a series of steps. Identification of proteins across serum and plasma. Pearson correlations were conducted in the TARC sub-sample across serum and plasma proteins to determine which markers were comparable across mediums. Model-based clustering algorithm [21] (Mclust package in R) was used to empirically determine the optimal correlation cut-off that separated the highly correlated versus weakly correlated proteins. The optimal cut-score was 0.75, which identified 33 proteins with high correlation (≥ 0.75) between serum and plasma (see Figure 1). T-test analyses comparing the abundance of proteins between AD and controls identified 29 that were differentially expressed between groups ($p < 0.05$) in full the TARC cohort (training set). Eleven proteins were significantly different between AD and control participants and were found to be correlated ≥ 0.75 across serum and plasma. These 11 proteins are defined as protein biomarkers in this study. Figure 2 reflects a graphic representation of the methods. Development of Biomarker Diagnostic Model. Next, we used the 11 protein biomarkers to develop our prediction model using random forest (RF) method [22,23], implemented using R package *randomforest* (V 4.5) [22]. The TARC cohort was designated as the training sample in which the prediction model was derived. Validation of the Prediction Model. The protein biomarker-based RF prediction model derived from the TARC serum-based biomarker training set (TARC) was applied to the ADNI plasma-based dataset (test sample) to predict the risk score for each patient in the ADNI cohort. Of note, no ADNI data were utilized in (1) identification of serum-plasma comparable proteins or (2) development of the RF prediction model. This was done to avoid the overfitting or other possible confounds across medium and/or cohorts. Diagnostic Accuracy. Diagnostic accuracy was evaluated by examining the area under the receiver operating characteristic (ROC) curves (AUC). Our approach to creating a blood-based diagnostic algorithm for AD is to combine the predicted biomarker risk score from the RF model with demographic and clinical lab data via a multivariate logistic regression model. Demographic data incorporated into the algorithm was age, gender, level of education, and presence of *APOE*E4* genotype (homozygous or heterozygous) while clinical lab data included glucose, triglycerides, total cholesterol, and homocysteine. These variables were included as they were (1) available from both cohorts and (2) have been linked to AD. Lastly, the likelihood ratios of having AD based on a positive test finding (LR+), the likelihood ratio of not having AD based on the algorithm (LR-) and the odds ratio of AD were calculated in the ADNI cohort.

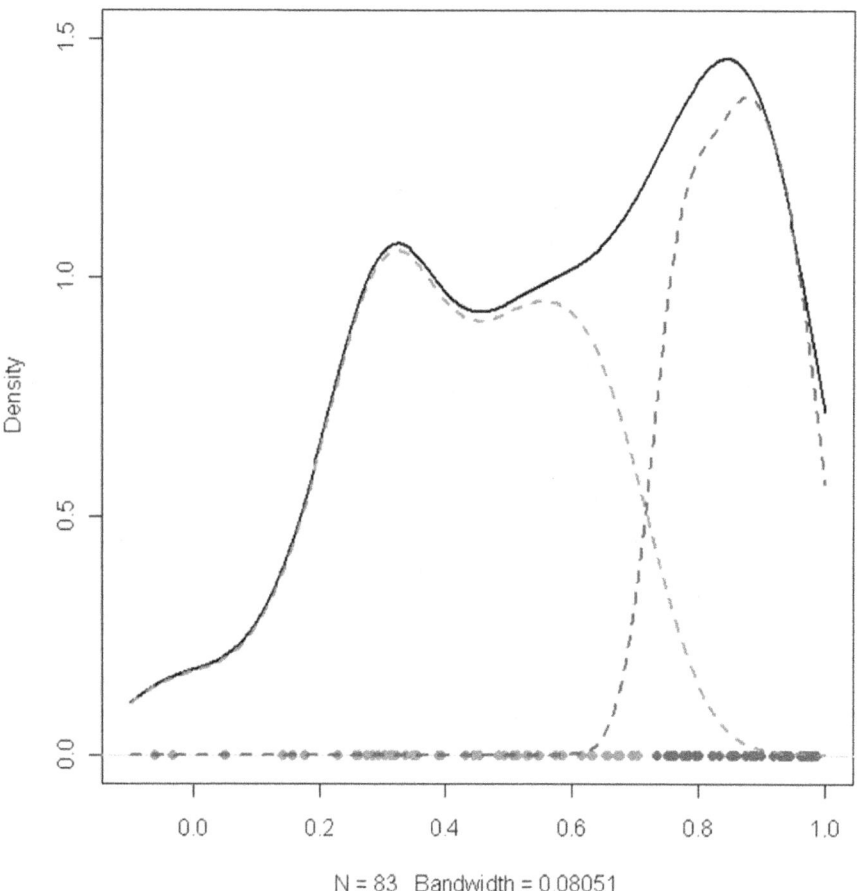

N = 83   Bandwidth = 0.08051

Figure 1. The density plot the Pearson's correlation coefficients between serum and plasma in TARC cohort. We used Mclust (model-based clustering algorithm [21]) package in R to fit the data and discovered two clusters in the correlation coefficients: one (red) corresponding to low correlation and the other (blue) corresponding to high correlation. The threshold value that separated these two clusters most effectively is 0.75. The black line is the density plot of all biomarkers. The dots represent the correlation coefficients of the biomarkers and the color indicates the cluster membership.
doi:10.1371/journal.pone.0028092.g001

Results

Demographic characteristics of the samples are provided in Table 1. Eleven proteins met our criteria of (1) having a correlation coefficient ≥0.75 between serum and plasma in the same participant and (2) being associated with disease status p<0.05. The 11 proteins were as follows: C-reactive protein, adiponectin, pancreatic polypeptide, fatty acid binding protein, interleukin 18, beta 2 microglobulin, tenascin C, T lymphocyte secreted protein 1.309, factor VII, vascular cell adhesion molecule 1, and monocyte chemotactic protein 1. See Table 2 for correlations among serum and plasma for these 11 proteins as well as the mean differences between cases and control groups of these biomarkers and clinical lab data across cohorts.

The optimal cut-score for the RF biomarker risk score from the test sample (ADNI) was 0.51 which obtained AUC of 0.70 with a sensitivity (SN) and specificity (SP) of 0.54 and 0.78, respectively. For comparison purposes, the ADNI CSF t-tau/Aβ_{1-42} ratio yielded a superior diagnostic accuracy with an observed AUC = 0.92, SN = 0.84, and SP = 1.00. However, as with our prior approach, when the biomarker risk score was combined with demographic and clinical lab data [2,5], the precision improved substantially. Our combined algorithm yielded a much better diagnostic accuracy with an observed AUC = 0.88, SN = 0.75, and SP = 0.91. Of note, the diagnostic accuracy of our serum-plasma based algorithm was comparable to that

obtained from ADNI CSF analyses. See Table 3 and Figure 3. The likelihood ratio positive (LR+) was 7.03 (SE = 1.17; 95% CI = 4.49–14.47), the likelihood ratio negative (LR−) was 3.55 (SE = 1.15; 2.22–5.71), and the odds ratio (OR) was 28.70 (1.55; 95% CI = 11.86–69.47). The misclassification rate was 14% (95% CI = 9–21%). If we set SN at 0.80 for our full algorithm, the resulting SP was 0.81, which also meets the criteria for the Consensus Report of the Working Group on Molecular and Biochemical Markers of AD [24].

Discussion

In the current study we demonstrate that (1) there are proteins that are highly correlated in plasma and serum and are associated with AD status across blood fractions, (2) these findings are replicable across independent cohorts, and (3) using these proteins, we generated a prediction model in the TARC cohort that, when combined with demographic and clinical lab data, yielded clinically significant classification accuracy in the ADNI cohort. To date, this is the first blood-based screener for AD developed that has been cross-validated in an independent large-scale cohort that also works across blood fractions. This work not only further supports the notion that an accurate blood-based screening tool for AD can be generated, but also that such an algorithm can be applied across serum and plasma mediums. Our 11-protein serum-plasma risk score alone yielded an AUC of 0.70 accuracy that was

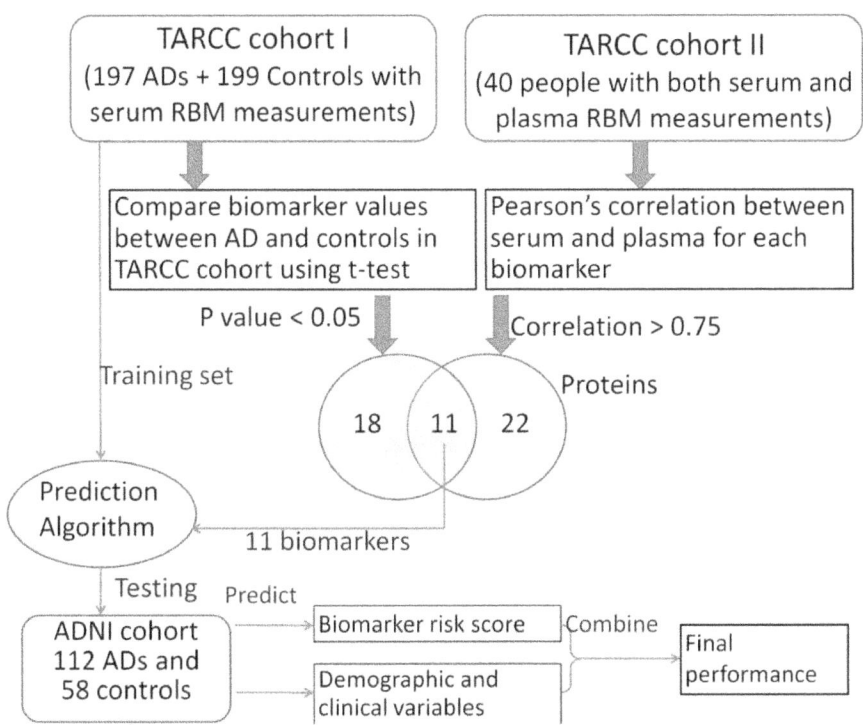

Figure 2. Outline of methods.
doi:10.1371/journal.pone.0028092.g002

enhanced by the addition of demographic (i.e. age, gender, education, *APOE*E4* status) and clinical lab (i.e. glucose, triglycerides, total cholesterol, and homocysteine) data. In Table 3, the addition of clinical lab data did not improve the overall accuracy of the algorithm beyond demographic information, which is largely driven by the *APOE*E4* rates in the ADNI cohort. However, in our prior work [5], the use of clinical lab data improved overall accuracy and will likely contribute to the robustness of our approach as it is applied to other cohorts. It is certainly possible that inclusion of additional markers, not available in the current analyses, would increase the accuracy of that risk score, which is an additional advantage of our approach as it can be expanded or reduced as necessary to support the accuracy and cost-effectiveness of the algorithm. A single biomarker algorithm that works across both serum and plasma will offer laboratories options that may be preferable for a variety of reasons.

There are several implications for the current findings. There are a number of previously conducted research projects with stored blood biospecimens; however, there is little consistency between what medium was stored. The current findings open up the possibility of utilizing samples from such studies to further validate and refine our algorithm. Additionally, it is likely that the components of diagnostic algorithms will be different from the components of algorithms for progression and different from those predicting long-term risk. Our findings offer a novel approach to each of these questions as well. These findings also support the need for standard protocols to be generated for blood-based AD biomarker research as is currently underway for the CSF markers.

These results also support the robustness of our methodological approach. In our initial serum-based algorithm, the biomarker risk score alone yielded an AUC of 0.91 whereas the serum-plasma algorithm in the current study yielded an AUC of 0.70. While impressive, this overall accuracy is not clinically adequate.

Table 1. Demographic characteristics of the cohorts.

	TARC – serum sample			TARC – plasma sample	ADNI		
	AD (N = 197)	Control (N = 198)	p-value	AD (n = 40)	AD (n = 112)	Control (n = 58)	p-value
Gender (male)	34.5%	31.3%	0.52	40%	42%	48%	0.52
Age (years, mean/sd)	77.4(8.3)	70.4(8.9)	<0.001	75.7(1.6)	75.2(8.1)	75.5(5.8)	0.63
Education (years, mean/sd)	14.0(3.5)	15.5(2.7)	<0.001	14.5(0.6)	15.1(3.2)	15.6(2.7)	0.38
APOE*E4 positive	59.3%	26.5%	<0.001	50%	68%	9%	<0.001

Note: TARC = Texas Alzheimer's Research Consortium; ADNI = Alzheimer's Disease Neuroimaging Initiative. Fisher exact test was used for categorical outcomes (Gender, APOE*E4 positive) and Wilcoxon test was used for continuous outcomes (Age, Education).
doi:10.1371/journal.pone.0028092.t001

Table 2. Biomarkers and Clinical Labs Across Cohorts.

Marker	Pearson correlation for serum vs. plasma (TARC cohort)	Mean difference in TARCC	Mean difference in ADNI
C Reactive Protein	0.97	−3.35	−2.07
Adiponectin	0.95	1.88	1.79
Pancreatic polypeptide	0.89	4.29	2.78
Fatty Acid Binding Protein	0.88	1.72	−0.79
IL 18	0.86	−1.87	0.51
Beta 2 Microglobulin	0.85	3.14	2.09
Tenascin C	0.85	4.56	2.93
I.309	0.8	1.12	−1.68
Factor VII	0.8	−2.78	−1.26
VCAM 1	0.78	3.00	2.82
MCP 1	0.75	−2.74	−0.30
Total Cholesterol	–	0.13	0.78
Triglycerides	–	−0.63	1.59
Homocysteine	–	3.99	1.06

Note: Mean difference reflects the mean difference between cases and controls divided by the its standard deviation.
doi:10.1371/journal.pone.0028092.t002

However, as with our prior approach, the combination of clinical lab data and demographic variables into the algorithm increased the precision substantially (AUC = 0.88). In our prior work, the training and test sample were both based on serum assays and were from the larger TARC cohort; however, the derivation of the algorithm in the TARC cohort and validation in the ADNI cohort supports the robustness of this method. As we have previously argued, using only age, gender, education and *APOE*E4* status, one can accurately classify a large number of AD cases when compared to controls. Therefore, consideration of such factors should be considered when examining biomarkers of AD status. We are not the first to demonstrate that inclusion of these factors into an algorithm can improve overall accuracy as others have suggested that a multi-marker approach is superior to single-marker approaches [25,26]. As an example, Vemuri and colleagues found that including demographic factors with structural MRI added to the overall accuracy of disease-prediction models even when cases and controls were matched by these variables [27]. This is important given that the TARC cohort did not match cases and controls whereas ADNI samples were matched. The robustness of our methodology may also provide an explanation for the lack of cross-validation of prior work [6,7]. The utility of our algorithm for separating MCI cases from normal controls (and/or AD) remains unknown at present.

The current markers overlap with our prior serum-only based algorithm [2,5] though they do not overlap with those found by Ray and colleagues [6], which may be due to the significant differences in assay platforms utilized. However, there is an existing literature directly or indirectly linking each of the 11 proteins identified in this study to AD. As with our prior work, many of the markers in the algorithm are inflammatory in nature, which we propose as evidence of an inflammatory endophenotype of AD [2,28]. We, and others, have documented a link between CRP and AD [28]. Based on the available data, we proposed that the link between CRP and the risk of AD changes over the life course with midlife elevations in CRP increasing risk for AD, but that this risk declines as one ages with decreased CRP related to AD status though elevations in CRP are still related to increased disease severity among cases [28]. Adiponectin, an adipocytokine, is related to obesity, insulin resistance, metabolic syndrome, type 2 diabetes, and cardiovascular disease [29] and was recently found to be elevated in plasma among MCI and AD cases [30].

Table 3. Diagnostic accuracy of the serum-plasma algorithm.

	AUC (95% CI)	SN (95% CI)	SP (95% CI)
biomarker + clinical + demographic	0.88 (0.83–0.93)	0.75 (0.67–0.83)	0.91 (0.80–0.96)
biomarker + demographic	0.88 (0.83–0.93)	0.79 (0.71–0.86)	0.87 (0.75–0.93)
Biomarker + clinical	0.71 (0.63–0.79)	0.73 (0.64–0.81)	0.60 (0.47–0.72)
biomarker risk score alone	0.70 (0.62–0.78)	0.54 (0.45–0.63)	0.78 (0.65–0.87)
clinical variables alone	0.59 (0.50–0.68)	0.53 (0.43–0.62)	0.72 (0.58–0.82)
demographic variables alone	0.81 (0.75–0.88)	0.70 (0.61–0.78)	0.92 (0.82–0.97)
CSF tau/abeta ratio	0.92 (0.87–0.96)	0.84 (0.76–0.90)	1.00 (0.93–1.00)

Note: AUC = area under the receiver operating characteristic curve; SN = sensitivity; SP = specificity; CI = confidence interval; demographic = age, gender, education, *APOE*E4* status (presence/absence); clinical = glucose, triglycerides, total cholesterol, homocysteine.
doi:10.1371/journal.pone.0028092.t003

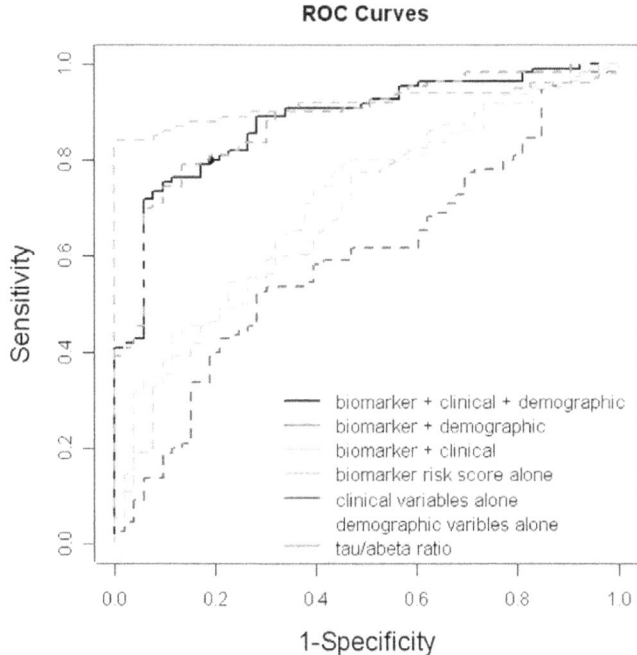

ROC Curves

- biomarker + clinical + demographic
- biomarker + demographic
- biomarker + clinical
- biomarker risk score alone
- clinical variables alone
- demographic varibles alone
- tau/abeta ratio

Figure 3. ROC curve for serum-plasma based biomarker algorithm. Each line represents the AUC of the respective portions of the algorithm with the yellow line reflecting chance.
doi:10.1371/journal.pone.0028092.g003

Therefore, adiponectin levels may be related to the documented links between changes in body composition (e.g. weight loss) seen in prodromal and early stage AD. Pancreatic polypeptide is also linked with diabetes and obesity [31,32] and may provide a clue into the biological link between these conditions and AD. Fatty acid binding proteins, cytosolic proteins found in all cells utilizing fatty acids, are rapidly released into circulation following cell damage [33]. Serum levels fatty acid binding proteins have been shown to be elevated among AD and other dementia cases as compared to normal controls [33,34]. A recent meta-analysis showed a significant up-regulation in blood concentrations of IL-18 (as well as IL-6, TNFα, IL1, transforming growth factor, IL-12) among AD cases [35]. β2 microglobulin is an amyloid protein [36] that has been found to be elevated in the CSF of AD cases [37,38]. Tenascin-C, an extracellular matrix glycoprotein, is involved in a number of biological processes that have been linked to AD including inflammation and angiogenesis [39], which may provide a biological mechanism linking AD to a broad spectrum of cardiovascular diseases and risk factors. The human cytokine I-309, a small glycoprotein, was recently found to be elevated in a proteomic study of CSF among AD cases and was also related to scores on a test of global cognitive functioning (i.e. Mini Mental State Examination [MMSE]) [40]. Factor VII is a protein in the coagulation cascade that is required for thrombin generation, which has also been linked to AD [41]. VCAM-1 is a member of the immunoglobulin superfamily that has been found elevated in plasma of AD cases [42]. It has been proposed that MCP-1 plays a dominant role in the chronic inflammation seen in AD [43] and has been found to be elevated in serum of patients diagnosed with MCI and mild AD [44].

Given the sheer volume of elders worldwide who are at risk for AD, there is an urgent need for a multi-stage approach to screening and diagnosis. There are insufficient numbers of dementia experts to meet the needs of all individuals at risk for the disease and prior work has demonstrated that non-experts are not completely accurate in diagnosing the disease [45], particularly in the earlier stages [46]. Our blood-based screener fits into the existing medical infrastructure where screen positives can be referred for confirmatory diagnosis using clinical, imaging, and/or CSF analysis. As with any screening measure, one must consider acceptable levels of false positive and false negative rates of the instrument as well as overall disease base rates of the setting when deciding on appropriate cut-scores on any instrument [47]. Therefore it is important that additional work be conducted to determine how this algorithm (and other previously published biomarkers) performs in community-based settings (e.g. primary care offices) as both the TARC and ADNI are clinic-based cohort studies. While sensitivity and specificity are not base rate dependent, accuracy of diagnosis (prediction of disease status present/absent) is a function of base rates of the disease within a given population therefore, overall accuracy of AD presence (i.e. true positives) will increase with advancing age while accuracy of AD absence (i.e. true negatives) will be higher with younger ages. As with age, *APOE*E4* genotype, gender, and/or years of education are also important considerations, which is why these variables are included in the algorithm itself.

The independent cohorts strongly support the validity of the findings. These observations also justify further analysis examining a broader range of markers across serum and plasma to determine if the biomarker risk score can be further refined. Our results also suggest that further work in the field should specifically examine the performance of blood-based protein panels across serum and plasma.

Acknowledgments

TARC. We would like to thank Dr. Christie Ballantyne and his lab at Baylor College of Medicine for measuring the clinical lab data of glucose, tryglicerides, total cholesterol, and homocysteins. We also would like to thank the people of Texas and the research participants for making this work possible. Funding acknowledgments are available online.

Investigators from the Texas Alzheimer's Research Consortium: Baylor College of Medicine: Susan Rountree, Christie Ballantyne, Eveleen Darby, Aline Hittle, Aisha Khaleeg; Texas Tech University Health Science Center: Paula Grammas, Benjamin Williams, Andrew Dentino, Gregory Schrimsher, Kuo Chuang Wu, Parastoo Momeni, Larry Hill; University of North Texas Health Science Center: Janice Knebl, Lisa Alvarez, Douglas Mains, Thomas Fairchild, James Hall; University of Texas Southwestern Medical Center: Joan Reisch, Perrie Adams, Roger Rosenberg, Ryan Huebinger, Janet Smith, Mechelle Murray, Tomequa Sears; University of Texas Health Sciences Center – San Antonio: Donald Royall, Raymond Palmer.

Data used in the preparation of this article were obtained from the Alzheimer's Disease Neuroimaging Initiative (ADNI) database (www.loni.ucla.edu/ADNI). As such, the investigators within the ADNI contributed to the design and implementation of ADNI and/or provided data, but did not participate in analysis or writing of this report. ADNI investigators include (complete listing available at www.loni.ucla.edu/ADNI/Collaboration/ADNI_Manuscript_Citations.pdf).

Author Contributions

Conceived and designed the experiments: SEO GX RB RD RDA. Performed the experiments: SEO GX RB KW RD RDA. Analyzed the data: SEO GX RB RH KW ME NGR RD RDA. Contributed reagents/materials/analysis tools: SEO GX RB KW RD RDA. Wrote the paper: SEO GX RB RH KW ME NGR RD RDA.

References

1. Thal LJ, Kantarci K, Reiman EM, Klunk WE, Weiner MW, et al. (2006) The role of biomarkers in clinical trials for Alzheimer disease. Alzheimer Disease & Associated Disorders 20: 6–15.
2. O'Bryant SE, Xiao G, Barber R, Reisch J, Doody R, et al. (2010) A serum protein-based algorithm for the detection of Alzheimer disease. Archives of Neurology 67: 1077–1081.
3. O'Bryant S, Xiao G, Barber R, Reisch J, Doody R, et al. for the Texas Alzheimer's Research Consortium (in press) A serum protein-based algorithm for the detection of Alzheiemr's disease. Arch Neurol.
4. Schneider P, Hampel H, Buerger K (2009) Biological marker candidates of alzheimer's disease in blood, plasma, and serum. CNS Neuroscience and Therapeutics 15: 358–374.
5. O'Bryant S, Xiao G, Barber R, Reisch J, Hall J, et al. (2011) A blood based algorithm for the detection of Alzheimer's disease. Dementia and Geriatric Cognitive Disorders 32: 55–62.
6. Ray S, Britschgi M, Herbert C, Takeda-Uchimura Y, Boxer A, et al. (2007) Classification and prediction of clinical Alzheimer's diagnosis based on plasma signaling proteins. Nature Medicine 13: 1359–1362.
7. Soares HD, Chen Y, Sabbagh M, Rohrer A, Schrijvers E, et al. (2009) Identifying early markers of alzheimer's disease using quantitative multiplex proteomic immunoassay panels. pp 56–67.
8. Buerger K, Ernst A, Ewers M, Uspenskaya O, Omerovic M, et al. (2009) Blood-Based Microcirculation Markers in Alzheimer's Disease-Diagnostic Value of Midregional Pro-atrial Natriuretic Peptide/C-terminal Endothelin-1 Precursor Fragment Ratio. Biological Psychiatry 65: 979–984.
9. Reddy MM, Wilson R, Wilson J, Connell S, Gocke A, et al. (2011) Identification of candidate IgG biomarkers for alzheimer's disease via combinatorial library screening. Cell 144: 132–142.
10. Mayeux R, Honig LS, Tang MX, Manly J, Stern Y, et al. (2003) Plasma A[beta]40 and A[beta]42 and Alzheimer's disease: relation to age, mortality, and risk. Neurology 61: 1185–1190.
11. Luis CA, Abdullah L, Paris D, Quadros A, Mullan M, et al. (2009) Serum β-amyloid correlates with neuropsychological impairment. Aging, Neuropsychology, and Cognition 16: 203–218.
12. Laske C, Stransky E, Leyhe T, Eschweiler GW, Wittorf A, et al. (2006) Stage-dependent BDNF serum concentrations in Alzheimer's disease. Journal of Neural Transmission 113: 1217–1224.
13. O'Bryant SE, Hobson V, Hall JR, Waring SC, Chan W, et al. (2009) Brain-Derived Neurotrophic Factor Levels in Alzheimer's Disease. Journal of Alzheimer's Disease 17: 1051–1055.
14. O'Bryant SE, Hobson VL, Hall JR, Barber RC, Zhang S, et al. (2010) Serum Brain-Derived Neurotrophic Factor Levels Are Specifically Associated with Memory Performance among Alzheimer's Disease Cases. Dementia and Geriatric Cognitive Disorders 31: 31–36.
15. Komulainen P, Pedersen M, Hanninen T, Bruunsgaard H, Lakka TA, et al. (2008) BDNF is a novel marker of cognitive function in ageing women: the DR's EXTRA Study. Neurobiology of Learning & Memory 90: 596–603.
16. Waring S, O'Bryant SE, Reisch JS, Diaz-Arrastia R, Knebl J, et al. (2008), for the Texas Alzheimer's Research Consortium (2008) The Texas Alzheimer's Research Consortium longitudinal research cohort: Study design and baseline characteristics. Texas Public Health Journal 60: 9–13.
17. McKhann D, Drockman D, Folstein M, et al. (1984) Clinical diagnosis of Alzheimer's disease: Report of the NINCDS-ADRDA Work Group. Neurology 34: 939–944.
18. Vemuri P, Wiste HJ, Weigand SD, Shaw LM, Trojanowski JQ, et al. (2009) MRI and CSF biomarkers in normal, MCI, and AD subjects: Diagnostic discrimination and cognitive correlations. Neurology 73: 287–293.
19. R Development Core Team (2009) R: A language and environment for statistical computing. Vienna, Austria.
20. Osborne J (2010) Improving your data transformations: Applying the Box-Cox transformation. Practical Assessment Research Evaluation 15: 2.
21. Fraley CR, AE (2002) Model-based clustering, discriminat analysis, and density estimation. Journal of the American Statistical Association 97: 611–631.
22. Breiman L (2001) Random forests. Machine Learning 45: 5–32.
23. Breiman L Manual on setting up, using, and understanding random forests V3.1.
24. Anonymous (1998) Consensus report of the Working Group on: "Molecular and Biochemical Markers of Alzheimer's Disease". The Ronald and Nancy Reagan Research Institute of the Alzheimer's Association and the National Institute on Aging Working Group.[see comment][erratum appears in Neurobiol Aging 1998 May–Jun;19(3):285]. Neurobiology of Aging 19: 109–116.
25. Zhang D, Wang Y, Zhou L, Yuan H, Shen D (2011) Multimodal classification of Alzheimer's disease and mild cognitive impairment. NeuroImage.
26. Brys M, Glodzik L, Mosconi L, Switalski R, De Santi S, et al. (2009) Magnetic resonance imaging improves cerebrospinal fluid biomarkers in the early detection of Alzheimer's disease. Journal of Alzheimer's Disease 16: 351–362.
27. Vemuri P, Gunter JL, Senjem ML, Whitwell JL, Kantarci K, et al. (2008) Alzheimer's disease diagnosis in individual subjects using structural MR images: Validation studies. NeuroImage 39: 1186–1197.
28. O'Bryant SE, Waring SC, Hobson V, Hall JR, Moore CB, et al. (2010) Decreased C-reactive protein levels in alzheimer disease. Journal of Geriatric Psychiatry and Neurology 23: 49–53.
29. Gustafson DR (2010) Adiposity hormones and dementia. Journal of the Neurological Sciences 299: 30–34.
30. Une K, Takei YA, Tomita N, Asamura T, Ohrui T, et al. (2011) Adiponectin in plasma and cerebrospinal fluid in MCI and Alzheimer's disease. European Journal of Neurology 18: 1006–1009.
31. Cui Y, Andersen DK (2011) Pancreatogenic diabetes: Special considerations for management. Pancreatology 11: 279–294.
32. Zhang L, Bijker MS, Herzog H (2011) The neuropeptide y system: Pathophysiological and therapeutic implications in obesity and cancer. Pharmacology and Therapeutics 131: 91–113.
33. Steinacker P, Mollenhauer B, Bibl M, Cepek L, Esselmann H, et al. (2004) Heart fatty acid binding protein as a potential diagnostic marker for neurodegenerative diseases. Neuroscience Letters 370: 36–39.
34. Teunissen CE, Veerhuis R, De Vente J, Verhey FRJ, Vreeling F, et al. (2011) Brain-specific fatty acid-binding protein is elevated in serum of patients with dementia-related diseases. European Journal of Neurology 18: 865–871.
35. Swardfager W, Lanctt K, Rothenburg L, Wong A, Cappell J, et al. (2010) A meta-analysis of cytokines in Alzheimer's disease. Biological Psychiatry 68: 930–941.
36. Gejyo F, Yamada T, Odani S, Nakagawa Y, Arakawa M, et al. (1985) A new form of amyloid protein associated with chronic hemodialysis was identified as β2-microglobulin. Biochemical and Biophysical Research Communications 129: 701–706.
37. Abdi F, Quinn JF, Jankovic J, McIntosh M, Leverenz JB, et al. (2006) Detection of biomarkers with a multiplex quantitative proteomic platform in cerebrospinal fluid of patients with neurodegenerative disorders. Journal of Alzheimer's Disease 9: 293–348.
38. Zellner M, Veitinger M, Umlauf E (2009) The role of proteomics in dementia and Alzheimer's disease. Acta Neuropathologica 118: 181–195.
39. Midwood KS, Hussenet T, Langlois B, Orend G (2011) Advances in tenascin-C biology. Cellular and Molecular Life Sciences 68: 3175–3199.
40. Hu WT, Chen-Plotkin A, Arnold SE, Grossman M, Clark CM, et al. (2010) Novel CSF biomarkers for Alzheimer's disease and mild cognitive impairment. Acta Neuropathologica 119: 669–678.
41. Akiyama H, Ikeda K, Kondo H, McGeer PL (1992) Thrombin accumulation in brains of patients with Alzheimer's disease. Neuroscience Letters 146: 152–154.
42. Ewers M, Mielke MM, Hampel H (2010) Blood-based biomarkers of microvascular pathology in Alzheimer's disease. Experimental Gerontology 45: 75–79.
43. Sokolova A, Hill MD, Rahimi F, Warden LA, Halliday GM, et al. (2009) Monocyte chemoattractant protein-1 plays a dominant role in the chronic inflammation observed in alzheimer's disease. Brain Pathology 19: 392–398.
44. Galimberti D, Fenoglio C, Lovati C, Venturelli E, Guidi I, et al. (2006) Serum MCP-1 levels are increased in mild cognitive impairment and mild Alzheimer's disease. Neurobiology of Aging 27: 1763–1768.
45. Boustani M, Callahan CM, Unverzagt FW, Austrom MG, Perkins AJ, et al. (2005) Implementing a screening and diagnosis program for dementia in primary care. Journal of General Internal Medicine 20: 572–577.
46. Doody R, Ferris S, Salloway S, Meuser TM, Murthy A, et al. (in press) Inter-rater reliability between expert and nonexpert physicians in the diagnosis of amnestic MCI in the community setting. Clinical Drug Investigation.
47. O'Bryant SE, Humphreys JD, Smith GE, Ivnik RJ, Graff-Radford NR, et al. (2008) Detecting dementia with the mini-mental state examination in highly educated individuals. Archives of Neurology 65: 963–967.

Plasma Biomarkers of Brain Atrophy in Alzheimer's Disease

Madhav Thambisetty[1]*, Andrew Simmons[2], Abdul Hye[2], James Campbell[3], Eric Westman[2], Yi Zhang[4], Lars-Olof Wahlund[5], Anna Kinsey[2], Mirsada Causevic[2], Richard Killick[2], Iwona Kloszewska[6], Patrizia Mecocci[7], Hilkka Soininen[8], Magda Tsolaki[9], Bruno Vellas[10], Christian Spenger[4], Simon Lovestone[1] for the AddNeuroMed consortium

1 Laboratory of Behavioral Neuroscience, National Institute on Aging, National Institutes of Health, Baltimore, Maryland, United States of America, 2 King's College London, Institute of Psychiatry, London, United Kingdom, 3 Proteome Sciences plc, Coveham House, Cobham, United Kingdom, 4 Department of Clinical Science, Intervention and Technology, Division of Radiology, Karolinska Institutet, Stockholm, Sweden, 5 Department of Neurobiology, Care Sciences and Society, Section of Clinical Geriatrics, Karolinska Institutet, Stockholm, Sweden, 6 Department of Old Age Psychiatry and Psychotic Disorders, Medical University of Lodz, Lodz, Poland, 7 Section of Gerontology and Geriatrics, Department of Clinical and Experimental Medicine, University of Perugia, Perugia, Italy, 8 Department of Neurology, University of Eastern Finland and University Hospital, Kuopio, Finland, 9 Department of Neurology, Aristotle University of Thessaloniki, Thessaloniki, Greece, 10 Department of Internal and Geriatrics Medicine, Hôpitaux de Toulouse, Toulouse, France

Abstract

Peripheral biomarkers of Alzheimer's disease (AD) reflecting early neuropathological change are critical to the development of treatments for this condition. The most widely used indicator of AD pathology in life at present is neuroimaging evidence of brain atrophy. We therefore performed a proteomic analysis of plasma to derive biomarkers associated with brain atrophy in AD. Using gel based proteomics we previously identified seven plasma proteins that were significantly associated with hippocampal volume in a combined cohort of subjects with AD (N = 27) and MCI (N = 17). In the current report, we validated this finding in a large independent cohort of AD (N = 79), MCI (N = 88) and control (N = 95) subjects using alternative complementary methods—quantitative immunoassays for protein concentrations and estimation of pathology by whole brain volume. We confirmed that plasma concentrations of five proteins, together with age and sex, explained more than 35% of variance in whole brain volume in AD patients. These proteins are complement components C3 and C3a, complement factor-I, γ-fibrinogen and alpha-1-microglobulin. Our findings suggest that these plasma proteins are strong predictors of in vivo AD pathology. Moreover, these proteins are involved in complement activation and coagulation, providing further evidence for an intrinsic role of these pathways in AD pathogenesis.

Citation: Thambisetty M, Simmons A, Hye A, Campbell J, Westman E, et al. (2011) Plasma Biomarkers of Brain Atrophy in Alzheimer's Disease. PLoS ONE 6(12): e28527. doi:10.1371/journal.pone.0028527

Editor: John C. S. Breitner, McGill University/Douglas Mental Health University Institute, Canada

Received September 20, 2011; Accepted November 9, 2011; Published December 21, 2011

Funding: This study was supported by InnoMed (Innovative Medicines in Europe), an Integrated Project funded by the European Union of the Sixth Framework program priority FP6-2004-LIFESCIHEALTH-5, Life Sciences, Genomics and Biotechnology for Health. Madhav Thambisetty held an Alzheimer's Society Research Fellowship at the Institute of Psychiatry, King's College London, and was an Emanoel Lee medical research fellow at St. Cross College, Oxford. AS and SL were supported by funds from the National Institute for Health Research Biomedical Research Centre for Mental Health at South London (www.nihr.ac.uk) and Maudsley National Health Service Foundation Trust and Institute of Psychiatry, King's College London. The funders had no role in study design, data collection and analysis, decision to publish, or preparation of the manuscript.

Competing Interests: As detailed below, intellectual property has been registered on the use of plasma proteins for use as biomarkers for AD by King's College London and Proteome Sciences, with Drs. Lovestone, Campbell, and Thambisetty named as inventors. Dr. Campbell was a full-time employee of Proteome Sciences, London, U.K., at the time of his contribution to the work described in this manuscript. This does not alter the authors' adherence to all the PLoS ONE policies on sharing data and materials. Patent Title Methods and Compositions Relating to Alzheimer's Disease Subject Covers utility of around 30 proteins, specifically listing 16 in the Dependent claims for diagnosis of Alzheimer's disease Filing Proteome Sciences with King's Business UK Priority GB0421639.6 dated 29/09/2004 PCT Application PCT/GB2005/003756 dated 29/09/2005 Application in Europe, Japan, US, Australia, and Canada, dated 15/03/2007 to 16/10/2007.

* E-mail: thambisettym@mail.nih.gov

Introduction

There is an urgent need for biomarkers of Alzheimer's disease (AD); especially to detect the early stages of disease. Such biomarkers have considerable potential in both clinical practice and research where they may accelerate the development of novel disease-modifying treatments [1]. In both the United States and Europe public/private consortia are conducting trials to discover such biomarkers [2,3]. Strategies for biomarker discovery in AD are well advanced using neuroimaging and assays of candidate proteins in cerebrospinal fluid (CSF). However these methods may

not be widely available for use in large, community based, multicentre studies or in the routine clinical care of large numbers of frail elderly people.

Approaches to biomarker discovery in AD have traditionally focused on demonstrating the power of candidate biomarkers to discriminate between cases and controls and have therefore relied upon standard sensitivity and specificity measures to evaluate the clinical utility of such biomarkers. We have previously used this strategy in a large proteomic analysis of plasma to derive a panel of proteins differentiating AD from age-matched healthy control subjects [4]. Employing two dimensional gel electrophoresis

(2DGE) followed by liquid chromatography tandem mass spectrometry (LC/MS/MS), we identified 15 plasma proteins whose concentrations were significantly different in AD compared to control subjects. Using semi-quantitative Western blotting, we subsequently validated two proteins; complement factor-H (CFH) and alpha2-macroglobulin (A2M) as AD-specific plasma biomarkers.

Although the above standard approach relying upon the binary distinction of differentiating disease from control may be useful, it may not be suitable for the identification of biomarkers accurately reflecting or measuring *in vivo* disease pathology in subjects with early or established AD. This attribute is in turn a key criterion for an AD biomarker [5] and one that might be especially useful in the setting of clinical trials for the enrichment of patient populations with varying severities of disease pathology. Case versus control approaches to biomarker discovery in AD also ignore the considerable overlap of pathologies such as those underlying vascular injury which are commonly observed in post mortem studies of AD patients [6]. An alternative approach is to therefore seek novel markers based primarily on their association with established metrics of disease pathology. We have successfully used this approach recently to identify plasma clusterin concentration as a marker of pathology in AD [7]. In the current study, we report the validation of a panel of plasma proteins associated with brain atrophy in AD.

Methods

Subjects and samples

We recruited 262 subjects (AD, N = 79); MCI, N = 88; and control N = 95) as part of AddNeuroMed, a multi-centre European study for the identification of AD biomarkers. Assessment, imaging and diagnostic procedures have been previously reported [8] [2].

Ethics committee approval

This study was approved by the South London and Maudsley NHS Foundation Trust ethics committee. Ethics committee approval was also obtained at each of the participating centres in accordance with the Alzheimer's Association's published recommendations [9].

MRI Data Acquisition

The primary outcome measure for validation was whole brain volume; chosen as an *in vivo* measure of pathology [10,11]. Whole-brain sagittal three-dimensional MP-RAGE images (TR = 8.6, TE = 3.8, 256×192 acquisition matrix, 180×1.2 mm slices) were obtained from all subjects on a 1.5T MR system at each of the 6 participating centres. Whole brain volumes, consisting of grey and white matter with CSF excluded and normalised to intracranial volume, were determined using an artificial neural network classifier [12]. Quality control of the MR systems was performed using the ADNI test object [13] and comparability between centres assured by repeat scanning of two volunteers on each system (whole brain volume coefficient of variation = 1.7%).

Selection of candidate biomarkers associated with brain atrophy

The selection of candidate plasma proteins for quantitative immunoassays in this report was based upon an earlier discovery-phase study in a separate cohort of AD (N = 27) and MCI (N = 17) subjects that identified the concentrations of seven plasma proteins as being significantly associated with hippocampal volume. These seven proteins were complement C3, γ-fibrinogen (Fibrinogen

gamma chain), serum albumin, complement factor-I (CFI), clusterin, α1-microglobulin, and serum amyloid-P (SAP). The detailed description of these discovery-phase 2DGE and LC/MS/MS experiments has been previously reported [7]. Briefly, the discovery-phase studies used optical densities of silver-stained protein spots in 2DGE gels and examined their association with hippocampal volumes estimated by manual tracing. Of these seven proteins, we recently validated plasma clusterin concentration as a candidate AD biomarker by reporting its association with disease severity, pathology and progression [7]. In the present report, our main aim was to examine the association with AD pathology of all the other plasma proteins (except clusterin and albumin) identified in our previous discovery-phase study. We therefore selected complement C3 and its cleavage product C3a, γ-fibrinogen, complement factor-I (CFI), α1-microglobulin, and serum amyloid-P (SAP) for validation in the current report using alternative methods in a large independent cohort of AD (N = 79), MCI (N = 88) and control (N = 95) subjects. We employed quantitative immunoassays to measure protein concentrations and automated estimates of whole brain volume using MRI images for measurement of brain atrophy.

Immunoassays

We used ELISA-based immunoassays where available (C3, C3a, and α-1-microglobulin) and semi-quantitative Western blotting in the remainder (CFI, SAP, γ-fibrinogen) (table S1 and table S2). All samples were run in quadruplicate except α-1-microglobulin which was run in duplicate. For Western blots, a reference plasma sample (consisting of at least 15 combined plasma samples from individuals collected in different centres) was run in duplicate on every gel and signals for CFI, SAP and γ-fibrinogen were normalised to the mean value of this sample.

Statistics

Inter-group differences in age, sex and education were tested by univariate general linear models. Differences in neuroimaging measures, MMSE and plasma concentrations of candidate biomarkers were tested by univariate general linear models after covarying for age. In order to account for the effects of age and sex, we first included these two variables alone as predictors of variance in whole brain volume in each of the AD, MCI and control groups using partial least squares (PLS) regression. Subsequently, the plasma protein concentrations of the candidate biomarkers were scaled to unit variance and together with age and sex, were entered into PLS regression analyses to derive models predictive of whole brain volume in each group (unit variance scaling gives both high and low variance variables equal importance in the model). In exploratory analyses, education was included as a covariate in all the PLS regression models. As it was found not to contribute to variance in whole brain volume, it was excluded from the final optimal PLS model.

The predictive ability of the PLS model was assessed using a seven-fold cross validation procedure and summarised as the root mean square error of prediction (RMSEP):

$$\text{RMSEP} = \sqrt{\frac{\sum_{i=1}^{n}(\hat{y}i - yi)^2}{n}}$$

where $\hat{y}_i$-y_i represents the residuals between predicted and actual values of whole brain volume. The RMSEP is analogous to a standard deviation of the differences between predicted and actual values of whole brain volume.

Table 1. Sample characteristics of AD, MCI and control participants in this study.

	AD (n = 79)	MCI (n = 88)	Control (n = 95)
Sex (M/F)	28/51	42/46	43/52
Age (years)	76.0 (6.0)*	74.6 (5.9)	73.1 (7.0)
Education (years)	7.9 (4.0)[†]	9.2 (4.3)[††]	10.8 (4.8)
Disease duration (years)	3.9 (2.4)		
MMSE	20.9 (4.6)[§]	27.3 (1.6)[§§]	29 (1.2)
Whole brain volume normalised to total ICV.	0.82 (0.03)[¶,¶¶]	0.85 (0.03)	0.86 (0.030)

Values are expressed as mean ± (SD).
*Differs from control; $p = 0.007$.
[§]Differs from control; $p < 0.001$.
[§§]Differs from control; $p < 0.001$.
[¶]differs from control; $p < 0.001$.
[¶¶]differs from MCI; $p < 0.001$.
[†]Differs from control; $p < 0.001$.
[††]Differs from control; $p < 0.02$.
doi:10.1371/journal.pone.0028527.t001

Results

We have previously reported the gel-based proteomics discovery of candidate plasma proteins associated with hippocampal atrophy in AD [7]. Having previously identified a set of proteins associated with hippocampal volume in disease state, we set out, in the current study, to validate these findings using alternative methods in a larger, independent cohort of subjects. We established, *a priori*, outcome criteria for validation; the primary outcome being association with whole brain volume, chosen both as an excellent discriminator of disease state [10,11] and a measure of atrophy readily suitable for analysis of MRI data obtained from a multi-centre study with fewer problems of rater-variability than manual estimates of hippocampal volume. Secondary outcomes were differences in concentrations of markers between diagnostic groups and/or correlation with clinical measures of disease severity (MMSE for cognition and Clinical Dementia Rating for global severity).

Subject characteristics

Patients with AD (N = 79; 75.6±6.0 years) were slightly older than both MCI (N = 88; 74.6±7.0 years; non-significant) and control subjects (N = 95; 73.1±6.7 years; $p = 0.005$; LSD post-hoc test). There were no significant differences in gender between the groups. Whole brain volume was significantly decreased in the AD group compared to both control ($p < 0.001$) and MCI ($p < 0.001$)

subjects (table 1). Table 2 shows the mean plasma concentrations of the assayed proteins with the corresponding standard errors.

Partial least squares regression of whole brain volume against predictor variables

In initial exploratory analyses, we first examined unadjusted univariate associations between concentrations of the six plasma proteins and whole brain volume in the AD group (table 3). Age and sex together accounted for 19.7% of variance in whole brain volume in the AD group. Single component PLS models were then fitted to whole brain volume wherein the predictor variables included age, sex, concentrations of the six plasma proteins and the ratio of complement C3:C3a. The latter measure was included as a predictor variable as it is an accepted marker of complement activation [14]. The model explaining the greatest variance in whole brain volume was in the AD group, where a single-component PLS model explained 37.7% of the variance (R2Y) in brain volume (Q2 provides an estimate of how well the model predicts the Y data and R2X denotes variance explained in the predictor variables) (table 2). A further refinement of this model was achieved by eliminating those predictor variables contributing the least to explaining variance in whole brain volume. Inspection of the variable influence on projection (VIP) plot showed that the ratio of C3:C3a and SAP concentration contributed least to explaining variance in whole brain volume in AD and these

Table 2. Plasma concentrations of assayed candidate biomarkers with their corresponding standard errors.

	AD	MCI	Control
C3 (µg/µl)	1588.0 (170.7)	1282.1 (110.5)	1167.1 (65.2)
C3a (ng/ml)	2653.3 (134.5)	2629.9 (136.2)	3064.0 (118.4)
A1M (mg/l)	16.7 (0.94)	17.27 (0.93)	15.58 (1.0)
CFI*	0.86 (0.01)	0.86 (0.01)	0.88 (0.01)
Gamma-fibrinogen*	0.92 (0.01)	0.96 (0.01)	0.94 (0.01)
SAP*	1.12 (0.05)	1.1 (0.04)	1.12 (0.05)

CFI, Gamma fibrinogen and SAP were assayed by Western blotting and their concentrations are in arbitrary units of optical density*.
doi:10.1371/journal.pone.0028527.t002

Table 3. Univariate associations between plasma concentrations of assayed candidate biomarkers and whole brain volume in AD; R = Pearson correlation coefficient; p = 2-tailed statistical significance.

Plasma protein	R/p
C3	0.31/0.006
C3a	0.27/0.02
A1M	−0.23/0.04
CFI	0.24/0.04
Gamma-fibrinogen	0.24/0.03
SAP	0.05/0.65

doi:10.1371/journal.pone.0028527.t003

A
VIP
2,0
1,5
1,0
0,5
0,0
-0,5
Age
C3
Gender
C3a
γ Fibrinogen
CFI
α -1-microglobulin
SAP
C3C3a
B
Observed WBV
0,92
0,90
0,88
0,86
0,84
0,82
0,80
0,78
0,76
0,74
0,73 0,74 0,75 0,76 0,77 0,78 0,79 0,80 0,81 0,82 0,83 0,84 0,85 0,86 0,87 0,88 0,89 0,90 0,91 0,92
Predicted WBV
C
R2Y and Q2Y
R2
Q2
0,9
0,8
0,7
0,6
0,5
0,4
0,3
0,2
0,1
0,0
-0,1
0,0 0,1 0,2 0,3 0,4 0,5 0,6 0,7 0,8 0,9 1,0
Correlations coefficient between original and permuted WBV

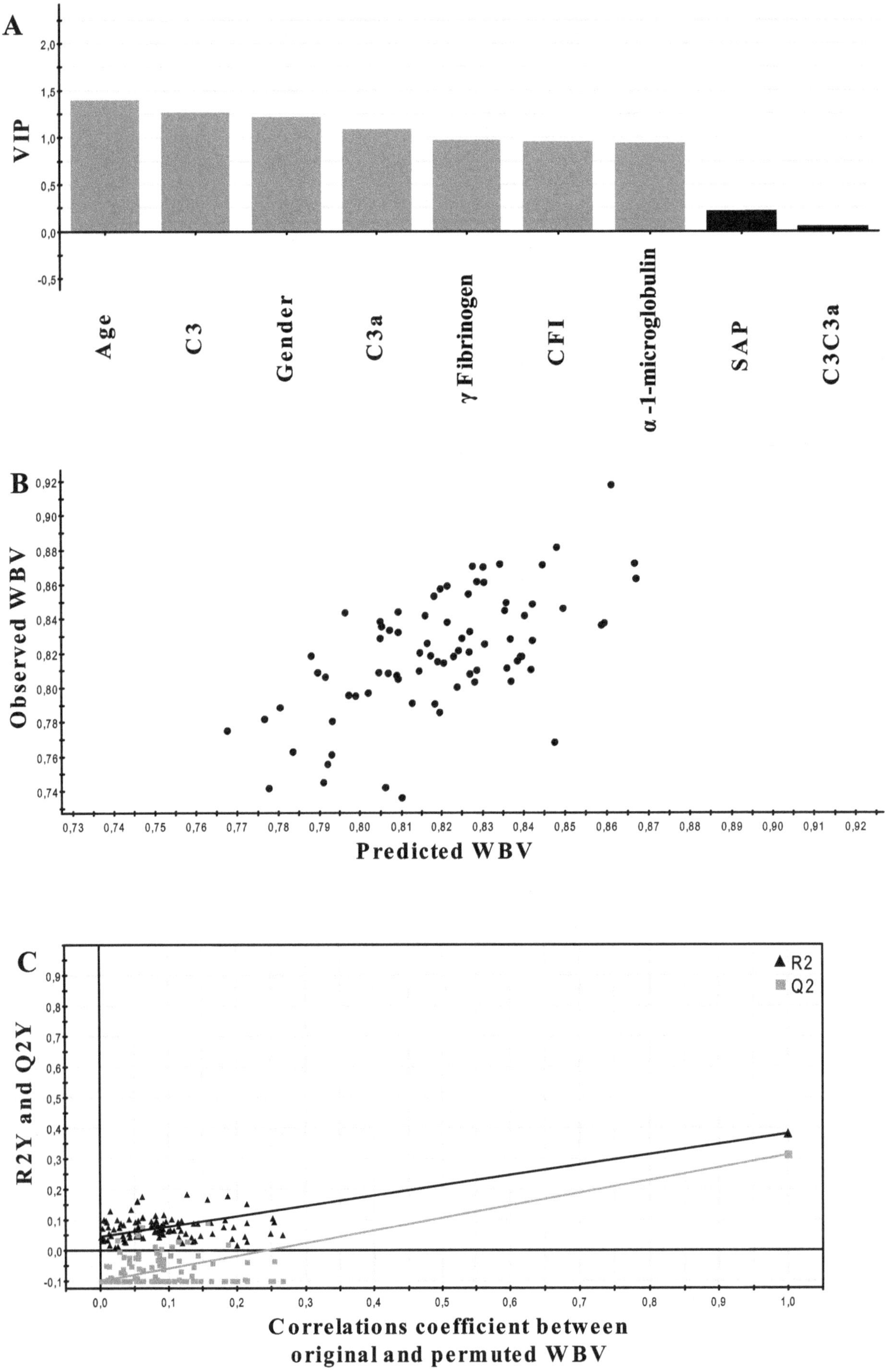

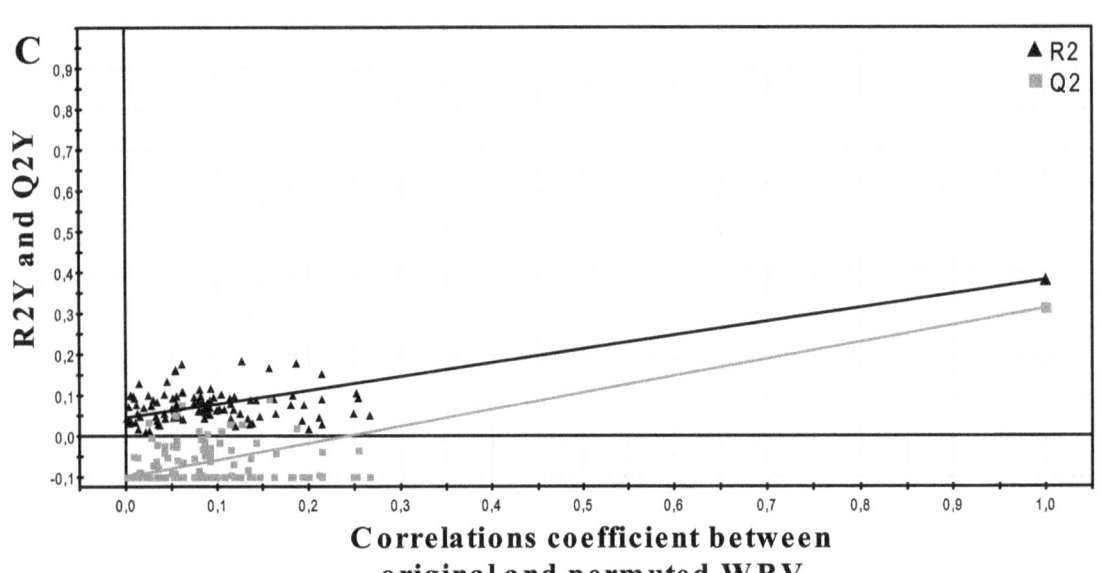

Figure 1. Plasma proteins associated with whole brain volume in Alzheimer's disease. A. Variable influence on projection (VIP) plot summarising the overall contribution of each predictor variable to the PLS model for brain volume in AD, summed over all components and weighted according to the Y variation accounted for by each component. Black bars represent variables contributing the least (SAP and C3:C3a) to variance in the brain volume and therefore eliminated in the final PLS model. **B**. The result of a seven-round cross validation exercise in which every point represents test data not used in the model-building. Plots of observed versus predicted values of normalised whole brain volume (WBV) in AD patients using a single-component PLS model constituted by age, sex, C3a, C3, γ-fibrinogen, α-1-microglobulin and CFI (regression line is represented by the equation: observed value = $[1.00 \pm 0.126 \times \text{predicted value}] + 0.0004 \pm 0.102$; root mean square error of predictions = 0.027). **C**. Internal validation of the final PLS model predicting whole brain volume in AD demonstrating clear decreases in model performance as the whole brain volume data are permuted relative to the predictor variables. R2Y (black triangles) describes how well the derived model fits the data and is the proportion of the sum of squares explained by the model. Q2 (red squares) describes the predictive ability of the derived model and is the cross validated R2Y. The pair of R2 and Q2 values at the extreme right represent the optimal PLS model constituted by age, sex, C3a, C3, γ-fibrinogen, α-1-microglobulin and CFI. The cluster of R2 and Q2 values at the left represent the PLS models derived by permutating the whole brain volume data relative to the predictor variables and show a clear decline in performance.
doi:10.1371/journal.pone.0028527.g001

variables were therefore eliminated (figure 1A). This refinement led to deriving a final optimal single-component PLS model with age, sex, complement C3, C3a, γ-fibrinogen, α-1-microglobulin and CFI that could together explain 38.2% of variance in whole brain volume in subjects with AD (table 4).

Cross validation of PLS model of plasma proteins predicting brain volume

The final PLS model for whole brain volume in AD consisting of age, sex, C3a, C3, γ-fibrinogen, α-1-microglobulin and CFI gave a low RMSEP value of 0.027 indicating good predictive power (figure 1B).

Internal validation of the PLS model for whole brain volume in AD

Further 'internal' model validation was effected by randomising the positions of the Y data in relation to their corresponding rows in the X matrix (typically 100 separate row permutations were performed) and observing the effect of this randomisation on the R2Y and Q2 values. Randomisation of the Y data considerably reduced R2Y and Q2 (figure 1C) in comparison to the original model, thereby indicating its validity. Furthermore, the results of this response permutation testing suggest that the likelihood of deriving a model with comparable predictive ability purely by chance was less than 1%, further indicating the robustness of the PLS model for whole brain volume in AD.

Clinical correlations with plasma biomarkers

We also examined the plasma concentrations of these proteins in relation to diagnosis and clinical measures of severity as secondary outcomes. Plasma C3 was significantly elevated in AD ($p = 0.03$) patients relative to controls. We also observed a trend for association between plasma C3 concentration and MMSE score in the combined group of AD and MCI subjects ($r = -0.14$, p = 0.07). Plasma γ-fibrinogen was significantly increased in MCI subjects versus AD ($p = 0.03$).

Discussion

We have adopted a novel approach to the discovery of biologically relevant plasma biomarkers in early AD. Our aim was to identify peripheral markers of AD by their association with established neuroimaging measures of pathology and then to validate these by alternative quantitative methods in a large and independent test population.

Multiple lines of evidence suggest that peripheral fluids such as plasma may be a rich source of biomarkers in AD. Such markers might reflect a systemic metabolic signature of AD or be a change in plasma secondary to a disease-specific process in the brain [15]. We have previously used a proteomic approach to identify plasma proteins differentially expressed in established AD [4]. Others have used arrays of candidate proteins, finding remarkably high sensitivity and specificity for diagnosis of established AD versus controls [16]. Both candidate and 'data-driven' approaches (proteomics, transcriptomics etc) tend to use disease status, either case versus control or control/MCI progression to case, as the primary outcome variable in discovery studies. Where the discovery paradigm uses large scale or array-based technologies, this can result in the identification of potential biomarkers with no known, or at best, uncertain, involvement in disease. Furthermore this binary distinction (disease/no disease) may result in the discovery of biomarkers that show excellent diagnostic or predictive characteristics but lack sensitivity in relation to disease progression or severity. To avoid these problems, we sought to discover, using proteomics, biomarkers where the primary outcomes were associations with well-established neuroimaging measures of disease pathology.

In the discovery-phase proteomics study which led us to the candidate plasma proteins of interest in the current report, we used hippocampal atrophy as a measure of disease pathology [7]. For validation of candidate markers in the present study, we chose an alternative measure of brain atrophy to overcome some of the limitations of manual hippocampal volumetry. The chief advantage of whole brain over manual estimates of hippocampal volume

Table 4. Summary of the partial least squares (PLS) models fitted to whole brain volume in AD; R2X-variance explained in the predictor variables; R2Y-variance explained in the response variable i.e. whole brain volume; Q2-goodness of prediction of the PLS model.

Number of components	Predictor variables	R2X	R2Y	Q2
1	Age, Sex	0.53	0.197	0.187
1	Age, Sex, C3, C3a, C3:C3a, CFI, SAP, γ-fibrinogen, α1-microglobulin	0.186	0.377	0.295
1*	Age, Sex, C3, C3a, CFI, γ-fibrinogen, α1-microglobulin	0.277	0.382	0.311

*Denotes final optimal PLS model, after eliminating those variables contributing the least to explaining variance in whole brain volume.
doi:10.1371/journal.pone.0028527.t004

is that the automated calculation of whole brain volume is not subject to inter-rater variability and is therefore readily utilisable in large multi-centre studies such as ours.

Moreover, like hippocampal atrophy, whole brain atrophy is also an early event in the disease, an excellent discriminator of disease state and correlates closely with longitudinal measures of atrophy [10,11,17]. Automated cross-sectional measurements of normalised whole brain volume have also been compared with longitudinal measures of rates of whole brain atrophy [11]. These studies have reported that the cross-sectional measurement of whole brain volume is nearly as powerful a discriminant between AD patients and controls as longitudinal observations on rates of whole brain atrophy. Equally importantly, there is a highly significant correlation between cross-sectional and longitudinal measures of whole brain atrophy in AD. The latter has also been used as a neuroimaging biomarker in a clinical trial of AD [18]. Cross-sectional measurement of whole brain volume was recently shown to differentiate between MCI subjects progressing to AD and those that remained stable [10]. In subjects with MCI and established AD, there was also a highly significant association between baseline whole brain volume and CSF $A\beta_{1-42}$, levels, further suggesting that this neuroimaging measure reflects an integral feature of AD neuropathology [19].

Our previous discovery-phase study demonstrated that seven plasma proteins were significantly associated with hippocampal volume in a combined cohort of AD and MCI subjects [7]. In the current report, we confirmed a significant association between these plasma proteins and whole brain volume in AD. Five proteins from the original panel of candidate biomarkers explained 18% of variance in brain volume in the AD group. Together with age and sex, these proteins could explain more than 35% of variance in brain volume in AD patients. Further cross validation and response permutation testing confirmed a robust predictive power of this PLS model for whole brain volume in AD.

Our results demonstrate that we have identified a panel of plasma proteins that are predictors of current disease severity as measured by well-established neuroimaging markers of pathology. Moreover, their association with core neuropathological features of AD suggests that these proteins are not merely non-specific markers of disability in the elderly, but biologically relevant proteins accurately reflecting disease pathology.

Most of the plasma proteins associated with neuroimaging measures of disease pathology in this study are components or regulators of the complement system and coagulation pathway. Multiple lines of evidence support a role for the complement system in the pathogenesis of AD [20,21] and recent proteomic studies have implicated complement proteins in the CSF, including C3a both as biomarkers of established AD [22] as well as predictors of conversion to AD in MCI subjects [23]. Fibrinogen is yet another candidate biomarker common to findings in the current report and a recent proteomic analysis in CSF that identified biomarkers discriminating AD from control samples [24]. It must be noted that very few studies have directly addressed the associations between peripheral concentrations of complement modulating proteins and their levels in the central nervous system. This is an important consideration in the interpretation of blood biomarker studies and their relevance to brain pathology in AD. We have recently attempted to address this question and reported that the plasma concentration of clusterin, a known complement modulator is significantly associated with its expression in brain regions vulnerable to AD pathology [25]. A significant association between γ-fibrinogen and brain volume

observed in the current report is also interesting in the light of data demonstrating an increased risk of dementia in subjects with elevated plasma levels of fibrinogen [26].

Our present study suggesting that complement regulators and complement-related proteins are candidate biomarkers of AD also extends findings from our previous proteomic analysis of plasma implicating complement factor-H (CFH) as an AD-specific plasma biomarker [4,27].

A limitation of the present study that must be acknowledged is its cross-sectional design. Therefore, while our results strongly suggest that we have identified a panel of biomarkers that reflect current disease status by their association with *in vivo* disease pathology, we have not yet extended these findings to examine the utility of these proteins in measuring disease progression. However, our findings merit independent confirmation by other groups and if replicated, are likely to be rapidly extended to longitudinal studies that examine their utility as markers of disease progression or treatment response in clinical trials. It must also be noted that the use of MRI-derived brain volume estimates in this and the majority of other AD biomarker studies may ignore the significant contribution of ischemic microvascular pathology to AD pathogenesis. This issue merits consideration in the interpretation of these studies, especially because of the paucity of reliable imaging biomarkers of microvascular brain injury [28].

In summary, we combined a proteomic and neuroimaging approach to the discovery of biologically relevant biomarkers in AD. Variation in just five plasma proteins, together with age and sex accounts for more than a third of the variance in brain volume suggesting that these proteins are likely to be strong predictors of pathology *in vivo*. We therefore suggest that plasma markers have the potential for future use in large scale community based settings – either in clinical practice or research. Furthermore, these findings add weight to the growing evidence implicating the complement and coagulation pathways in AD pathogenesis.

Supporting Information

Table S1   Details of reagents used in Western Blot assays.
(DOC)

Table S2   Details of reagents used in ELISA assays.
(DOC)

Acknowledgments

We are grateful to Vaksha Patel for expert technical assistance with the 2DGE experiments and to the following for work on the AddNeuroMed project, including assessment of research participants: Nicola Dunlop, Catherine Tunnard, Rufina Leung and Nicola Archer (London); Emma Reynish (Toulouse); Tomasz Sobow (Lodz); Niki Day and Simon Beaulah (BioWisdom); Seija Hynynen (Kuopio); Penelope Mauredaki (Thessaloniki); Emanuela Costanzi, Roberto Tarducci and Roberta Cecchetti (Perugia), Eva-Lena Engman, Dagmawi Elehu, Johan O. Bengtsson and Tony Segerdahl (Karolinska Institutet, Stockholm); and Per Julin (AstraZeneca).

Author Contributions

Conceived and designed the experiments: Madhav Thambisetty AS SL. Performed the experiments: Madhav Thambisetty AS AH AK MC RK. Analyzed the data: AS Madhav Thambisetty EW JC YZ. Contributed reagents/materials/analysis tools: L-OW IK PM HS Magda Tsolaki BV CS SL. Wrote the paper: Madhav Thambisetty AS SL.

References

1. Cummings JL, Doody R, Clark C (2007) Disease-modifying therapies for Alzheimer disease: challenges to early intervention. Neurology 69: 1622–1634.

2. Lovestone S, Francis P, Strandgaard K (2007) Biomarkers for disease modification trials–the innovative medicines initiative and AddNeuroMed. J Nutr Health Aging 11: 359–361.

3. Mueller SG, Weiner MW, Thal LJ, Petersen RC, Jack CR, et al. (2005) Ways toward an early diagnosis in Alzheimer's disease: the Alzheimer's Disease Neuroimaging Initiative (ADNI). Alzheimers Dement 1: 55–66.

4. Hye A, Lynham S, Thambisetty M, Causevic M, Campbell J, et al. (2006) Proteome-based plasma biomarkers for Alzheimer's disease. Brain 129: 3042–3050.

5. The Ronald and Nancy Reagan Research Institute of the Alzheimer's Association and the National Institute on Aging Working Group (1998) Consensus report of the Working Group on: "Molecular and Biochemical Markers of Alzheimer's Disease". Neurobiol Aging 19: 109–116.

6. Schneider JA, Arvanitakis Z, Bang W, Bennett DA (2007) Mixed brain pathologies account for most dementia cases in community-dwelling older persons. Neurology 69: 2197–2204.

7. Thambisetty M, Simmons A, Velayudhan L, Hye A, Campbell J, et al. (2010) Association of plasma clusterin concentration with severity, pathology, and progression in Alzheimer disease. Arch Gen Psychiatry 67: 739–748.

8. Simmons A, Westman E, Muehlboeck S, Mecocci P, Vellas B, et al. (2011) The AddNeuroMed framework for multi-centre MRI assessment of Alzheimer's disease: experience from the first 24 months. Int J Geriatr Psychiatry 26: 75–82.

9. Alzheimer's Association (2004) Research consent for cognitively impaired adults: recommendations for institutional review boards and investigators. Alzheimer Dis Assoc Disord 18: 171–175.

10. Karas G, Sluimer J, Goekoop R, van der Flier W, Rombouts SA, et al. (2008) Amnestic mild cognitive impairment: structural MR imaging findings predictive of conversion to Alzheimer disease. AJNR Am J Neuroradiol 29: 944–949.

11. Smith SM, Rao A, De Stefano N, Jenkinson M, Schott JM, et al. (2007) Longitudinal and cross-sectional analysis of atrophy in Alzheimer's disease: cross-validation of BSI, SIENA and SIENAX. Neuroimage 36: 1200–1206.

12. Zijdenbos AP, Forghani R, Evans AC (2002) Automatic "pipeline" analysis of 3-D MRI data for clinical trials: application to multiple sclerosis. IEEE Trans Med Imaging 21: 1280–1291.

13. Jack CR, Jr., Bernstein MA, Fox NC, Thompson P, Alexander G, et al. (2008) The Alzheimer's Disease Neuroimaging Initiative (ADNI): MRI methods. J Magn Reson Imaging 27: 685–691.

14. Stove S, Welte T, Wagner TO, Kola A, Klos A, et al. (1996) Circulating complement proteins in patients with sepsis or systemic inflammatory response syndrome. Clin Diagn Lab Immunol 3: 175–183.

15. Mattila KM, Frey H (1995) Two-dimensional analysis of qualitative and quantitative changes in blood cell proteins in Alzheimer's disease: search for extraneuronal markers. Appl Theor Electrophor 4: 189–196.

16. Ray S, Britschgi M, Herbert C, Takeda-Uchimura Y, Boxer A, et al. (2007) Classification and prediction of clinical Alzheimer's diagnosis based on plasma signaling proteins. Nat Med 13: 1359–1362.

17. Murphy DG, DeCarli CD, Daly E, Gillette JA, McIntosh AR, et al. (1993) Volumetric magnetic resonance imaging in men with dementia of the Alzheimer type: correlations with disease severity. Biol Psychiatry 34: 612–621.

18. Fox NC, Black RS, Gilman S, Rossor MN, Griffith SG, et al. (2005) Effects of Abeta immunization (AN1792) on MRI measures of cerebral volume in Alzheimer disease. Neurology 64: 1563–1572.

19. Wahlund LO, Blennow K (2003) Cerebrospinal fluid biomarkers for disease stage and intensity in cognitively impaired patients. Neurosci Lett 339: 99–102.

20. Bonifati DM, Kishore U (2007) Role of complement in neurodegeneration and neuroinflammation. Mol Immunol 44: 999–1010.

21. Shen Y, Meri S (2003) Yin and Yang: complement activation and regulation in Alzheimer's disease. Prog Neurobiol 70: 463–472.

22. Finehout EJ, Franck Z, Choe LH, Relkin N, Lee KH (2007) Cerebrospinal fluid proteomic biomarkers for Alzheimer's disease. Ann Neurol 61: 120–129.

23. Simonsen AH, McGuire J, Hansson O, Zetterberg H, Podust VN, et al. (2007) Novel panel of cerebrospinal fluid biomarkers for the prediction of progression to Alzheimer dementia in patients with mild cognitive impairment. Arch Neurol 64: 366–370.

24. Craig-Schapiro R, Kuhn M, Xiong C, Pickering EH, Liu J, et al. (2011) Multiplexed immunoassay panel identifies novel CSF biomarkers for Alzheimer's disease diagnosis and prognosis. PLoS One 6: e18850.

25. Thambisetty M, An Y, Kinsey A, Koka D, Saleem M, et al. (2012) Plasma clusterin concentration is associated with longitudinal brain atrophy in mild cognitive impairment. Neuroimage 59: 212–217.

26. van Oijen M, Witteman JC, Hofman A, Koudstaal PJ, Breteler MM (2005) Fibrinogen is associated with an increased risk of Alzheimer disease and vascular dementia. Stroke 36: 2637–2641.

27. Thambisetty M, Hye A, Foy C, Daly E, Glover A, et al. (2008) Proteome-based identification of plasma proteins associated with hippocampal metabolism in early Alzheimer's disease. J Neurol 255: 1712–1720.

28. Mills S, Cain J, Purandare N, Jackson A (2007) Biomarkers of cerebrovascular disease in dementia. Br J Radiol 80 Spec No 2: S128–145.

Evaluation of a Previously Suggested Plasma Biomarker Panel to Identify Alzheimer's Disease

Maria Björkqvist[1]*, Mattias Ohlsson[2], Lennart Minthon[3,4], Oskar Hansson[3,4]

1 Brain Disease Biomarker Unit, Department of Experimental Medical Science, Wallenberg Neuroscience Center, Lund University, Lund, Sweden, 2 Computational Biology and Biological Physics, Lund University, Lund, Sweden, 3 Clinical Memory Research Unit, Department of Clinical Sciences Malmö, Lund University, Malmö, Sweden, 4 Neuropsychiatric Clinic, Skåne University Hospital, Malmö, Sweden

Abstract

There is an urgent need for biomarkers in plasma to identify Alzheimer's disease (AD). It has previously been shown that a signature of 18 plasma proteins can identify AD during pre-dementia and dementia stages (Ray et al, Nature Medicine, 2007). We quantified the same 18 proteins in plasma from 174 controls, 142 patients with AD, and 88 patients with other dementias. Only three of these proteins (EGF, PDG-BB and MIP-1δ) differed significantly in plasma between controls and AD. The 18 proteins could classify patients with AD from controls with low diagnostic precision (area under the ROC curve was 63%). Moreover, they could not distinguish AD from other dementias. In conclusion, independent validation of results is important in explorative biomarker studies.

Citation: Björkqvist M, Ohlsson M, Minthon L, Hansson O (2012) Evaluation of a Previously Suggested Plasma Biomarker Panel to Identify Alzheimer's Disease. PLoS ONE 7(1): e29868. doi:10.1371/journal.pone.0029868

Editor: Michelle L. Block, Virginia Commonwealth University, United States of America

Received July 11, 2011; **Accepted** December 5, 2011; **Published** January 18, 2012

Funding: This work was supported by the Swedish Research Council, the Swedish Brain Power, the Regional Agreement on Medical Training and Clinical Research (ALF) between Skåne County Counsil and Lund University and the Torsten and Ragnar Söderberg Foundation. MB is supported by BenteRexed foundation. The funders had no role in study design, data collection and analysis, decision to publish, or preparation of the manuscript.

Competing Interests: The authors have declared that no competing interests exist.

* E-mail: maria.bjorkqvist@med.lu.se

Introduction

Alzheimer's disease (AD) is the major cause of dementia and a great medical and socioeconomic problem worldwide. As populations get older, the prevalence of AD will increase considerably during the coming decades [1]. The pathological characteristics of AD are senile plaques and neurofibrillary tangles, containing aggregated amyloid β (Aβ) and hyperphosphorylated tau protein, respectively [1,2]. Aβ accumulation is thought to start many decades before symptoms occur [3]. During the last few years, it has become more apparent that disease-modifying therapies for AD are more likely to be successful if initiated during the early stages of the disease when neurodegeneration is not yet too severe [4,5]. Therefore, biomarkers are urgently needed to correctly identify subjects affected by AD before they have developed dementia [5,6]. Cerebrospinal fluid biomarker can identify prodromal AD with acceptable accuracy [7–9]. However, plasma is much easier obtained than cerebrospinal fluid. Therefore, it was a major breakthrough when Ray and collaborators found that a pattern of 18 proteins in plasma could classify samples from AD and controls with almost 90% accuracy [10]. The same plasma proteins could also predict the patients with mild cognitive impairment who would later develop AD. The study comprised of 259 plasma samples obtained from in total 7 clinical centres [10].

In the present study, we evaluated the diagnostic value of the same 18 proteins as Ray et al [10], using 433 plasma samples obtained at Skåne University Hospital, Sweden, from 174 controls, 142 patients with AD, 29 patients with depression, and 88 patients with other types of dementia than AD (i.e 37 with Lewy Body dementia, 11 with Parkinson's disease with dementia, 22 with frontotemporal dementia, 18 with vascular dementia).

Materials and Methods

Collection and processing of human plasma samples

The study population was recruited at the memory disorder clinic, Skåne University Hospital, Malmö, Sweden. The patients underwent thorough standard examinations conducted by a trained physician, including neurological, physical and psychiatric examinations. The patients who during clinical follow-up received a diagnosis of AD had to meet the DSM-IIIR criteria of dementia [11] and the criteria of probable AD defined by NINCDS-ADRDA [12]. Subjects who were diagnosed as having vascular dementia (VaD) fulfilled the DSM-IIIR criteria of dementia and the requirements for probable VaD by NINDS-AIREN [13] or the recommendations by Erkinjuntti and co-workers for VaD of the subcortical type [14]. For patients who developed dementia with Lewy bodies (DLB) or frontotemporal dementia, the consensus criteria by McKeith and collaborators [15] and McKhann and colleagues were used [16], respectively. The healthy volunteers had no memory complaints or other cognitive symptoms, preservation of general cognitive function, and no active neurological or psychiatric diseases.

The study was conducted in accordance with the Helsinki Declaration and approved by the ethics committee of Lund University, Sweden. All subjects gave informed written consent.

Non-fasting plasma was collected between 9 and 11 am. After venipuncture, blood was collected in tubes prepared with EDTA to prevent coagulation. Samples were centrifuged, and plasma was removed from the tubes leaving 1 ml of plasma to avoid contamination of plasma with blood cells including trombocytes. Within one hour from venipuncture the plasma was frozen in polypropylene tubes at −80°C until biochemical analysis.

Analysis of plasma proteins

Quantibody® Human Costum Cytokine Antibody Array was performed by RayBiotech (as per company description) on blinded samples for the following markers; ANG-2I, CAM-1, IGFBP-6, PARC, PDGF-BB, RANTES, EGF, G-CSF, GDNF, IL-1a, IL-3, IL-8, IL-11, MCP-3, M-CSF, MIP-1δ, TNFa, and TRAIL R4. A positive control (four biotin-labelled bovine IgG spot) was included on each array and used for inter- and intra-slide normalization. For a quadruplicate spot, outliers as value above 30% over the median, was excluded. All samples were analyzed in a single run to minimize variation.

Selected cytokines (M-CSF and TNF-α) were quantified in triplicates using Meso Scale Discovery (MSD®, Gaithersburg, MD) electrochemoluminescence assays using a modification of the manufacturer's protocol. 30 ul was used as the sample volume and a 10-point standard curve was used, ranging from 2500 pg/ml to 0 pg/ml. The sample and calibrator were incubated on the MSD plate for 3 h (instead of 2 h), followed by a wash (as per manufacturer's recommendation). The MSD plate was then incubated with detection antibody solution for 3 h (instead of 2 h) before wash and read as per manufacturer's recommendation. Results were analyzed on a SECTOR™ 6000 instrument (MSD).

The operator was unaware of the disease state of each sample during processing and statistical analysis was performed independently.

Statistical analysis

The statistical analyses were accomplished using SPSS for Windows, version 18.0.1 (SPSS Inc/IBM, Chicago, IL, USA). To compare demographic and plasma data between groups, non-parametric Kruskal-Wallis tests were performed followed by Mann-Whitney U-tests for continuous variables. Pearson's x^2 test was used for dichotomous variables.

To assess the ability of the plasma data to separate groups (AD vs. Controls or AD vs. other dementia) multiple logistic regression [17], artificial neural network (ANN) [18] and nearest shrunken centroid [19] classification models were used. The latter was the method used by Ray et al. Bagging ensembles [20] of standard multi-layer perceptrons with one hidden layer were used in the ANN models. The size of the ensemble was set to 30 and the number of hidden nodes of the individual networks in the ensemble was two. No effort was made to tune these parameters. The nearest shrunken centroid method was implemented using the R package *pamr*. The area under the ROC curve (AUC) was used

Table 1. Subject demographics and plasma protein levels.

	Controls (n = 174)	Depr (n = 29)	AD (n = 142)	FTD (n = 22)	VaD (n = 18)	PDD (n = 11)	DLB (n = 37)
Mean age (range)	74 (62–99)	59 (42–76)	76[a,b] (56–87)	62 (43–78)	76 (56–84)	72 (62–81)	74 (54–85)
Women	117	15	40[c]	11	14	5	26
MMSE	29±0,1	28±0,4	21±0,4[d,e]	22±1,1	22±0,8	20±2,0	21±0,9
ANG-2	2444±143	1710±232	2306±284	2043±320	2410±527	1789±535	2335±341
ICAM-1	224±9	250±31	216±9	222±28	220±22	162±16	204±15
IGFBP-6	382±13	366±21	377±13	337±19	373±40	391±51	379±17
PARC (CCL18)	43±2,7	40±6,0	40±2,4	38±5,1	39±7,9	33±5,3	41±3,9
PDGF-BB	4385±288	6339±1122	5701±427[f]	5896±706	9302±3278	8557±3513	5798±1431
RANTES (CCL5)	18±0,7	20±1,5	20±0,7	20±1,3	23±3,2	19±2,3	18±1,3
EGF	541±31	665±65	706±32[g]	825±79	799±158	907±117	580±49
G-CSF	54±3,1	41±5,1	57±6	56±10	53±12	56±13	42±3,9
GDNF	103±33	86±34	322±262	79±15	41±11	34±12	45±6,5
IL-1a	13±2,4	11,2±3,2	26±17	11±1,7	8,5±1,9	10±2,0	9,5±1,3
IL-3	44±15	29±9,1	87±63	32±6,3	14±3,8	15±4,1	22±6,0
IL-8 (CXCL8)	11±1,0	8,5±0,8	10±0,5	12±1,9	10±1,4	11±1,2	10±0,8
IL-11	236±27	185±78	249±34	249±53	260±74	158±563	263±49
MCP-3 (CCL7)	51±4,8	47±6,4	82±30	51±6,8	52±12	67±8,2	42±6,1
M-CSF	1,0±0,2	1,3±0,7	1±0,3	1,2±0,37	0,77±0,51	1,2±0,5	1,0±0,4
MIP-1d (CCL15)	2361±85	2322±229	2845±142[h]	2452±200	2383±312	3154±453	3144±348
TNF-a	23±4,6	15±2,5	17±1,3	17±2,6	15±2,8	16±2,6	16±2,0
TRAILR4	36±15	12±4,3	169±157	17±7,1	13±9,1	3,1±2,3	9,5±3,3

Table 1. Values are given in ng/L, except for ICAM-1, IGFBP-6, PARC and RANTES for which concentrations are given in µg/L.
When comparing AD vs 1) Controls, 2) Depression and 3) other dementias the following significant changes were observed:
[a]AD vs control p = 0.01,
[b]AD vs depression p<0.001, AD vs other dementias p = 0.01.
[c]AD vs depression p = 0.034.
[d]AD vs control p<0.001,
[e]AD vs depression p = 0.001.
[f]AD vs control p = 0.004.
[g]AD vs control p<0.001.
[h]AD vs control p = 0.011 (Kruskal–Wallis one-way analysis of variance by ranks followed by Mann-Whitney U test).
Abbreviations: Depr, depression; AD, Alzheimers disease; FTD, frontotemporal lobe dementia; VaD, vascular dementia; PDD, Parkinson's disease with dementia; DLB = dementia with Lewy bodies.
doi:10.1371/journal.pone.0029868.t001

to measure the performance of the classification models. For all three models, 10-fold cross-validation was used to estimate true AUC values. The cross-validation procedure was repeated 100 times, with random 10-fold splits each time, in order to decrease random fluctuations.

Results

In table 1 we present the demographic data and levels of the 18 plasma proteins obtained when using Quantibody® Human Costum Cytokine Antibody Array (RayBiotech). The subjects affected by AD were slightly older than the controls and the group affected by other forms of dementias ($p \leq 0.01$). Only three proteins of the 18 proteins, (EGF, PDG-BB and MIP-1δ), were found to be significantly altered in plasma from AD patients when compared to controls (table 1). None of the proteins differed between the AD group and the group with other dementias than AD. Analyses of two cytokines (M-CSF and TNF-a) with ELISA technology verified that there were no statistical differences between AD and control plasma samples (in control plasma, n = 148, M-CSF levels were 21.82 ± 0.87 ng/L and TNF-a levels were 1.90 ± 0.14 ng/L, in AD plasma, n = 148, the corresponding levels were 24.03 ± 0.71 and 1.85 ± 0.06 ng/L respectively).

When classifying the AD group from the controls, the cross-validation AUC for the logistic regression model was 0.60 using all 18 proteins. The corresponding AUC for the ANN model and the nearest shrunken centroid classifier was 0.63. When only using the three proteins that differed significantly between groups (i.e. EGF, PDG-BB and MIP-1δ), as inputs to the classifiers, the AUC increased to 0.66 for all three models.

A worse performance was obtained when classifying the group with AD from the group with other forms of dementia than AD. Using all plasma proteins the cross-validation AUC was below 0.5 indicating no classification ability at all. This was true for all three models. The best individual protein in terms of AUC performance was TRAIL-R4 with an AUC of 0.61 (cross-validation result).

To further illustrate the limitation of the 18 plasma protein panel to differentiate AD from the controls and other dementia groups, multidimensional scaling (MDS) plots were produced (figure 1). These plots show a large degree of overlap between the diagnostic groups.

Discussion

Characterizing protein markers in plasma has created optimism for finding detectable disease-specific pattern of changes. A biomarker panel of eighteen plasma proteins were shown in 2007 to classify blinded samples from AD and control subjects with close to 90% accuracy and to identify patients who had mild cognitive impairment that progressed to Alzheimer's disease [10]. The study was comprised of 259 plasma samples obtained from in total seven different clinical centres.

Interestingly, when re-analysing the same data set, originally obtained from the Ray et al study, a subset of plasma proteins (as z-scores of plasma proteins) resulted in good diagnostic accuracy [21]. However, following up on these results, using bead-based multiplex technology, Soares and co-workers have shown that when using a subset of the proteins included in the original 18 protein panel a diagnostic accuracy of only 61% was obtained when differentiating cases with AD from controls [22]. Later Rocha de Paula et al. proposed, using the original data set provided by Ray et al, that including pair-wise differences of z-score values to the mathematical method, could collectively provide a good discrimination value [23].

In the present study we found that the 18 plasma protein panel could classify samples from AD and controls with an AUC of only 63%, indicating that this protein panel cannot be used in the clinical diagnostic work-up of AD. The same protein panel could not distinguish cases with AD from subjects affected by other forms of dementia. In addition, the pattern of protein changes observed in the present study was not the same as in Ray et al. More specifically, in the training set described in the study by Ray

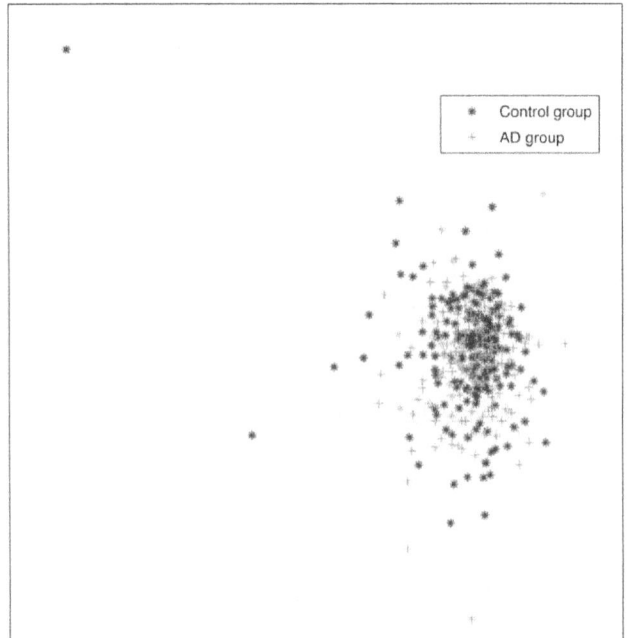
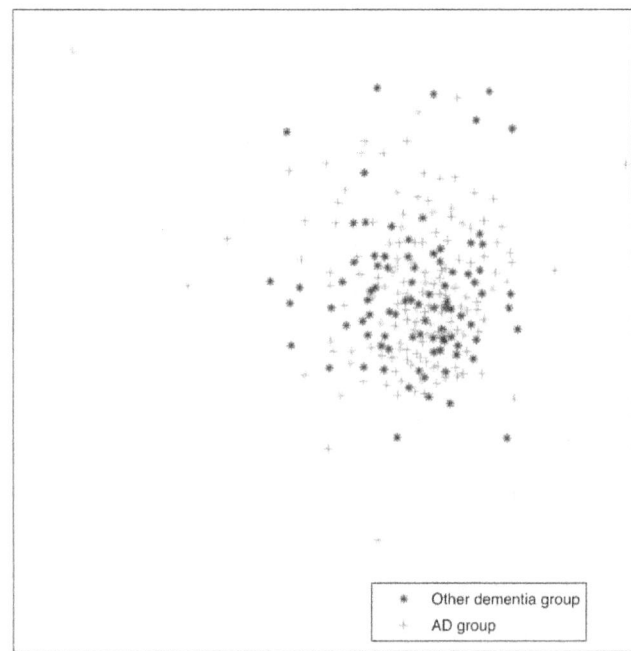

Figure 1. Multidimensional scaling plots (MDS) for the data. The left figure shows a MDS projection to 2 dimensions, using all 18 proteins, for the AD and the Control groups. The right figure is the corresponding plot for the AD and the other dementias group.

doi:10.1371/journal.pone.0029868.g001

et al [10], plasma z- levels of PDGF-BB, EGF and MIP-1δ were seen to be reduced in AD cases. In contradiction to this, in the present study the plasma levels of these proteins were increased in the AD cases. Similarly, Marksteiner et al have found that plasma MIP-1δ and EGF are increased in AD patients when compared to patients affected by depression [24].

Several of the 18 proteins included in the biomarker panel are involved in the immune response [10]. There are, however, important caveats to the use of plasma immune markers as biomarkers of disease progression or diagnostic predictors. AD is a slowly progressive disorder and systemic changes in the blood are likely to be subtle and difficult to monitor. There are also technical limitations in assaying low abundant cytokines and many factors likely influence plasma immune markers, such as concomitant infection and inflammatory illness. Furthermore, many cytokines has been shown to display diurnal variation [25] and different handlings as well as storage of samples are known to affect the levels of many biomarkers. Therefore, standardization of pre-analytical procedures is vital to obtain reproducible results. To increase the possibility of successful reproduction of biomarker studies in the future the handling of samples should be carefully described, including data describing the time from venipuncture to minus 80 freezer storage, time of day that venipuncture was performed and if samples were collected fasting or non-fasting. Moreover, when using samples from different clinical centres all diagnostic groups (including controls) need to be obtained from each clinical centre in order to be able to investigate potential variations in biomarker levels between different clinical sites.

A limitation of this study is that the array-based method used is a potentially unreliable tool to disprove the original study by Ray et al, who also used a similar and non-validated method. However, in the present study we selected two cytokines for confirmation measurements with a standardized ELISA method, and again found no statistical differences between control and AD samples.

Our results indicate that multiplex platforms might be important for biomarker discovery, but validation of the results using new patient cohorts as well as other analytical techniques are vital. At least two patient-control cohorts with all important diagnostic groups present in each will likely be needed to verify obtained data. Importantly, recent data show that highly cited biomarker studies often report larger effect estimates than are reported in subsequent meta analyses [26]. This further strengthens our notion that validation is crucial in biomarker research.

Acknowledgments

We thank Professor Carsten Peterson for valuable discussions.

Author Contributions

Conceived and designed the experiments: MB OH MO. Performed the experiments: MB MO. Analyzed the data: MB MO OH. Contributed reagents/materials/analysis tools: MB OH MO. Wrote the paper: MB OH MO LM.

References

1. Blennow K, de Leon MJ, Zetterberg H (2006) Alzheimer's disease. Lancet 368: 387–403.
2. Querfurth HW, LaFerla FM (2010) Alzheimer's disease. N Engl J Med 362: 329–344.
3. Jack CRJ, Knopman DS, Jagust WJ, Shaw LM, Aisen PS, et al. (2010) Hypothetical model of dynamic biomarkers of the Alzheimer's pathological cascade. Lancet Neurology 9: 119–128.
4. Perrin RJ, Fagan AM, Holtzman DM (2009) Multimodal techniques for diagnosis and prognosis of Alzheimer's disease. Nature 461: 916–922.
5. Blennow K, Hampel H, Weiner M, Zetterberg H (2010) Cerebrospinal fluid and plasma biomarkers in Alzheimer disease. Nat Rev Neurol 6: 131–144.
6. Hampel H, Frank R, Broich K, Teipel SJ, Katz RG, et al. (2010) Biomarkers for Alzheimer's disease: academic, industry and regulatory perspectives. Nat Rev Drug Discov 9: 560–574.
7. Mattsson N, Zetterberg H, Hansson O, Andreasen N, Parnetti L, et al. (2009) CSF biomarkers and incipient Alzheimer disease in patients with mild cognitive impairment. JAMA 302: 385–393.
8. Hansson O, Zetterberg H, Buchhave P, Londos E, Blennow K, et al. (2006) Association between CSF biomarkers and incipient Alzheimer's disease in patients with mild cognitive impairment: a follow-up study. Lancet Neurol 5: 228–234.
9. Shaw LM, Vanderstichele H, Knapik-Czajka M, Clark CM, Aisen PS, et al. (2009) Cerebrospinal fluid biomarker signature in Alzheimer's disease neuroimaging initiative subjects. Ann Neurol 65: 403–413.
10. Ray S, Britschgi M, Herbert C, Takeda-Ushimara, Boxer A, et al. (2007) Classification and prediction of clinical Alzheimer's diagnosis based on plasma signaling proteins. Nat Med 13: 1359–1362.
11. Association AP (1987) Diagnostic and Statistical Manual of Mental Disorders. third, revised ed. Washington DC: American Psychiatric Association.
12. McKhann G, Drachman D, Folstein M, Folstein M, Katzman R, et al. (1984) Clinical diagnosis of Alzheimer's disease: report of the NINCDS-ADRDA Work Group under the auspices of Department of Health and Human Services Task Force on Alzheimer's Disease. Neurology 34: 939–944.
13. Roman GC, Tatemichi TK, Erkinjuntti T, Cummings JL, Masde JC, et al. (1993) Vascular dementia: diagnostic criteria for research studies. Report of the NINDS-AIREN International Workshop. Neurology 43: 250–260.
14. Erkinjuntti T, Inzitari D, Pantoni L, Wallin A, Scheltens P, et al. (2000) Research criteria for subcortical vascular dementia in clinical trials. J Neural Transm Suppl 59: 23–30.
15. McKeith IG, Perry EK, Perry RH (1999) Report of the second dementia with Lewy body international workshop: diagnosis and treatment. Consortium on Dementia with Lewy Bodies. Neurology 53: 902–905.
16. McKhann GM, Albert MS, Grossman M, Miller B, Dickson D, et al. (2001) Clinical and pathological diagnosis of frontotemporal dementia: report of the Work Group on Frontotemporal Dementia and Pick's Disease. Arch Neurol 58: 1803–1809.
17. Hosmer D, Lemeshow S (1989) Applied logistic regression. New York: Wiley.
18. Bishop CM (1995) Neural Networks for Pattern Recognition. Oxford: Oxford University Press.
19. Tibshirani R, Hastie T, Narasimhan B, Chu G (2002) Diagnosis of multiple cancer types by shrunken centroids of gene expression. Proceedings of the National Academy of Sciences of the United States of America 99: 6567–72.
20. Breiman L (1996) Bagging predictors, Machine Learning 24: 123–140.
21. Gòmez Ravetti M, Moscato P (2008) Identification of a 5-protein biomarker molecular signature for predicting Alzheimer's disease. PLoS ONE 3: e3111.
22. Soares HD, Chen Y, Sabbagh M, Rohrer A, Schrijvers E, et al. (2009) Identifying Early Markers of Alzheimer's Disease using Quantitative Multiplex Proteomic Immunoassay Panels. Annals of the New York Academy of Sciences 1180: 56–67.
23. Rocha de Paula M, Gòmez Ravetti M, Berretta R, Moscato P (2011) Differences in abundances of cell-signalling proteins in blood reveal novel biomarkers for early detection of clinical alzheimer's disease. PLoS ONE 6(3): e17481. doi:10.1371/journal.pone.0017481.
24. Marksteiner J, Kemmler G, Weiss EM, Knaus G, Ullrich C, et al. (2011) Five out of 16 plasma signaling proteins are enhanced in plasma of patients with mild cognitive impairment and Alzheimer's disease. Neurobiology of aging 3: 539–40.
25. Knudsen LS, Christensen IJ, Lottenburger T, Svendsen MN, Nielsen L, et al. (2008) Pre-analytical and biological variability in circulating interleukin 6 in healthy subjects and patients with rheumatoid arthritis. Biomarkers 13: 59–78.
26. Ioannidis JP, Panagiotou OA (2011) Comparison of effect sizes associated with biomarkers reported in highly cited individual articles and in subsequent meta-analyses. JAMA 21: 2200–10.

Multi-Method Analysis of MRI Images in Early Diagnostics of Alzheimer's Disease

Robin Wolz[1,9], Valtteri Julkunen[2,9], Juha Koikkalainen[3], Eini Niskanen[2,4], Dong Ping Zhang[1], Daniel Rueckert[1], Hilkka Soininen[2,5], Jyrki Lötjönen[3*], the Alzheimer's Disease Neuroimaging Initiative[¶]

1 Biomedical Image Analysis Group, Department of Computing, Imperial College London, London, United Kingdom, 2 Department of Neurology, Kuopio University Hospital, Kuopio, Finland, 3 Knowledge Intensive Services, VTT Technical Research Centre of Finland, Tampere, Finland, 4 Department of Applied Physics, University of Eastern Finland, Kuopio, Finland, 5 Institute of Clinical Medicine, Neurology, University of Eastern Finland, Kuopio, Finland

Abstract

The role of structural brain magnetic resonance imaging (MRI) is becoming more and more emphasized in the early diagnostics of Alzheimer's disease (AD). This study aimed to assess the improvement in classification accuracy that can be achieved by combining features from different structural MRI analysis techniques. Automatically estimated MR features used are hippocampal volume, tensor-based morphometry, cortical thickness and a novel technique based on manifold learning. Baseline MRIs acquired from all 834 subjects (231 healthy controls (HC), 238 stable mild cognitive impairment (S-MCI), 167 MCI to AD progressors (P-MCI), 198 AD) from the Alzheimer's Disease Neuroimaging Initiative (ADNI) database were used for evaluation. We compared the classification accuracy achieved with linear discriminant analysis (LDA) and support vector machines (SVM). The best results achieved with individual features are 90% sensitivity and 84% specificity (HC/AD classification), 64%/66% (S-MCI/P-MCI) and 82%/76% (HC/P-MCI) with the LDA classifier. The combination of all features improved these results to 93% sensitivity and 85% specificity (HC/AD), 67%/69% (S-MCI/P-MCI) and 86%/82% (HC/P-MCI). Compared with previously published results in the ADNI database using individual MR-based features, the presented results show that a comprehensive analysis of MRI images combining multiple features improves classification accuracy and predictive power in detecting early AD. The most stable and reliable classification was achieved when combining all available features.

Citation: Wolz R, Julkunen V, Koikkalainen J, Niskanen E, Zhang DP, et al. (2011) Multi-Method Analysis of MRI Images in Early Diagnostics of Alzheimer's Disease. PLoS ONE 6(10): e25446. doi:10.1371/journal.pone.0025446

Editor: Celia Oreja-Guevara, University Hospital La Paz, Spain

Received July 12, 2011; **Accepted** September 5, 2011; **Published** October 13, 2011

Funding: This project is partially funded under the 7th Framework Programme by the European Commission (http://cordis.europa.eu/ist/). Data collection and sharing for this project was funded by the Alzheimer's Disease Neuroimaging Initiative (ADNI; Principal Investigator: Michael Weiner; NIH grant U01 AG024904). ADNI is funded by the National Institute on Aging, the National Institute of Biomedical Imaging and Bioengineering (NIBIB), and through generous contributions from the following: Pzer Inc., Wyeth Research, Bristol-Myers Squibb, Eli Lilly and Company, GlaxoSmithKline, Merck & Co. Inc., AstraZeneca AB, Novartis Pharmaceuticals Corporation, Alzheimer's Association, Eisai Global Clinical Development, Elan Corporation, plc, Forest Laboratories, and the Institute for the Study of Aging, with participation from the U.S. Food and Drug Administration. Industry partnerships are coordinated through the Foundation for the National Institutes of Health. The grantee organization is the Northern California Institute for Research and Education, and the study is coordinated by the Alzheimer's Disease Cooperative Study at the University of California San Diego. ADNI data are disseminated by the Laboratory of Neuro Imaging at the University of California Los Angeles. Data used in the preparation of this article were obtained from the ADNI database (www.loni.ucla.edu/ADNI). As such, the investigators within the ADNI contributed to the design and implementation of ADNI and/or provided data but did not participate in analysis or writing of this report. ADNI investigators include (complete listing available at http://adni.loni.ucla.edu/wp-content/uploads/how_to_apply/ADNI_Authorship_List.pdf).

Competing Interests: The authors have declared that no competing interests exist.

* E-mail: jyrki.lotjonen@vtt.fi

9 These authors contributed equally to this work.

¶ For information on the Alzheimer's Disease Neuroimaging Initiative please see the Acknowledgments section.

Introduction

Alzheimer's disease (AD) is the most common cause of dementia globally and one of the major healthcare issues of the future. It has been estimated that during the next four decades the prevalence of AD will quadruple from 27 to 106 million by which time 1 in 85 persons worldwide will be living with the disease [1]. Even a modest delay of one year in disease onset and progression could reduce the number of cases by 9 million [1]. Interventions are postulated to be most effective when directed at patients at the earliest stages of the disease, which underlines the importance of early diagnosis of AD [2]. Mild cognitive impairment (MCI) is a heterogeneous syndrome that increases the risk of developing AD markedly [3]. However, not all MCI subjects convert to AD and some may even return to normal cognition [4].

The search for reliable biomarkers of AD-type pathology and predictors of disease progression among MCI subjects is ongoing. AD is characterized by neurofibrillary tangles and amyloid plaques in the brain [5]. Degenerative changes in the human neurotransmitter system lead to atrophy in selected brain regions [6]. The most promising candidate biomarkers are the ones derived from structural and functional neuroimaging as well as those measured in cerebrospinal fluid (CSF) and plasma [7]. Amyloid-based measures like the CSF-peptide $A\beta_{42}$ and the uptake of the PiB tracer on positron emission imaging (PET) show the earliest AD-type changes [7]. However, there is evidence that the number of amyloid plaques reach their saturation levels already by the time patients have clinically apparent symptoms of cognitive impairment [8,9], whereas atrophy, neuronal loss, synaptic loss, and the number of tangles increase with severity of illness [10]. These findings suggest that, although amyloid-based biomarkers may be used as longitudinal markers of AD type pathology, they seem to offer only limited insight into which MCI subjects will most likely convert to AD in the near future. In a recently published dynamic model of biomarker behavior in the AD spectrum, biomarkers based on structural magnetic resonance imaging (MRI) have been shown to be correlated with a progression from MCI to AD [11]. Such biomarkers could therefore improve the accuracy of early AD diagnostics and reduce especially the amount of false positive diagnoses. Besides providing chance for a more focused and earlier intervention, structural MRI biomarkers of AD could also aid the development of new disease-modifying drugs by acting as surrogate markers of disease progression, reduce the number of subjects needed to detect significant drug effect and provide quantitative measures of treatment benefits [12].

It has been shown that the early diagnostics of AD can be improved by using multiple different biomarkers simultaneously. Usually these studies have combined MRI-based markers with biomarkers based on positron emission tomography (PET) [13,14], cerebrospinal fluid (CSF) [15,16] or both [17–19]. Achieved results vary from no additional benefit [15,17] to significant improvement [13,14,16,20]. However, availability of all three biomarkers (CSF, PET, MRI) is not very common in clinical practice since obtaining all measures is laborious for the patient and clinician, induces delays and increases the costs of the diagnosis significantly. Furthermore, measurements obtained from CSF and PET are considered invasive. Recent studies focusing on only structural MRI have reached correct classification accuracys (CCR) of 76–94% in identifying healthy controls (HC) from patients with AD and 64–82% in predicting which MCI subjects will convert to AD in the imminent future [21–27]. The high variation in these results can be attributed to differences in study populations as well as evaluation designs. With the Alzheimer's Disease Neuroimaging Study (ADNI) [28], a large multi-center study on MR imaging in AD has been established that is available to the wider research community. Based on a large sub-group of ADNI subjects, Cuingnet et al. [29] presented a comparison of ten MRI-based feature extraction methods and their ability to discriminate between clinically relevant subject groups. The ten methods evaluated comprise five voxel-based methods, three methods based on cortical thickness and two methods based on the hippocampus. Best sensitivity/specificity values reported are 81%/95% for AD vs HC, 70%/61% for S-MCI vs P-MCI and 73%/85% for HC vs P-MCI.

In this paper we use the ADNI database to evaluate the ability of the combination of different MR-based features to increase classification accuracy. We evaluate the power of hippocampal volume (HV), cortical thickness (CTH), tensor-based morphometry (TBM) and features extracted from a recently proposed manifold-based learning (MBL) framework to discriminate healthy controls from subjects with AD and to predict conversion from MCI to AD. For evaluation we used all 834 ADNI baseline images that were available from the ADNI webpage. Compared to previous work this paper aims at establishing the improvement in accuracy and stability that can be achieved by combining more than one MR-based feature. To the best of our knowledge it is the first comprehensive study that analyzes MRI-derived features for the full ADNI dataset. For direct comparison with the work by Cuingnet et al. [29] we also evaluated all results on the subset used in their work.

To test the influence of the classification method used, we utilized both support vector machines (SVMs) and a linear discriminant analys (LDA) to evaluate classification accuracy (CCR), sensitivity (SEN) and specificity (SPE) in each experiment.

Materials and Methods

Subjects

In the ADNI study, brain MR images were acquired at regular intervals after an initial baseline scan from approximately 200 cognitively normal older subjects (HC), 400 subjects with mild cognitive impairment (MCI), and 200 subjects with early AD. Detailed inclusion/exclusion criteria used for the different subject groups in ADNI are defined in [30]. The AD group has scores between 20–26 (inclusive) on the Mini-Mental State Examination (MMSE) [31], and a Clinical Dementia Rating (CDR) [32] of 0.5 or 1.0. Furthermore, these subjects fulfil the NINCDS/ADRDA criteria for probable AD [33]. MCI subjects included have MMSE scores between 24–30 (inclusive), a memory complaint, have objective memory loss measured by education adjusted scores on Wechsler Memory Scale Logical Memory II, a CDR of 0.5, absence of significant levels of impairment in other cognitive domains, essentially preserved activities of daily living, and an absence of dementia [30]. Healthy subjects have MMSE scores between 24–30 (inclusive), a CDR of 0, are non-depressed, non MCI, and nondemented. A more detailed description of the ADNI study is given in Appendix S1.

All 834 ADNI subjects (231 HC, 238 S-MCI, 167 P-MCI, 198 AD) for which a 1.5T T1-weighted MRI scan at baseline was available were included in this study. 167 subjects in the MCI group converted to AD as of July 2011. We therefore independently analysed progressive MCI (P-MCI) subjects and subjects with a stable diagnosis of MCI (S-MCI).

Table 1 shows the demographics for the 834 study subjects. Statistically significant differences in the demographics and clinical variables between the study groups were assessed using Student's unpaired t-test. In this work, the difference was considered statistically significant if $p < 0.05$ if not stated otherwise. There were more men than women in all other groups besides the AD group. MMSE scores were significantly different in the pairwise comparisons between all study groups. CDR scores of the HC and AD groups are significantly different to the ones of the two MCI groups. Healthy subjects had a significantly lower Geriatric Depression Scale (GDS) compared to all other groups. Compared to all other groups, AD subjects had significantly shorter education.

MRI Acquisition

Standard 1.5T screening/baseline T1-weighted images obtained using volumetric 3D MPRAGE protocol with resolutions

Table 1. Subjects.

Group	HC	S-MCI	P-MCI	AD
N	231	238	167	198
Men	52%	66%	62%	52%
Age	76.02 (5.0)	74.85 (7.8)	74.6 (7.0)	75.68 (7.7)
MMSE	29.1* (1.0)	27.3* (1.8)	26.6* (1.7)	23.3* (2.0)
CDR	0 (0)	0.49 (0.05)	0.50 (0)	0.75 (0.25)
GDS	0.83* (1.14)	1.60 (1.42)	1.53 (1.30)	1.67 (1.42)
Education	16.0 (2.8)	15.6 (3.1)	15.7 (2.9)	14.7* (3.1)
APOE4 status ($\varepsilon 3\varepsilon 4/\varepsilon 4\varepsilon 4$)	23%/2%	31%/8%	50%/16%	42%/18%
Months to conversion			18.2 (10.1)	

*means statistically significant different from all other groups.
doi:10.1371/journal.pone.0025446.t001

ranging from 0.9 mm × 0.9 mm × 1.20 mm to 1.3 mm × 1.3 mm × 1.20 mm were included from the ADNI database. For detailed information of the MRI protocols and preprocessing steps see [34].

Feature extraction

All fully automated feature extraction methods described below were applied to images that were preprocessed by the ADNI pipeline.

Hippocampal volume. Baseline hippocampal volumes were measured using an approach based on fast and robust multi-atlas segmentation [35,36]. In this approach, multi-atlas label propagation is applied in combination with atlas selection to obtain the hippocampus segmentation. A set of hippocampus atlases is selected from a pool of atlas images according to image similarity with the query image. After registering all atlases to the query image, a spatial prior is generated from the multiple label maps. This spatial prior is then used to obtain a final segmentation based on an expectation maximization (EM) segmentation algorithm [37].

Cortical thickness. CTH is measured in the baseline T1-weighted structural MR images by using an automated computational surface-based method developed at the McConnell Brain Imaging Centre, Montreal Neurological Institute, McGill University, Montreal, Canada (http://www2.bic.mni.mcgill.ca/) [38]. Individual MRI volumes were registered to standard space using the ICBM152 template [39]. Intensity non-uniformities were corrected [40] before the final brain mask was calculated [41]. Tissues were segmented into white matter (WM), grey matter (GM) and cerebrospinal fluid (CSF) using the INSECT-algorithm [42] and the magnitude of PVE was estimated by using the trimmed minimum covariance determinant (TMCD) method [43]. The brains were divided automatically into two separate hemispheres and the inner and outer surfaces of the cortex were extracted according to intersections between WM and GM (white matter surface, WMS) as well as GM and CSF (grey matter surface, GMS) using the Constrained Laplacian-Based Automated Segmentation with Proximities (CLASP) algorithm [44]. The inner surface was first formed by deforming an ellipsoid polygon mesh to the shape of the WMS. GMS was obtained by further expanding the inner surface. Each polygon mesh surface consisted of 81,920 polygons and 40,962 nodes per hemisphere. The thickness of the cortex was defined at each linked node as the distance between the two concentrically linked polygon meshes on the WMS and the GMS. This t-link metric has been proven to be the simplest yet most precise way to determine cortical thickness [38]. Although MR images were transformed to standard space to allow for group analysis, thickness calculations were performed in each subject's native space. Finally, cortical thickness maps were smoothed with a 20 mm FWHM diffusion smoothing kernel to improve the signal-to-noise ratio and statistical power [45]. The described toolbox did not achieve satisfactory results on some study subjects because of i) failure in tissue segmentation and brain masking (48 subjects) and ii) failure in partial volume effect estimation (59 subjects). As a result the pipeline crashed and CTH measures were not obtained for 76 subjects (24 control, 35 MCI, 17 AD). Also the cortical model of 31 subjects (10 control, 13 MCI, 8 AD) was completely deformed and thus unusable. For these 107 subjects the CTH features were considered as missing values. CTH features used in the classification experiments are introduced below.

Tensor-based morphometry. The TBM analysis was performed using a multi-template approach [46,47]. In TBM, a template image is non-rigidly registered to a study image, and, typically, the determinant of the Jacobian matrix ('the Jacobian') of the deformation is used to measure the voxel-level morphometry.

Instead of using just one template image, we used 30 randomly selected images (10 controls, 10 MCIs, and 10 ADs) from the ADNI database as template images. The template images were used also in the classification analysis to maximize the number of subjects. Each template image was registered to a study image, and Jacobian maps were computed for each template image. To combine the results of multiple templates, all template images were registered to the mean anatomical template generated from the 30 images, and all the results were normalized to this reference space [47]. The combination of the results was performed by averaging the ROI-wise feature values of all the templates as described in detail below.

Manifold-based learning. In this machine learning approach, non-linear dimensionality reduction with Laplacian eigenmaps [48] is used to learn features to discriminate between different subject groups. Laplacian eigenmaps estimates the low-dimensional representation of a set of input images based on a similarity graph that is defined with pairwise image similarities [48]. The hypothesis is that such a low-dimensional representation captures the variability in the dataset in a more compact way than pairwise image similarities directly. We estimate pairwise image similarities from the intensity appearance in a region around hippocampus and amygdala since both structures are known to be affected by AD in an early stage. All images are aligned in a template space using a coarse non-rigid registration (10 mm B-spline control-point spacing, [49]). Such a coarse non-rigid alignment ensures that corresponding brain structures are aligned but still allows to measure subject-specific differences. After performing dimensionality reduction, the first 20 dimensions of the resulting manifold are used as features to perform classification with the different methods used. More details on the theory and application of this manifold learning approach can be found in [20,50]. Figure 1 exemplarily shows a 2D embedding of a set of ADNI images acquired from healthy controls and subjects with AD. It can be seen that even two embedding dimensions give a relatively good separation between both groups. In our experiments we used a higher dimensional space allowing better discrimination.

ROI-wise features for CTH and TBM

Both CTH and TBM analyses produce local (point-wise) information, either on cortical thickness or the volume. Thus, the number of original features is enormous, and to make the classification more efficient and robust, the number of features has to be reduced. We evaluated both features in a statistical region of interest (ROI) defined as detailed in Appendix S2. Figures 2 and 3 show t-values for statistically significant differences between study groups for TBM and CTH respectively. A detailed description of the definition of these statistical ROIs is given in Appendix S2.

Study design

Table 2 presents an overview on the features calculated for all 834 available ADNI baseline images. All feature values were corrected for age and gender using a linear regression model where control subjects were used as the training set, i.e., the normal, not disease-related, age and gender related differences in the classification features were removed. Feature selection was then carried out on the corrected feature sets using stepwise regression [51].

We used two subsets to perform classification:

I. All 834 available baseline images described in the subjects section

II. 509 baseline images used by Cuingnet et al. [29] and detailed in their publication.

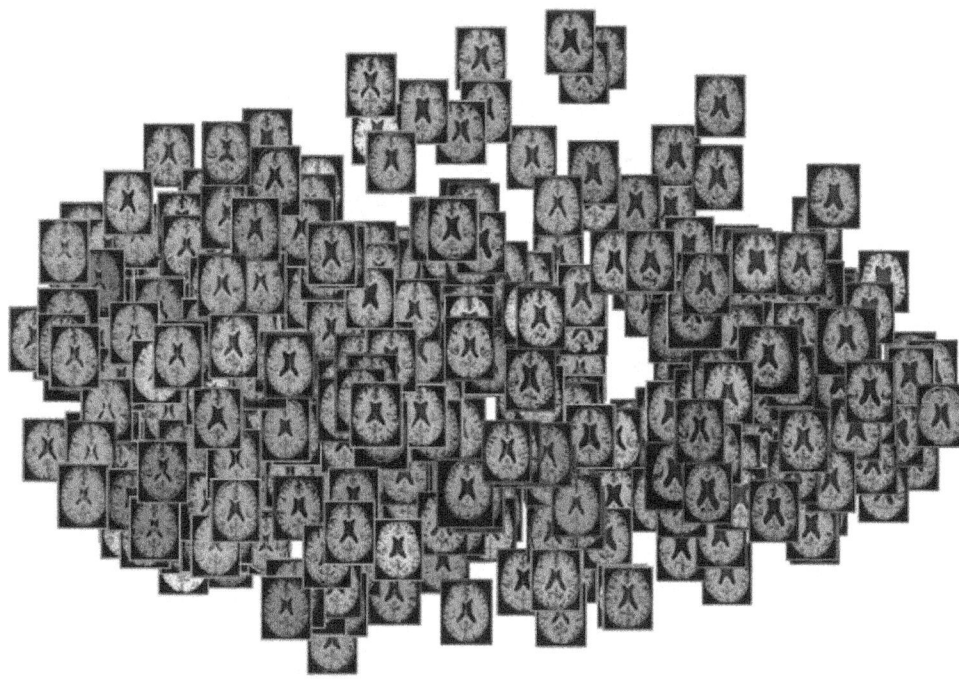

Figure 1. 2D manifold embedding of a set of images acquired from healthy controls (red) and subjects with AD (blue).
doi:10.1371/journal.pone.0025446.g001

The following sections describe the definition of the statistical ROIs and evaluation strategy used for the two datasets respectively.

Dataset I. In order to perform the study using cross-validation in the full dataset, it was divided into three equally sized parts. One part was used to perform the statistical tests for the CTH and TBM features, and the remaining two parts were used to evaluate the classification accuracy. This was repeated three times so that each part was once used to perform the statistical tests. Afterwards, the results of the three repetitions were averaged. The classification accuracy was evaluated using leave-N-out cross validation on those subjects not included in the statistical tests. Five percent of the evaluation subjects were regarded as the test set, and the remaining 95% of the subjects were used to train a classifier which was then applied to the test set. This was repeated table-1-caption100 times, each time selecting randomly the test set subjects. Finally, the results of the 100 repetitions were averaged.

Consequently, in overall, the classification evaluation was performed using 300 (3×100) repetitions, and the results presented in this paper are the average values of all these classifications.

Dataset II. Statistical ROIs for CTH and TBM feature extraction were calculated from the 325 baseline images that are not part of dataset II. In order to allow direct comparison of classification accuracy with the work by Cuingnet et al. [29], separate training and testing sets for the different comparisons were defined using the exact sub-groups reported in their manuscript. Around 50% of all subjects are used to train the different types of classifiers and the reported results are based on classifying the remaining subjects.

Classification methods

We used two different widely used methods to perform classification based on individual features and their combination:

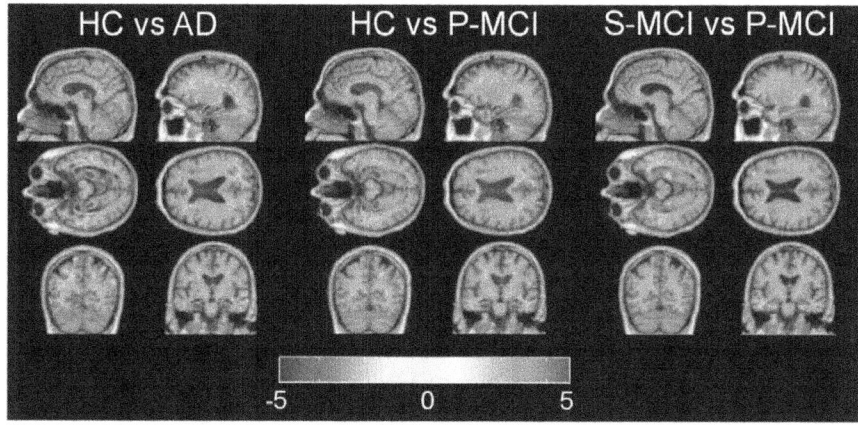

Figure 2. Results for voxelwise t-tests for statistically significant group differences with features extracted from TBM.
doi:10.1371/journal.pone.0025446.g002

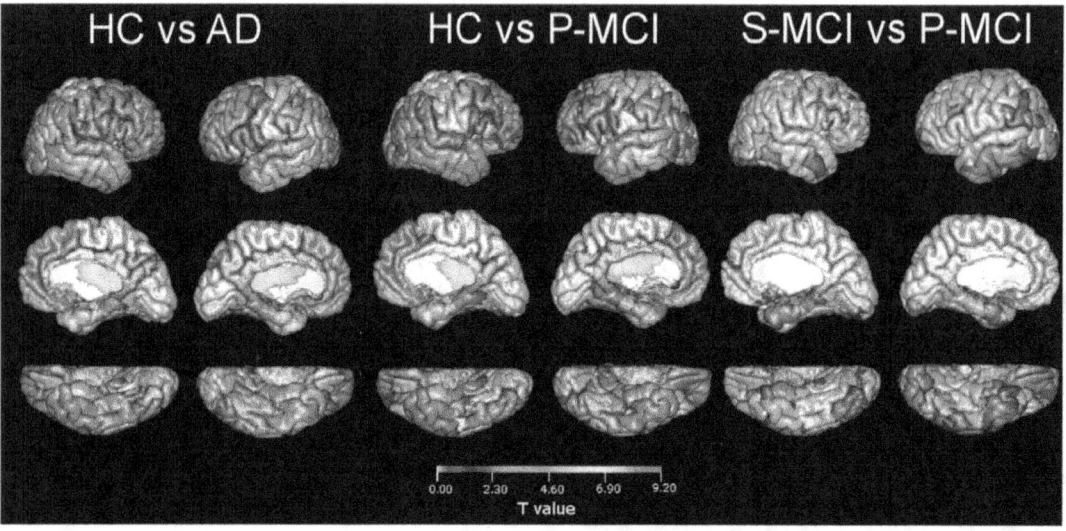

Figure 3. Results for t-tests for statistically significant group differences based on cortical thickness measurements.
doi:10.1371/journal.pone.0025446.g003

Linear discriminant analysis (LDA). Linear discriminant analysis (LDA) is a widely used technique to find a linear combination of features to best separate several classes [52]. In this work we used LDA as implemented in the *classify* function in Matlab with a multivariate normal density model with uninformative priors (p = 0.5).

Support vector machines (SVM). Support vector machines use training data to find a separating hyperplane in the n-dimensional training space that best separates two subject groups [53]. Test subjects are then classified according to their position relative to the defined hyperplane in the n-dimensional feature space. We used the libSVM library to perform the analysis. The radial basis function kernel was selected based on the guidelines provided by the libSVM library (Software available 2.3.2011 at http://www.csie.ntu.edu.tw/cjlin/libsvm).

Results

We used both classification methods to measure classification accuracy based on individual features as well as the combination of all features. The results for the comparisons HC vs AD, HC vs P-MCI and S-MCI vs P-MCI in the full ADNI database are presented in Tables 3, 4 and 5 respectively. Presented are classification accuracy (CCR), sensitivity (SEN) and specificity (SPE). Furthermore, the 95% confidence interval for the classification accuracy is estimated based on the multiple classification runs. Statistically

significant improvements achieved when combining all features are marked with † (p < 0.0001). To test for significance, unpaired t-tests were carried out between distribution estimates for the corresponding classification rates based on the multiple runs. All estimated distributions passed a normality test using a Kolmogorov-Smirnov test at α = 0.05.

For direct comparison with work presented by Cuingnet et al. [29], we performed classification based on the training- and testing sets defined in their manuscript as described above. S-MCI and P-MCI groups are defined in the same way as in the original publication. Sensitivity and specificity values for the classification in all three clinical pairings are reported in Table 6. Following the clear advantage for LDA in the performance on the full dataset, we only report results with this classifier for dataset II.

Discussion

In this study we assessed the automatic diagnostic capabilities of 4 structural MRI features (MBL, HC, CTH, TBM) separately and combined in 834 baseline images acquired in the ADNI study. When applied separately, TBM provided the overall best results, closely followed by MBL. Combining all features improved the results in all study experiments. Our results show how a combination of different MRI-based features can improve results based on only one measurement, resulting in a more powerful and stable classifier. The most significant improvement of the combination

Table 2. Features used in the study.

Method	No of features	Description
Hippocampal volume (HV)	1	total volume of left and right hippopcampus
Cortical thickness (CTH)	9 (HC vs AD)	average cortical thickness within a ROI defined based on group-level statistical analysis
	7 (HC vs P-MCI)	
	8 (S-MCI vs P-MCI)	
Tensor-based morphometry (TBM)	84	average Jacobian of atrophic voxels within a ROI, weighted based on voxel-wise p-values
Manifold-based learning (MBL)	20	coordinates of a subject in a low-dimensional manifold space learned from pairwise image similarities

doi:10.1371/journal.pone.0025446.t002

Table 3. Classification results for HC vs AD.

Feature	LDA			SVM		
	CCR [95% CI]	SEN	SPE	CCR [95% CI]	SEN	SPE
MBL	85† [64 100]	87	83	85 [64 100]	87	83
HV	81† [57 100]	81	79	81† [57 100]	84	77
CTH	81† [64 100]	89	71	82† [57 100]	90	73
TBM	87† [71 100]	90	84	87 [71 100]	89	84
All	89 [71 100]	93	85	86 [71 100]	94	78

†means statistically significant different from the combined results with p < 0.0001. CCR = Correct classification rate, SEN = Sensitivity, SPE = Specificity.
doi:10.1371/journal.pone.0025446.t003

Table 5. Classification results for S-MCI vs P-MCI.

Feature	LDA			SVM		
	CCR [95% CI]	SEN	SPE	CCR [95% CI]	SEN	SPE
MBL	65† [36 86]	64	66	65† [43 86]	77	48
HV	65† [36 86]	63	67	62 [36 86]	83	33
CTH	56† [29 86]	63	45	59 [36 79]	96	03
TBM	64† [36 86]	65	62	64† [36 86]	77	44
All	68 [43 93]	67	69	60 [36 86]	92	14

†means statistically significant different from the combined results with p < 0.0001.
doi:10.1371/journal.pone.0025446.t005

over the best individual feature can be observed for HC vs P-MCI with 5% units followed by 3 and 2% units for S-MCI vs P-MCI and HC vs AD, respectively. These improvements lead to 20, 12 and 9 subjects more being correctly classified respectively when using the combined feature set as compared to the best single feature for every comparison. Comparing two classification approaches based on LDA and SVMs resulted in a clear advantage of the former.

Several studies reported classification results using single MRI methods for the HC/AD classification (Table 7). Liu et al. [24] reported SEN/SPE of 92/90 in the classification of HC/AD subjects using regional cortical volumes in the AddNeuroMed dataset. McEvoy et al. [26] report a CCR of 89 on images from the ADNI database using features from cortical thickness and structural volumes. Vemuri et al. [54] present a SEN/SPE of 86/86 on 380 subjects using the STAND score. In our study the results obtained with single methods are lower (71–90) but almost identical when the methods were combined. It should be noted, however, that Liu and colleagues did not use cross-validation or separate training/testing sets when producing the results which could lead to overestimation of the results in a dataset outside the study cohort. Gerardin et al. [23] acquired a high SEN/SPE of 96/92 by using hippocampal shape analysis, but the number of subjects (25 HC, 23 AD) was quite low in order to produce results with good generalizability. Westman et al. [55] reported a CCR of 82 for HC vs AD classification and 73 for HC vs P-MCI classification by using various regional brain volumes. Our results are substantially more accurate, the group sizes are larger and clinical follow-up time is one year longer. Chupin et al. [21] reported SEN/SPE of 75/77 (hippocampal volume) and Querbes et al. [27] a CCR of 85 (cortical thickness), both lower than the

results acquired with the combination of features or TBM features independently in our study.

Varying results concerning AD prediction (S-MCI/P-MCI classification using baseline measurements) have been published (Table 7): Querbes et al. [27] reported a CCR of 73, Liu et al. [25] a SEN/SPE of 76/68, Chupin et al. [21] reported a SEN/SPE of 60/65 and Davatzikos et al. [15] SEN/SPE of 95/38. Our results with separate and combined baseline features lie in the range of these results (SEN/SPE 63/67, 64/66 and 67/69 when using HV, MBL and the combined features, respectively).

There can be several explanations for the variation in the reported results. A majority of the studies in this field have used different statistical methods and MRI feature extraction strategies on different datasets, which makes a comparison of the results complicated. Also the variation in the size of the study samples and the use (or ignoring) of cross-validation or separate training/testing sets are important factors, which both have crucial impact on the reliability and generalizability of the results. In Lötjönen et al. [36], we demonstrated that choosing from a population of 350 cases several times 2/3 for the training set and 1/3 for the test set and using hippocampus volume as a classification feature can lead to any classification accuracy between 53% and 77%. This observation is also confirmed by the high confidence intervals for the classification accuracies reported in Tables 3, 4 and 5. This shows that a fair comparison of methods based on the classification accuracy is difficult if not exactly the same data and classification approaches are used. Furthermore, since the ADNI study is still ongoing, several subjects labeled as S-MCI will progress in the future to the P-MCI group.

A recent study with a subset of ADNI subjects assessed the classification performance of several structural MRI methods in experiments comparable to our investigation [29]. Reported

Table 4. Classification results for HC vs P-MCI.

Feature	LDA			SVM		
	CCR [95% CI]	SEN	SPE	CCR [95% CI]	SEN	SPE
MBL	78† [54 100]	81	75	77† [54 92]	84	69
HV	76† [54 92]	77	76	78 [54 92]	83	71
CTH	77† [54 100]	85	65	77 [54 100]	89	62
TBM	79† [62 100]	82	76	80† [62 100]	85	74
All	84 [62 100]	86	82	82 [62 100]	93	67

†means statistically significant different from the combined results with p < 0.0001.
doi:10.1371/journal.pone.0025446.t004

Table 6. Classification results based on a subset of ADNI that was previously used for classification by Cuingnet et al. [29].

Feature	HC vs AD		HC vs P-MCI		S-MCI vs P-MCI	
	SEN	SPE	SEN	SPE	SEN	SPE
MBL	90	74	84	92	55	76
HV	80	69	75	76	63	70
CTH	85	75	86	59	72	35
TBM	93	76	90	84	63	59
All	94	76	94	89	69	54

doi:10.1371/journal.pone.0025446.t006

Table 7. Classification results of healthy control (HC), mild cognitive impairment (MCI) and Alzheimer's disease subjects reported in the recent literature.

Study	N	Features	HC vs AD			HC vs P-MCI			S-MCI vs P-MCI		
			CCR	SEN	SPE	CCR	SEN	SPE	CCR	SEN	SPE
Liu et al. [24]	333	Cortical volumes	91	92	90	-	-	-	-	-	-
Gerardin et al. [23]*	70	Hippocampus shape	94	96	92	-	-	-	-	-	-
Chupin et al. [21]*	605	Hippocampus volume	76	75	77	-	-	-	64	60	65
Querbes et al. [27]*	382	Cortical thickness	85	-	-	-	-	-	73	75	68
Liu et al. [25]	312	Amygdala/caudate volumes	-	-	-	-	-	-	69	76	68
Davatzikos et al. [15]*	356	SPARE-AD index	-	-	-	-	-	-	56	95	38
Cuingnet et al. [29]*	509	Various	-	81	95	-	73	85	-	62	69
Hinrichs et al. [14]*	159	MRI & PET	81	-	-	60	92	14	-	-	-
Westman et al. [55]	351	Various volumes	82	-	-	73	-	-	-	-	-
McEvoy et al. [26]*	398	Cortical thickness/various volumes	89	83	93	-	-	-	-	-	-
Vemuri et al. [54]	380	STAND score	-	86	86	-	-	-	-	-	-

N = Number of study subjects,
* = ADNI dataset.
doi:10.1371/journal.pone.0025446.t007

SEN/SPE lie in the ranges 59/81–81/95 (HC vs AD) and 70/73–73/85 (HC vs P-MCI). While most methods tested did not exceed the accuracy of a random classifier for the discrimination between S-MCI and P-MCI, the best results reported for this task were a SEN/SPE of 62/69 when using hippocampal volume. To allow a direct comparison of the results reported by Cuingnet et al. [29], we evaluated our features on the exact same training- and testing sets used in their paper. This direct comparison shows that our results compare favourably to other, established methods in neuroimaging. For HC vs AD classification, individual features in our study give more sensitive but less specific results than most methods in the previous publication. Combining all features gives an overall better classification accuracy than the majority of previously tested methods. Our results on the combined feature set furthermore outperform the majority of methods tested by Cuingnet et al. [29] when predicting MCI conversion as well as all methods for the classification between HC and P-MCI. A significant difference in classification accuracy can be observed between the full ADNI dataset and this smaller subset used for comparison with previous work. Reasons may include a strict separation into trainin- and testing sets which may result in less generalisability as well as the shorter follow-up period that was considered to define progression to AD.

Some studies have also combined different biomarkers (CSF, MRI, PET) with the idea of measuring different aspects of AD pathology and thus improve the classification accuracy. Hinrichs et al. [14] improved their HC/AD classification CCR by a few % units to 81 by combining MRI and PET. Eckerström et al. [16] studied the separation of a unified HC/S-MCI group from P-MCI group with CSF proteins and manual hippocampal volumes. They found CSF to be superior to MRI (SEN/SPE of 95/79 vs 86/66) while the combination performed best (SEN/SPE 90/91). However, it should be noted that the study sample in that particular study was small (a total of 68 subjects) and neither cross-validation or separate training/testing sets were used in order to ensure good generalizability of the results. In Kohannim et al. [17], the improvement from using multiple biomarkers was not significant and Davatzikos et al. [15] reported marginal improvements which, however, may be related to the fact that results with only one biomarker were not very good to begin with.

Considering solely the classification accuracies of the present study and those reported in literature, it seems questionable if the collection of several biomarkers is worth the effort and resource. A combination of different features extracted from a single MRI seems to provide results that are comparable or better than those obtained with other or multiple biomarkers. In a clinical point of view, this is interesting since it means that a single MRI scan provides not only aid to differential diagnostics of cognitive impairment, but also reliably describes a persons phase in the HC/AD continuum. MRI is also widely available, non-invasive and often useful in the differential diagnostics of memory problems thus making it a compelling option as the first biomarker that would be obtained from a patient with mild memory problems. However, a comprehensive differential diagnostics between AD and non-AD cognitive impairments will still require assessment of various different biomarkers. Also, it should be noted that the computational techniques used in this paper are not widely available in the clinical environment and thus limit their usage in the clinical work at present.

Strengths of the presented study are i) the use of multiple features extracted from one imaging modality, ii) large groups, iii) rigorous validation process of the results using cross-validation, and iv) results comparable or better than the ones published so far.

Our study has also some limitations that should be mentioned. The results are obtained from a single (although collected from multiple sites) cohort and should be also validated in other cohorts. A longer clinical follow-up time would be needed to see if the classification results of S-MCI/P-MCI experiment changed when more of the MCI subjects converted to AD. Furthermore, the ADNI study does not provide postmortem pathological confirmation of the clinical status. With this limitation, individual subjects might be wrongly categorized. Although a rigorous validation process was used, optimally we need to establish standardized cut-offs that would be well generalizable to other cohorts outside ADNI. That is, however, beyond the possibilities of this study and will require vast standardization and validation procedures. Also, the CTH pipeline had problems especially with severely atrophied brains or MRI scans with poor image quality. A more robust pipeline would be desirable in order to guarantee a more reliable feature extraction.

Supporting Information

Appendix S1 The Alzheimer's Disease Neuroimaging Initiative. (DOCX)

Appendix S2 ROI-wise features for CTH and TBM. (DOCX)

Acknowledgments

Data used in the preparation of this article were obtained from the ADNI database (www.loni.ucla.edu/ADNI). As such, the investigators within the ADNI contributed to the design and implementation of ADNI and/or provided data but did not participate in analysis or writing of this report. ADNI investigators include (complete listing available at http://adni.loni.ucla.edu/wp-content/uploads/how_to_apply/ADNI_Authorship_List.pdf).

Author Contributions

Conceived and designed the experiments: RW VJ JK DR HS JL. Performed the experiments: RW VJ JK EN DPZ. Analyzed the data: RW VJ JK. Contributed reagents/materials/analysis tools: RW JK DR JL. Wrote the paper: RW VJ.

References

1. Brookmeyer R, Johnson E, Ziegler-Graham K, Arrighi HM (2007) Forecasting the global burden of Alzheimer's disease. Alzheimer's and Dementia 3: 186–191.
2. Cummings J, Doody R, Clark C (2007) Disease-modifying therapies for alzheimer disease: challenges to early intervention. Neurology 69: 1622–1634.
3. Petersen R (2001) Practice parameter: early detection of dementia: mild cognitive impairment (an evidence-based review). Neurology 56: 1133.
4. Gauthier S, Reisberg B, Zaudig M, Petersen R, Ritchie K, et al. (2006) Mild cognitive impairment. Lancet 367: 1262–1270.
5. Braak H, Braak E (1991) Neuropathological stageing of Alzheimer-related changes. Acta Neuropathologica 82: 239–259.
6. Wenk G (2003) Neuropathologic changes in alzheimer's disease. Journal of Clinical Psychiatry 64 Suppl 9.
7. Hampel H, Brger K, Teipel SJ, Bokde AL, Zetterberg H, et al. (2008) Core candidate neurochemical and imaging biomarkers of alzheimer's disease. Alzheimer's and Dementia 4: 38–48.
8. Hyman BT, Marzloff K, Arriagada PV (1993) The lack of accumulation of senile plaques or amyloid burden in Alzheimer's disease suggests a dynamic balance between amyloid deposition and resolution. J Neuropathol Exp Neurol 52: 594–600.
9. Gmez-Isla T, Hollister R, West H, Mui S, Growdon J, et al. (1997) Neuronal loss correlates with but exceeds neurofibrillary tangles in alzheimer's disease. Ann Neurol 41: 17–24.
10. Ingelsson M, Fukumoto H, Newell KL, Growdon JH, Hedley-Whyte ET, et al. (2004) Early abeta accumulation and progressive synaptic loss, gliosis, and tangle formation in ad brain. Neurology 62: 925–31.
11. Jack C, Jr., Knopman D, Jagust W, Shaw L, Aisen P, et al. (2010) Hypothetical model of dynamic biomarkers of the alzheimer's pathological cascade. Lancet Neurology 27: 685–691.
12. Hampel H, Frank R, Broich K, Teipel S, Katz J, abd Hardy RG, et al. (2010) Biomarkers for alzheimer's disease: academic, industry and regulatory perspectives. NatRevDrug Discov 9: 560–574.
13. Fan Y, Resnick SM, Wu X, Davatzikos C (2008) Structural and functional biomarkers of prodromal alzheimer's disease: A high-dimensional pattern classification study. NeuroImage 41: 277–285.
14. Hinrichs C, Singh V, Xu G, Johnson S (2009) Mkl for robust multi-modality ad classification. In: MICCAI (II) Springer, volume 5762 of Lecture Notes in Computer Science. pp 786–794.
15. Davatzikos C, Bhatt P, Shaw LM, Batmanghelich KN, Trojanowski JQ (2010) Prediction of MCI to AD conversion, via MRI, CSF biomarkers, and pattern classification. Neurobiology of Aging In Press, Corrected Proof: -.
16. Eckerstrom C, Andreasson U, Olsson E, Rolstad S, Blennow K, et al. (2010) Combination of hippocampal volume and cerebrospinal uid biomarkers improves predictive value in mild cognitive impairment. Dement Geriatr Cogn Disord 29: 294–300.
17. Kohannim O, Hua X, Hibar DP, Lee S, Chou YY, et al. (2010) Boosting power for clinical trials using classifiers based on multiple biomarkers. Neurobiology of Aging 31: 1429–1442.
18. Landau S, Harvey D, Madison C, Reiman E, Foster N, et al. (2010) Comparing predictors of conversion and decline in mild cognitive impairment. Neurology 75: 230–8.
19. Walhovd KB, Fjell AM, Brewer J, McEvoy LK, Fennema-Notestine C, et al. (2010) Combining MR Imaging, Positron-Emission Tomography, and CSF Biomarkers in the Diagnosis and Prognosis of Alzheimer Disease. American Journal of Neuroradiology 31: 347–354+.
20. Wolz R, Aljabar P, Hajnal JV, Lotjonen J, Rueckert D (2011) Manifold learning combining imaging with non-imaging information. In: IEEE International Symposium on Biomedical Imaging. pp 960–963.
21. Chupin M, Hammers A, Liu R, Colliot O, Burdett J, et al. (2009) Automatic segmentation of the hippocampus and the amygdala driven by hybrid constraints: Method and validation. NeuroImage 46: 749–761.
22. Devanand DP, Pradhaban G, Liu X, Khandji A, De Santi S, et al. (2007) Hippocampal and entorhinal atrophy in mild cognitive impairment - Prediction of Alzheimer disease. Neurology 68: 828–836+.
23. Gerardin E, Chetelat G, Chupin M, Cuingnet R, Desgranges B, et al. (2009) Multidimensional classification of hippocampal shape features discriminates Alzheimer's disease and mild cognitive impairment from normal aging. NeuroImage 47: 1476–1486.
24. Liu Y, Paajanen T, Zhang Y, Westman E, Wahlund LO, et al. (2009) Combination analysis of neuropsychological tests and structural MRI measures in differentiating AD, MCI and control groups–The AddNeuroMed study. Neurobiology of Aging In Press, Corrected Proof: -.
25. Liu Y, Paajanen T, Zhang Y, Westman E, Wahlund LO, et al. (2010) Analysis of regional MRI volumes and thicknesses as predictors of conversion from mild cognitive impairment to Alzheimer's disease. Neurobiology of Aging 31: 1375–1385.
26. McEvoy L, Fennema-Notestine C, JC R, Hagler D, Holland D, et al. (2009) Alzheimer disease: quantitative structural neuroimaging for detection and prediction of clinical and structural changes in mild cognitive impairment. Radiology 251: 1950–205.
27. Querbes O, Aubry F, Pariente J, Lotterie JA, Dmonet JF, et al. (2009) Early diagnosis of alzheimer's disease using cortical thickness: impact of cognitive reserve. Brain 132: 2036–2047.
28. Mueller SG, Weiner MW, Thal IJ, Petersen RC, Jack C, et al. (2005) The Alzheimer's Disease Neuroimaging Initiative. Neuroimaging Clinics of North America 15: 869–877.
29. Cuingnet R, Gerardin E, Tessieras J, Auzias G, Lehricy S, et al. (2010) Automatic classification of patients with Alzheimer's disease from structural MRI: A comparison of ten methods using the ADNI database. NeuroImage In Press, Corrected Proof: -.
30. Petersen RC, Aisen PS, Beckett LA, Donohue MC, Gamst AC, et al. (2010) Alzheimer's Disease Neuroimaging Initiative (ADNI): clinical characterization. Neurology 74: 201–209.
31. Folstein MF, Folstein SE, McHugh PR (1975) Mini-mental state: A practical method for grading the cognitive state of patients for the clinician. Journal of Psychiatric Research 12(3): 189–198.
32. Morris J (1993) The Clinical Dementia Rating (CDR): current version and scoring rules. Neurology 43: 2412–2414.
33. McKhann G, Drachman D, Folstein M, Katzman R, Price D, et al. (1984) Clinical diagnosis of alzheimer's disease: report of the nincds-adrda work group under the auspices of department of health and human services task force on alzheimer's disease. Neurology 34: 939–944.
34. Jack CR, Jr., Bernstein MA, Fox NC, Thompson P, Alexander G, et al. (2008) The Alzheimer's disease neuroimaging initiative (ADNI): MRI methods. Journal of Magnetic Resonance Imaging 27: 685–691.
35. Lotjonen JM, Wolz R, Koikkalainen JR, Thurfjell L, Waldemar G, et al. (2010) Fast and robust multi-atlas segmentation of brain magnetic resonance images. NeuroImage 49: 2352–2365.
36. Lotjonen J, Wolz R, Koikkalainen J, Julkunen V, Thurfjell L, et al. (2011) Fast and robust extraction of hippocampus from mr images for diagnostics of alzheimer's disease. NeuroImage 56: 185–196.
37. Van Leemput K, Maes F, Vandermeulen D, Suetens P (1999) Automated model-based tissue classification of MR images of the brain. IEEE Transactions on Medical Imaging 18: 897–908.
38. Lerch J, Evans A (2005) Cortical thickness analysis examined through power analysis and a population simulation. NeuroImage 24: 163–173.
39. Mazziotta J, Toga A, Evans A, Fox P, Lancaster J, et al. (2001) A probabilistic atlas and reference system for the human brain: International Consortium for Brain Mapping (ICBM). Philos Trans R Soc Lond B Biol Sci 356: 1293–1322.
40. Sled JG, Zijdenbos AP, Evans AC (1998) A nonparametric method for automatic correction of intensity nonuniformity in MRI data. IEEE Transactions on Medical Imaging 17: 87–97.
41. Smith SM (2002) Fast robust automated brain extraction. Hum Brain Mapp 17: 143–155.
42. Zijdenbos AP, Forghani R, Evans AC (1998) Automatic quantification of MS lesions in 3D MRI brain data sets: Validation of INSECT. In: III WMW, Colchester ACF, Delp SL, eds. MICCAI Springer, volume 1496 of Lecture Notes in Computer Science. pp 439–448.
43. Tohka J, Zijdenbos A, Evans A (2004) Fast and robust parameter estimation for statistical partial volume models in brain mri. NeuroImage 23: 84–97.
44. Kim JS, Singh V, Lee JK, Lerch J, Ad-Dab'bagh Y, et al. (2005) Automated 3-d extraction and evaluation of the inner and outer cortical surfaces using a laplacian map and partial volume effect classification. NeuroImage 27: 210–221.
45. Chung M, Taylor J (2004) Diffusion smoothing on brain surface via finite element method. In: ISBI IEEE. pp 432–435.

46. Brun CC, Lepor N, Pennec X, Lee AD, Barysheva M, et al. (2009) Mapping the regional inuence of genetics on brain structure variability – a tensor-based morphometry study. NeuroImage 48: 37–49.

47. Koikkalainen J, Lotjonen J, Thurfjell L, Rueckert D, Waldemar G, et al. (2011) Multi-template tensor-based morphometry: Application to analysis of alzheimer's disease. NeuroImage 56: 1134–1144.

48. Belkin M, Niyogi P (2003) Laplacian eigenmaps for dimensionality reduction and data representation. Neural Computation 15: 1373–1396.

49. Rueckert D, Sonoda LI, Hayes C, Hill DLG, Leach MO, et al. (1999) Nonrigid registration using free-form deformations: Application to breast MR images. IEEE Transactions on Medical Imaging 18: 712–721.

50. Wolz R, Heckemann RA, Aljabar P, Hajnal JV, Hammers A, et al. (2010) Measurement of hippocampal atrophy using 4D graph-cut segmentation: Application to ADNI. NeuroImage 52: 1009–1018.

51. Draper NR, Smith H (1998) Applied Regression Analysis (Wiley Series in Probability and Statistics). Wiley.

52. Krzanowski WJ (1988) Principles of Multivariate Analysis: A User's Perspective Oxford University Press.

53. Cortes C, Vapnik V (1995) Support-vector networks. Machine Learning 20: 273–297.

54. Vemuri P, Gunter JL, Senjem ML, Whitwell JL, Kantarci K, et al. (2008) Alzheimer's disease diagnosis in individual subjects using structural mr images: Validation studies. NeuroImage 39: 1186–1197.

55. Westman E, Simmons A, Zhang Y, Muehlboeck JS, Tunnard C, et al. (2011) Multivariate analysis of mri data for alzheimer's disease, mild cognitive impairment and healthy controls. NeuroImage 54: 1178–1187.

Inflammatory Proteins in Plasma Are Associated with Severity of Alzheimer's Disease

Rufina Leung[1], Petroula Proitsi[2], Andrew Simmons[1,2], Katie Lunnon[2], Andreas Güntert[2], Deborah Kronenberg[1], Megan Pritchard[1], Magda Tsolaki[3], Patrizia Mecocci[4], Iwona Kloszewska[5], Bruno Vellas[6], Hilkka Soininen[7], Lars-Olaf Wahlund[8], Simon Lovestone[1,2]*

1 King's College London and National Institute for Health Research (NIHR), Biomedical Research Centres at South London and Maudsley NHS Foundation Trust and Guy's and St. Thomas' NHS Foundation Trust, London, United Kingdom, 2 King's College London, Institute of Psychiatry, London, United Kingdom, 3 3rd Department of Neurology, "G.Papanicolaou" Hospital, Aristotle University of Thessaloniki, Thessaloniki, Greece, 4 Institute of Gerontology and Geriatrics, University of Perugia, Perugia, Italy, 5 Department of Old Age Psychiatry and Psychotic Disorders, Medical University of Lodz, Lodz, Poland, 6 UMR INSERM 1027, Gerontopole, CHU Toulouse, University of Toulouse, Toulouse, France, 7 University of Eastern Finland and University Hospital of Kuopio, Kuopio, Finland, 8 Department of Neurobiology, Care Sciences and Society, Section of Clinical Geriatrics, Karolinska Institutet, Karolinska University Hospital, Huddinge, Stockholm, Sweden

Abstract

Markers of Alzheimer's disease (AD) are being widely sought with a number of studies suggesting blood measures of inflammatory proteins as putative biomarkers. Here we report findings from a panel of 27 cytokines and related proteins in over 350 subjects with AD, subjects with Mild Cognitive Impairment (MCI) and elderly normal controls where we also have measures of longitudinal change in cognition and baseline neuroimaging measures of atrophy. In this study, we identify five inflammatory proteins associated with evidence of atrophy on MR imaging data particularly in whole brain, ventricular and entorhinal cortex measures. In addition, we observed six analytes that showed significant change (over a period of one year) in people with fast cognitive decline compared to those with intermediate and slow decline. One of these (IL-10) was also associated with brain atrophy in AD. In conclusion, IL-10 was associated with both clinical and imaging evidence of severity of disease and might therefore have potential to act as biomarker of disease progression.

Citation: Leung R, Proitsi P, Simmons A, Lunnon K, Güntert A, et al. (2013) Inflammatory Proteins in Plasma Are Associated with Severity of Alzheimer's Disease. PLoS ONE 8(6): e64971. doi:10.1371/journal.pone.0064971

Editor: Ashley I. Bush, University of Melbourne, Australia

Received July 6, 2012; **Accepted** April 23, 2013; **Published** June 10, 2013

Funding: This research was conducted at, and part funded by, the National Institute for Health Research (NIHR) Mental Health Biomedical Research Centre and Dementia Biomedical Research Unit at South London and Maudsley NHS Foundation Trust and King's College London. The views expressed are those of the author(s) and not necessarily those of the NHS, the NIHR or the Department of Health. AddNeuroMed/InnoMed, (Innovative Medicines in Europe) is an Integrated Project funded by the European Union of the Sixth Framework program priority FP6-2004-LIFESCIHEALTH-5, Life Sciences, Genomics and Biotechnology for Health. The funders had no role in study design, data collection and analysis, decision to publish, or preparation of the manuscript.

Competing Interests: The authors have declared that no competing interests exist.

* E-mail: simon.lovestone@kcl.ac.uk

Introduction

Alzheimer's disease (AD) is the most common form of dementia and although progress is being made, the development of disease modification therapies is currently hampered by the lack of biomarkers. There are many potential types of biomarkers, but in particular, indicators of disease progression or disease state would find utility in clinical trials, to stratify participants or to measure change over time [1–3]. Currently, cerebrospinal fluid (CSF) levels of tau and amyloid beta (Aβ) are the most reliable and widely used protein markers for AD. However, there are practical drawbacks of using CSF as a sample medium, in addition to poor correlation between the protein levels and disease severity [4]. Several other potential protein-based AD markers have been explored during the past decade [5], these markers have most often been analyzed in relation to diagnosis rather than disease severity or clinical progression. In addition to fluid biomarkers, neuroimaging measures, including hippocampal volume analysis, have become widely used in clinical trials [6].

Considerable evidence suggests that inflammation plays a role in the pathogenesis of AD [7,8], and the central nervous system (CNS) contains many components of the immune system that are synthesized by astrocytes, microglia and neurons [9,10]. Fibrillar Aβ deposition is associated with the activation of microglia [10–12], itself a relatively early event in the pathogenesis of AD, and the formation of the Aβ/microglia complex in early stages of AD has been reported to precede extensive tau-related neurofibrillary pathology [4,13,14]. The immune response of the brain is orchestrated by microglial cells which, on activation, become phagocytes and secrete a wide range of inflammatory mediators, including cytokines and chemokines, growth factors, complement molecules and adhesion molecules [15]. An increased interest in the complex network of cytokines has identified a growing number of inflammatory cytokines involved in CNS disorders, with a number of studies identifying cytokine proteins able to predict clinical AD diagnosis with high accuracy [16–18].

Our aim was to investigate the inflammatory response to AD in plasma samples and to examine whether plasma cytokines are associated with disease severity or disease progression. We analyzed a panel of 27 cytokines in a cohort of 351 patients with neuroimaging data available using multiplex immunoassays. The cytokine profiles of AD, MCI and control cases were compared,

133

evaluated with respect to neuroimaging measures and to rate of decline.

Materials and Methods

AddNeuroMed Cohort

Samples used came from the AddNeuroMed study, a cross-European cohort for biomarker discovery. In this cohort, AD cases were assessed with a range of measures, including clinical at three monthly intervals in the first year and annually thereafter. MCI and control groups were assessed annually. The disease duration of AD cases were provided by their doctors, families and carers. All subjects were white Europeans recruited from the UK, France, Italy, Finland, Poland and Greece. The full standardized assessment in these studies includes demographic and medical information, cognitive assessment including the Mini-Mental State Examination (MMSE), Alzheimer's Disease Assessment Scale – cognitive (ADAS-Cog), Consortium to Establish a Registry for Alzheimer's Disease (CERAD) battery, and scales to assess function, behaviour and global levels of severity including the Clinical Dementia Rating (CDR) scale. The cohort has been previously described in [19,20].

Informed consent was obtained from all subjects according to the Declaration of Helsinki (1991) and protocols and procedures were approved by the relevant Institutional Review Board at each collection site. All participants, or their carers where capacity was compromised and gave written consent or assent according to the laws of the relevant country. The capacity for consent was assessed by a clinician with experience in capacity assessment in the context of dementia. Exclusion criteria included other neurological or psychiatric disease, significant unstable systemic illness or organ failure and alcohol or substance misuse.

Subjects

A total of 351 subjects were selected for this analysis grouped into 3 categories: 112 control subjects, 122 MCI patients and 117 AD patients. A second time point for biochemical analysis in relation to the progression of disease was used for this study (one year follow-up from baseline) with sample available from 104 of

the 117 AD patients. The age range for subjects in the AD, MCI and control group were comparable (Table 1).

MMSE and CDR assessments were available from all 351 subjects, and ADAS-cog assessment was performed in AD patients only.

Sample Preparation and Data Acquisition

All participants were required to fast for two hours before blood sample collection; only water or fluids containing no milk or sugar were allowed during the fasting period. Plasma samples were collected using EDTA coated tubes and centrifuged at 3000 rpm for 8 minutes at 4°C before being aliquoted and then frozen at −80°C.

Plasma samples were analyzed with a multiplex suspension array system using Bioplex Luminex 200 instrument (Bio-Rad Laboratories, Hercules, CA). The panel (Bio-Plex Human cytokine 27–Plex) consisted of the following 27 cyto- and chemokines: Interleukin (IL)-1β, IL-1ra, IL-2, IL-4, IL-5, IL-6, IL-7, IL-8, IL-9, IL-10, IL-12 (p70), IL-13,IL-15, IL-17, Eotaxin, fibroblast growth factor (FGF) basic, granulocyte-colony stimulating factor (G-CSF), granulocyte-macrophage colony stimulation factor (GM-CSF), Interferon-gamma (IFN-γ), interferon-inducible protein-10 (IP-10), monocyte chemotactic protein-1 (MCP-1), macrophage inflammatory protein (MIP)-1α, MIP-1β, platelet-derived growth factor (PDGF)-BB, Rantes, tumor necrosis factor (TNF)-α and vascular endothelial growth factor (VEGF). The overall detection concentration range according to the standard curves was 6,560–82,807 pg/ml.

The samples were prepared according to the manufacturer's instructions. All samples and standards were run in duplicate and were measured as pg/ml. The system running protocol was set according to manufacturer's guidelines: the protocol was set to a high RP1 (fluorescent channel) target value for CAL2 calibration and the acceptable recovery percent range to a range of 80–120%. The protocol was set to 100 beads per region and the sample volume adjusted to 50 µl. After the plate reading, the results files were generated using Bio-Plex Manager software 4 (Bio-Rad Laboratories, Hercules, CA).

Table 1. Demographic and clinical parameters of AD patients, MCI and control subjects.

Variables	Controls	MCI	AD
	Baseline N = 112	Baseline N = 122	Baseline N = 117 Year follow up N = 104
Gender (F/M)	60/52	60/62	78/39 (baseline) 70/34 (year follow up)
Age, (mean, SD)*	72.3, (6.72)	73.9, (5.63)	76.2, (6.09)
MMSE score (median), (±SD) ¥	29, (1.21)	27, (1.64)	20.37, (4.68)
CDR score (median), (±SD) ≠	0, (0.09)	0.5, (0.05)	1, (0.48)
ADAS-cog score (mean), (±SD)	N/A	N/A	24.9, (9.97)
APOε4 allele presence	N = 32	N = 35	N = 59 (baseline) N = 50 (year follow up)

Key:
MMSE = Mini-Mental State Examination; CDR = Clinical Dementia Rating; ADAS-cog = Alzheimer's Disease Assessment Scale-cognitive subscale; Year follow up = a year follow up from baseline.
SD = Standard Deviation.
*ANOVA F = 5.72 (2,329); p = 0.0036. Scheffe test: Control v MCI p = 0.480; Control v AD p = 0.004; MCI v AD p = 0.107.
¥ANOVA F = 221.29 (2,328); p<0.001. Scheffe test: Control v MCI p<0.001; Control v AD p<0.001; MCI v AD p<0.001.
≠ANOVA F = 1320.56 (2,214) p<0.0001. Scheffe test: Control v MCI p<0.001; Control v AD p<0.001; MCI v AD p<0.001.

doi:10.1371/journal.pone.0064971.t001

Table 2. Concentrations of analytes in plasma and association of analytes with diagnostic groups.

Cytokine	ACTUAL PROTEIN LEVELS (pg/ml)						LINEAR REGRESSION (ON TRANSFORMED DATA)									LINEAR REGRESSION (ON TRANSFORMED DATA) Whole Cohort comparison
	CTL		MCI		AD		Controls-MCI			Controls-AD			MCI-AD			
	Mean	Range	Mean	Range	Mean	Range	Beta (R²)	95% CI	p	Beta (R²)	95% CI	p	Beta (R²)	95% CI	p	p
IL-1b	3	0.99–11.97	3	1.05–9.26	3.3	1.21–13.03	0.09 (-0.004)	-0.094, 0.235	0.278	0.1 (-0.005)	-1.755, 0.74	0.257	0.01 (0)	-0.235, 0.094	0.921	0.757
IL-1ra	137.9	4.61–602.53	155.7	5.90–1698.63	221.7	6.13–5843.77	0.02 (0)	-0.285, 0.26	0.894	0.01 (-1.00E-04)	-1.403, 2.882	0.925	0 (0)	-0.26, 0.285	0.972	0.451
IL-2	10.5	0.51–50.59	11	1.52–37.93	14	0.91–192.57	0.16 (-0.004)	-0.225, 0.458	0.91	0.09 (-0.001)	-1.272, 3.084	0.51	-0.07 (-8.00E-04)	-0.458, 0.225	0.701	0.157
IL-4	3	0.65–10.52	3	0.44–12.10	2.9	0.49–8.77	-0.03 (-0.001)	-0.155, 0.175	0.679	-0.06 (-0.002)	-1.23, 1.409	0.457	-0.03 (-1.00E-04)	-0.175, 0.155	0.717	0.469
IL-5	4.8	1.04–24.57	4.4	0.83–15.17	4.3	1.00–15.82	-0.03 (-2.00E-04)	-0.3, 0.135	0.791	-0.05 (-0.001)	-1.93, 1.1	0.651	-0.02 (-1.00E-04)	-0.135, 0.3	0.841	0.988
IL-6	8.9	1.26–36.58	9.6	1.10–28.53	11.2	0.93–74.8	0.01 (0)	-0.181, 0.278	0.917	0.11 (-0.003)	-1.65, 2.512	0.342	0.1 (-0.003)	-0.278, 0.181	0.382	0.472
IL-7	6.2	1.21–23.92	6.5	1.29–28.05	6.9	0.98–37.49	0.03 (-2.00E-04)	-0.137, 0.315	0.798	0.06 (-0.001)	-3.376, 0.699	0.584	0.03 (-3.00E-04)	-0.315, 0.137	0.759	0.499
IL-8	8.3	1.92–31.34	7.5	0.93–32.89	7.5	0.63–20.14	-0.12 (-0.005)	-0.295, 0.116	0.203	-0.09 (-0.003)	-2.181, 0.936	0.362	0.03 (-3.00E-04)	-0.116, 0.295	0.732	0.642
IL-9	63.2	6.41–808.92	56.3	6.49–301.58	65.6	6.41–518.76	0.07 (-0.001)	-0.179, 0.345	0.601	0.09 (-0.002)	-1.764, 2.394	0.509	0.02 (-1.00E-04)	-0.345, 0.179	0.872	0.244
IL-10	10	0.97–37.62	9.8	0.97–42.18	12.1	1.02–49.73	0.06 (-0.001)	-0.252, 0.511	0.764	0.3 (-0.017)	-2.14, 2.977	0.134	0.25 (-0.011)	-0.511, 0.252	0.215	0.185
IL-12	15.4	1.99–128.57	14.3	1.31–41.65	18	1.24–238.34	-0.14 (-0.004)	-0.282, 0.246	0.272	-0.01 (0)	-4.147, -0.021	0.933	0.13 (-0.004)	-0.246, 0.281	0.299	0.857
IL-13	8.9	1.74–58.41	9.9	1.37–42.13	9	1.79–41.02	0.06 (-0.001)	-0.065, 0.353	0.559	-0.05 (-0.001)	-2.472, 0.749	0.62	-0.11 (-0.004)	-0.353, 0.065	0.265	0.475
IL-15	6.7	0.88–59.14	6.4	1.18–39.57	5.9	0.79–26.69	0.2 (-0.009)	-0.127, 0.59	0.276	0.13 (-0.004)	-3.568, 1.172	0.485	-0.07 (-0.001)	-0.591, 0.127	0.688	0.065
IL-17	65.1	2.90–253.32	63.9	3.09–258.41	59.5	3.42–237.07	-0.07 (-0.001)	-0.325, 0.309	0.641	-0.17 (-0.005)	-1.054, 4.228	0.265	-0.1 (-0.001)	-0.309, 0.325	0.498	0.287

Table 2. Cont.

Cytokine	ACTUAL PROTEIN LEVELS (pg/ml)						LINEAR REGRESSION (ON TRANSFORMED DATA)									LINEAR REGRESSION (ON TRANSFORMED DATA) Whole Cohort comparison
	CTL		MCI		AD		Controls-MCI			Controls-AD			MCI-AD			
	Mean	Range	Mean	Range	Mean	Range	Beta (R²)	95% CI	p	Beta (R²)	95% CI	p	Beta (R²)	95% CI	p	p
Eotaxin	79.5	11.15–291.31	77.9	7.14–318.78	87	15.25–384.91	−0.04 / −0.001	−0.294 / 0.131	0.706	0.16 / −0.009	−1.794 / 1.381	0.128	0.2 / −0.015	−0.131 / 0.294	0.045*	0.297
FGF	30.7	1.63–89.61	44.1	2.91–133.40	53.6	3.44–147.52	0.33 / −0.018	0.112 / 0.893	0.086	0.49 / −0.038	−0.732 / 3.641	0.012*	0.16 / −0.004	−0.893 / 0.112	0.387	0.298
G-CSF	73.6	16.30–143.37	74.4	11.35–187.81	73.7	19.31–168.61	−0.05 / −0.002	−0.137 / 0.147	0.501	−0.09 / −0.005	−1.554 / 0.656	0.231	−0.04 / −0.001	−0.147 / 0.137	0.576	0.404
GM-CSF	47.1	0.60–164.87	47.1	2.36–181.64	47.7	2.13–291.80	0.06 / −0.001	−0.23 / 0.312	0.674	−0.04 / 2.00E-04	−5.12 / −0.208	0.797	−0.1 / 0.002	−0.312 / 0.23	0.485	0.598
IFN-γ	170.6	13.18–1032.07	171	3.42–791.40	202.2	7.94–1884.05	0.03 / −1.00E-04	−0.214 / 0.308	0.825	−0.06 / −0.001	−3.04 / 1.8	0.654	−0.09 / −0.001	−0.308 / 0.214	0.488	0.625
IP-10	605.9	131.77–2105.65	567	25.40–2448.32	629.6	149.75–2203.04	−0.05 / −0.001	−0.208 / 0.1	0.535	−0.01 / 0	−1.81 / 0.991	0.924	0.04 / −0.001	−0.099 / 0.208	0.593	0.56
MCP-1	32.5	5.70–99.22	30.3	6.78–65.61	34.8	2.51–105.24	0.06 / −0.002	−0.166 / 0.187	0.465	0.14 / −0.009	−2.555 / 0.601	0.109	0.08 / −0.003	−0.187 / 0.166	0.365	0.72
PDGF	3205.2	49.84–15964.6	3353.5	33.96–15300.08	2989.9	54.40–10105.77	−0.17 / −0.004	−0.324 / 0.262	0.238	−0.25 / −0.008	−3.79 / 0.8	0.099	0.08 / −8.00E-04	−0.262 / 0.324	0.593	0.445
TNF-α	81.6	5.44–374.58	74.4	8.31–276.37	79.5	6.65–328.53	−0.12 / −0.004	−0.304 / 0.151	0.279	−0.09 / −0.002	−0.811 / 2.63	0.399	0.02 / −2.00E-04	−0.151 / 0.304	0.828	0.535

Whole cohort presents results for the whole cohort and was based on all three diagnostic groups. Plasma protein levels were generally higher in AD than in MCI or control with a few exceptions. The relationship between cytokines and diagnostic groups was assessed by linear regression adjusting for age, gender, collection site and presence of the *APOε4* allele. In this analysis beta values are for the log transformed data. Key: Beta = regression coefficient (slope) on log- transformed data; 95% CI = 95% confidence interval; $R^2 = R^2$ value (coefficient of determination) after adjusting for covariates; *$p < 0.05$.

doi:10.1371/journal.pone.0064971.t002

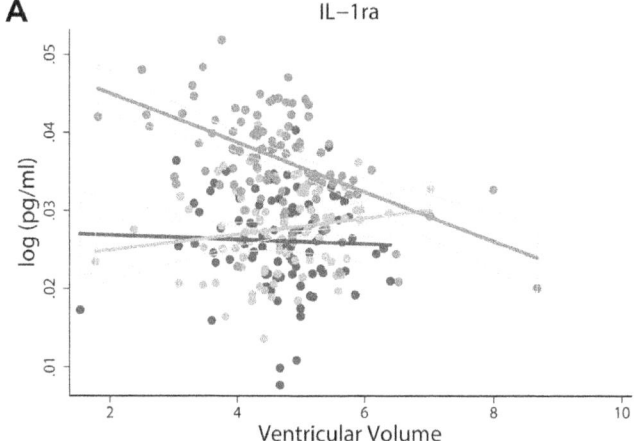

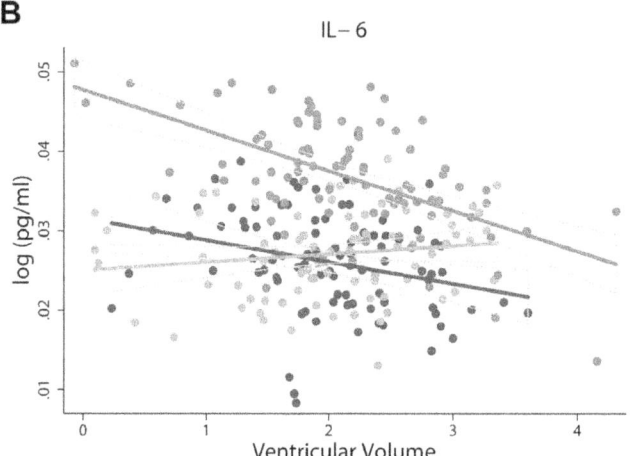

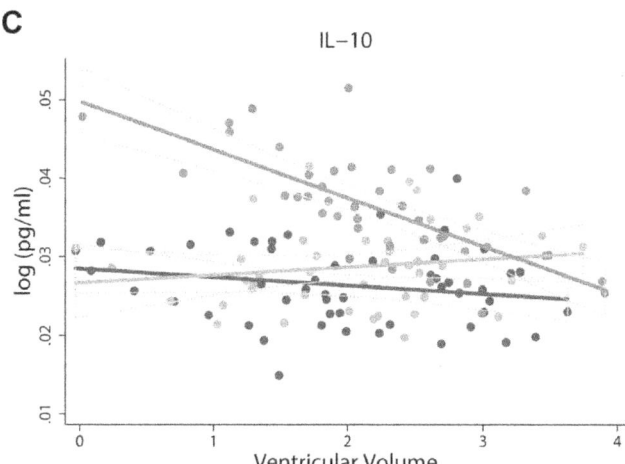

Figure 1. Association between inflammatory proteins levels measured in plasma versus ventricular volume. Scatter diagram with regression lines show the relationship between proteins levels of IL-1ra (N = 86) (figure 1A), IL-6 (N = 83) (figure 1B) and IL-10 (N = 38)(figure 1C)and ventricular volume in the three separate diagnostic groups. Keys: Blue line and dots denote control samples; orange line and dots denote MCI samples; red line and dots denote AD samples; brown dotted line denotes 95% CI.
doi:10.1371/journal.pone.0064971.g001

Data Processing

Some samples duplicate measures were excluded from further analysis. The exclusion was based on the observed concentration of standards that were not within the 80–120% recovery range. In order to screen outliers, we generated a correlation matrix with each subject for all 27 analytes. This gave us an output in the form of a correlation coefficient. Patients falling below an $r = 0.8$ correlation coefficient threshold were omitted from subsequent analysis.

Neuroimaging

Six different 1.5 T MR systems (4 General Electric, 1 Siemens and 1 Picker) were used for data collection. Data acquisition was designed to be compatible with the Alzheimer Disease Neuroimaging Initiative (ADNI) [21]. The imaging protocol was based on using a high resolution saggital 3D T1-weighted MPRAGE volume (voxel size $1.1 \times 1.1 \times 1.2$ mm3) and axial proton density/T2-weighted fast spin echo images. Full brain and skull coverage was required and a detailed quality control was carried out on all MR images according to the AddNeuroMed quality control procedure [20,22]. All MR images were examined by an on-site radiologist for exclusion of any subjects with non-AD related pathologies.

MR Image Analysis

The highly automated Freesurfer pipeline (version 4.5.0) was used to produce both regional cortical thickness measures and regional volume measures. Cortical reconstruction and volumetric segmentation included removal of non-brain tissue, automated Talairach transformation, intensity correction and segmentation of the subcortical white matter and deep gray matter volumetric structures (including hippocampus, amygdala, caudate, putamen, ventricles). Identification of the grey matter/white matter boundary was followed by surface inflation and registration to a spherical atlas which utilises individual cortical folding patterns to match cortical geometry across subjects and parcellation of the cerebral cortex into units based on gyral and sulcal structure. All regional volume measures from each subject were normalised by the subjects' intracranial volume. Cortical thickness measures were used in their raw form.

Statistical Analysis

Statistical analysis was performed in SPSS Version 15 (SPSS Inc., Chicago, USA) and STATA 10 (Stata Corporation, College Station, TX, USA). The Kolmogorov-Smirnov test was used to check for normal distribution of continuous outcomes. In cases of non-normality the natural log of each variable was used. Linear regression was used in order to compare baseline (visit 1) plasma cytokine levels between AD, MCI and control samples adjusting for age, gender, centre and presence of the *APOε4* allele. Multiple linear regression was also employed to investigate the relationship of neuroimaging measures, such as whole brain volume, hippocampus and entorhinal cortex with baseline cytokine levels adjusting for age, gender, centre, presence of the *APOε4* allele and disease status. Linear regression was also performed to assess the relationship of covariates (Table S1). To test whether the association of cytokines with disease status differed between subjects in different *APOε4* allele or gender strata, or whether the association of neuroimaging measures with cytokines was different amongst disease groups, we tested for interactions followed by likelihood ratio tests to compare a model assuming no interaction to a model with an interaction term. If significant interactions were identified, data was presented separately for different strata. Differences were considered significant if $p \leq 0.05$ (two-tailed).

Table 3. Summary statistics for the multiple linear regression model assessing the relationship between inflammatory proteins and ventricular volume.

Cytokine	Whole cohort			Controls			MCI			AD		
(pg/ml)	Beta (R²)	95% CI	p value	Beta (R²)	95% CI	p value	Beta (R²)	95% CI	p value	Beta (R²)	95% CI	p value
IL-1ra	2.00E-04	−0.002	0.77	0.003	−0.001	0.099	0.002	−0.001	0.223	−0.003	−0.006	0.021*
	(−0.008)	0.001		−0.032	0.006		−0.013	0.004		−0.068	−8.80E-04	
IL-6	−0.001	−0.003	0.151	−2.10E-03	−0.004	0.904	0.001	−0.002	0.405	−0.005	−0.009	0.018*
	−0.033	0.001		−0.028	0.004		−0.016	0.004		−0.101	−0.001	
IL-10	−0.001	−0.003	0.431	−1.10E-03	−0.004	0.809	0.001	−0.004	0.805	−0.006	−0.011	0.028*
	(−0.031)	0.001		−0.031	0.003		−0.059	0.005		−0.103	−0.001	

Whole cohort presents results for the whole cohort and was based on all three diagnostic groups with 255 subjects for IL-1ra, 250 subjects for IL-6 and 128 subjects for IL-10.

The relationship between cytokines and MRI measures was assessed by multiple linear regression adjusting for age, gender, collection site and presence of the *APOε4* allele.

Key: Beta = regression coefficient (slope) on log- transformed data; 95% CI = 95% confidence interval; $R^2 = R^2$ value (coefficient of determination) after adjusting for covariates;

*$p < 0.05$; Ventricular Volume is normalized to Intracranial Volume (ICV).

doi:10.1371/journal.pone.0064971.t003

Association of Cognitive Decline with Changes in Cytokine Levels

AD patients were grouped into slow, intermediate and fast declining patients, based on cognitive decline slope per year in MMSE, ADAS-cog and CDR. Cognitive decline slopes were calculated using mixed linear effects models. The average baseline cognitive outcome and the average change in the cognitive outcome over follow-up time was calculated for all subjects per day as a group (fixed effects) and subject-specific intercept and slope terms which reflected deviation from the group average (mixed linear effects) were calculated. The calculation included adjustment for age at baseline, disease duration at baseline, gender, cholinesterase inhibitors, antidepressants, antipsychotics, ethnicity/centre, education, being a widow/er, being in a nursing home and presence of *APOε4* allele. Covariates significant at the p<0.10 level were included in a final model for each cognitive model. The annual cognitive decline was obtained by multiplying the slope of cognitive decline measured using days with the average number of days per year (365.25). An annual MMSE, ADAS-cog and CDR score decline of 4 or more was considered as fast decline, whereas an annual MMSE score decline of 2–4 was considered as intermediate decline; and a score below 2 was considered as slow decline.

To assess change in cytokines as a function of cognition in people with dementia, we measured cytokines in subjects with AD at year 1 as well as at baseline. Mixed linear mixed effects models as described above were used to investigate the relationship between changes in cytokine levels measured at baseline and at year 1 and cognitive decline in AD. As before, the calculation included adjustment for age at baseline, disease at baseline, gender, cholinesterease inhibitors, antidepressants, antipsychotics, ethnicity/centre, education, being a widow/er, being in a nursing home and presence of *APOε4* allele. Only age at baseline, disease duration, centre and gender were robustly associated with cytokine changes between the two visits and were therefore used as covariates. A significant interaction between the cognitive decline group and the variable indicating when cytokine levels were

Table 4. Summary statistics for the multiple linear regression model assessing the relationship between inflammatory proteins and brain MRI measures (whole brain volume and left entorhinal cortex).

Cytokine	Whole cohort			Controls			MCI			AD		
(pg/ml)	Beta (R²)	95% CI	p value	Beta (R²)	95% CI	p value	Beta (R²)	95% CI	p value	Beta (R²)	95% CI	p value
WTNF-α	−0.005	−0.011	0.081	−0.001	−0.01	0.754	−0.003	−0.014	0.613	−0.01	−0.02	0.047*
	−0.008	0.001		(−0.042)	0.007		−0.002	0.008		−0.04	7.80E-03	
EIL-13	−1.00E-04	−6.50E-05	0.171	4.10E-04	−4.80E-05	0.389	−1.20E-05	9.10E-05	0.351	−9.00E-05	−1.80E-04	0.048*
	−0.005	3.30E-05		−0.008	1.30E-04		−0.01	6.70E-05		−0.048	4.70E-06	

The relationship between cytokines and MRI measures was assessed by multiple linear regression adjusting for age, gender, collection site and presence of the *APOε4* allele. Whole cohort result shows the model overall data and was based on all three diagnostic groups with 239 subjects for TNF-α and 241 subjects for IL-13.

Key: Beta = regression coefficient (slope) on transformed data; CI = 95% confidence interval; $R^2 = R^2$ value (coefficient of determination) after adjusting for covariates; *$p < 0.05$; W indicates whole brain volume (normalized to Intracranial Volume (ICV)); E indicates left entorhinal cortex(normalized to Intracranial Volume (ICV)).

doi:10.1371/journal.pone.0064971.t004

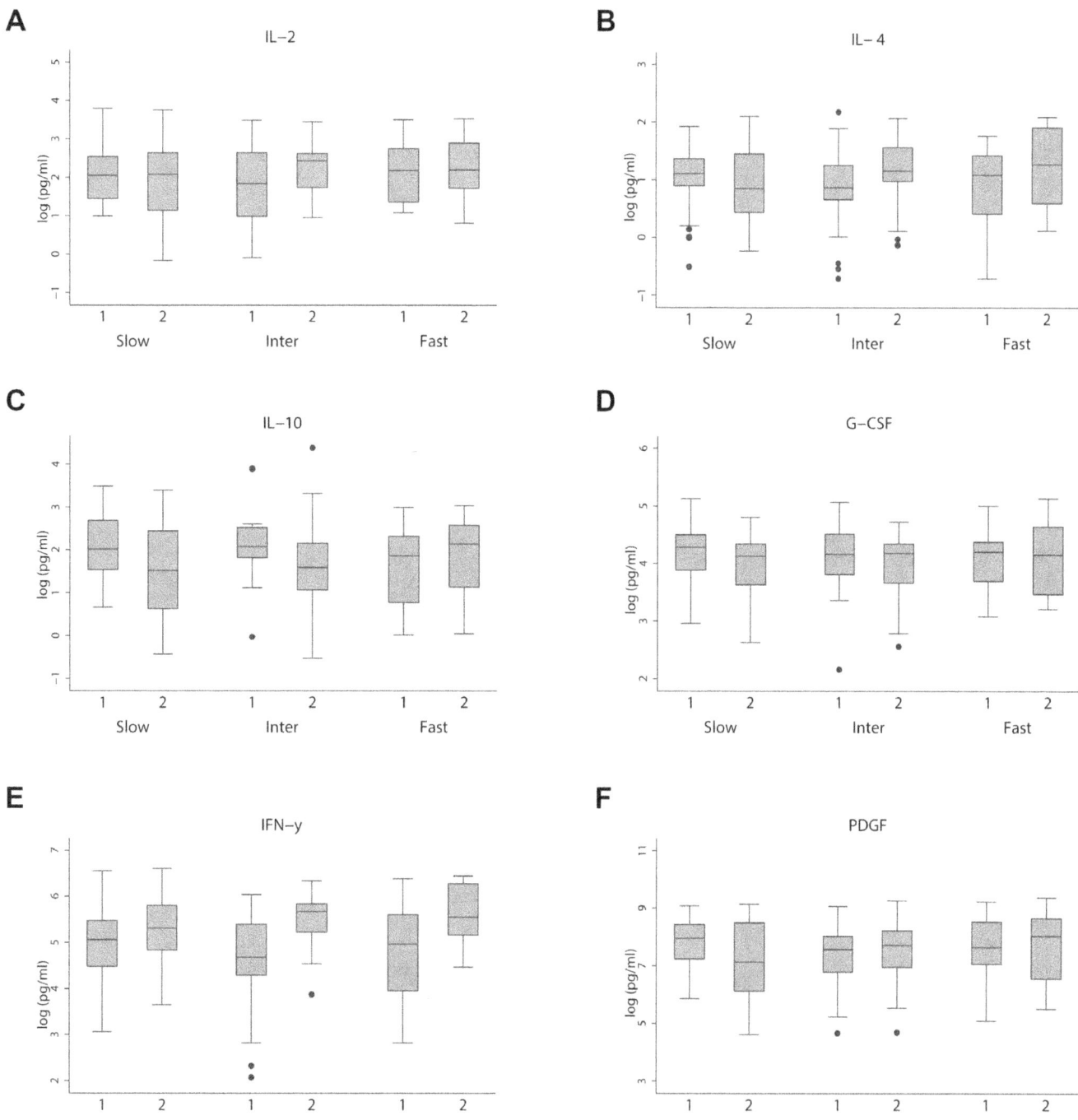

Figure 2. Inflammatory proteins levels at Visit 1 (baseline) and Visit 2 (one year follow up from baseline) for the three ADAS-cog cognitive decline groups. Linear mixed effects models indicated significant yearly changes in the log-transformed IL-2 (figure 2A), IL-4 (figure 2B), IL-10 (figure 2C), G-CSF (figure 2D), IFN-γ (figure 2E), and PDGF (figure 2F) (pg/ml) inflammatory protein levels between the three cognitive decline groups, after adjusting for covariates. Slow indicates slow decliner. Inter indicates intermediate decliner. Fast indicates fast decliner Key: 1– Visit 1(Baseline); 2– Visit 2 (one year follow up from baseline).
doi:10.1371/journal.pone.0064971.g002

measured (visit) would indicate differences between the change in cytokine levels and decline group.

Results

Exclusions

Four analytes, namely MIP-1α, MIP-1β, RANTES (CCL5) and VEGF, were excluded from analysis as more than 50% of the subjects fell below an $r = 0.8$ correlation coefficient threshold suggesting technical failure. In average, across the remaining 23 analytes a range of 1–14 subjects were excluded from analysis, as they fell below the $r = 0.8$ correlation coefficient threshold in the correlation matrix. The number of excluded subjects was similar across the three diagnostic groups. The demographics and clinical parameters of AD patients, MCI and control subjects are presented in Table 1 and Table 2 shows the results of the 23 detectable proteins in plasma.

Table 5. Summary of longitudinal changes in inflammatory protein levels between cognitive decline groups as measured by ADAS-cog.

Cytokine	ACTUAL PROTEIN LEVELS (pg/ml)						LINER MIXED EFFECTS MODEL					
	Slow		Intermediate		Fast		Slow versus Inter¥			Slow versus fast¥		
	ADAS-Cog Decliners		ADAS-Cog Decliners		ADAS-Cog Decliners							
	Mean (SD) [N]		Mean (SD) [N]		Mean (SD) [N]							
(pg/ml)	Baseline	Year 1	Baseline	Year 1	Baseline	Year 1	Beta	95% CI	p value	Beta	95% CI	p value
IL-2	11.73	9.64	9.82	11.86	19.45	12.17		0.105	0.021*		−0.511	
	−13.27	−8.09	−9.09	−7.74	−39.57	−69.55	0.691	1.278		0.086	0.683	0.777
	[77]	[83]	[44]	[47]	[23]	[22]						
IL-4	3.11	3.02	2.78	3.54	2.9	3.96		0.074	0.016*		0.051	
	(1.31)	−1.77	−1.73	−1.72	−1.55	−2.33	0.392	0.713		0.387	0.729	0.024*
	[114]	[91]	[64]	[51]	[31]	[24]						
IL-10	11.38	7.69	14.17	10.45	7.59	9.39		−0.654	0.724		0.037	
	−8.81	−7.65	−145.96	−18.1	−6.24	−6.2	0.143	0.941		0.825	1.627	0.040*
	[54]	[67]	[29]	[37]	[16]	[18]						
G-CSF	76.76	58.79	72.21	61.81	65.4	68.8		−0.036	0.084		0.006	
	−38.1	−28.14	−36.83	−26.26	−30.52	−39.29	0.265	0.564		0.316	0.627	0.046*
	[112]	[89]	[63]	[49]	[31]	[24]						
IFN-γ	209.12	241.6	178.56	270.62	235.41	319.21		0.086	0.018*		−0.069	
	−241.6	−146.43	−222.89	−132.29	(334.19)	−194.33	0.493	0.908		0.347	0.774	0.102
	[116]	[91]	[65]	[51]	[33]	[24]						
PDGF	3135.09	2536.81	2422.27	2823.29	3149.69	3628.44		0.065	0.031*		−0.057	
	−1969.2	−2481.5	−2079.5	−2769.5	−2760.1	−3668.9	0.731	1.399		0.62	1.3	0.073
	[111]	[85]	[64]	[46]	[32]	[23]						

The relationship between change in cytokine levels over one year and AD cognitive decline group was assessed by mixed effect model adjusting for age, gender, APOε4 allele, collection site and disease duration. Slow indicates slow decliner. Inter indicates intermediate decliner. Fast indicates fast decliner. Key: Beta = regression coefficient (slope) on transformed data; 95%CI = 95% confidence interval;N = number of sample; ¥ - coefficients represent the difference in the slopes for the given cytokine between cognitive decline groups across the two time points (i.e. interaction between time and the rate of decline groups).
*p<0.05.
doi:10.1371/journal.pone.0064971.t005

Peripheral Cytokine Levels Reflect the Inflammatory Process Associated with AD

First, in order to evaluate whether a different extent of inflammation in AD, MCI and controls is reflected in the respective plasma samples, baseline cytokine levels between the different groups were compared. The level of FGF (p = 0.012) was significantly different between AD and control subjects; whereas Eotaxin (p = 0.045) was significantly different between AD and MCI (Table 2).

Inflammatory Proteins in Plasma are Associated with Pathological Severity

Regression analyses were performed to examine the relationship between inflammatory cytokines and disease severity as measured by atrophy on MRI measures. We first assessed the relationship between multiple cytokine levels and neuroimaging measures of whole brain volume, entorhinal cortex, entorhinal cortex thickness, hippocampal volume and ventricular volume in the whole data set sample. There was no significant relationship between multiple cytokine levels and neuroimaging measures except for TNF-α (p = 0.045), which correlated with left hippocampal volume (data not shown).

We then examined whether association of cytokines with MRI measurements differed between the different diagnostic groups. Significant interactions in the ventricular volume, whole brain volume and entorhinal cortex were observed between four cytokines [IL-6 (p = 0.005), IL-10 (p = 0.025), IL-13 (p = 0.028) and IL-1ra (p = 0.002)] and clinical status (Table S2). Although we did not observe any associations between these cytokines and neuroimaging measurements for the whole cohort, significant associations between these five cytokines and neuroimaging measures were observed in AD patients (Table 3, 4). Specifically, three measures (IL-1ra, IL-6 and IL-10) significantly associated with ventricular volume in AD (Figure 1).

Inflammatory Proteins in Plasma are Associated with Rate of Cognitive Decline in AD

We then compared changes in the inflammatory signals between baseline and year 1 visit in participants with different rates of clinical decline, as measured with the MMSE, ADAS-cog and CDR. Overall, we observed significant changes in levels of a number of cytokines between patients with a fast or intermediate cognitive decline and patients with slow cognitive decline, particularly measured with the ADAS-cog. Specifically, we found a significant increase in the levels of IL-4 (p = 0.024), IL-10 (p = 0.040) and G-CSF (p = 0.046) in AD patients with a fast cognitive decline compared to slow cognitive decline in ADAS-cog over one year (Figure 2 and Table 5). AD patients with intermediate cognitive decline showed significantly higher levels of IL-2 (p = 0.021), IL-4 (p = 0.016), IFN-γ (p = 0.018) and PDGF (p = 0.031) compared to those with slow cognitive decline over one year (Figure 2 and Table 5).

Discussion

We investigated plasma levels of cytokines in AD, MCI and control samples to determine whether inflammatory proteins are associated with disease progression or disease severity as assessed by memory test scores or by neuroimaging data respectively. AD is characterized by early memory loss with the first sites of pathological change measurable in life being the hippocampus and the entorhinal cortex [23,24]. Around 80–90% of AD subjects show atrophy in both sites compared to only 5–10% of control subjects [25,26]. Our study identified a number of analytes that correlate with brain imaging data - five analytes being associated with ventricular, whole brain and entorhinal measures of atrophy. In addition, six analytes were associated with rates of decline in cognitive scores.

A number of studies have reported that Aβ deposition can activate microglia and induce the production of IL-1, IL-6, TNF-α and MCP-1 in the AD brain [7,27–32]. Aβ-induced secretion of IFN-γ and IL-1β has also been observed [33]. Grammas & Ovase demonstrated a high level of production of IL-1β, IL-6, MCP-1 and TNF-α in AD brain microvessels compared to control [34]. McGeer & Zhao showed IL-10 can be produced by microglia [35,36]. Moreover, Soares's study observed an elevation of IL-13 level was associated with APOε4 allele; a known risk factor for AD [37]. The elevation of these inflammatory proteins in AD brain microvessels suggest that these proteins may play a role in neuronal damage.

Our study finds IL-6, TNF-α and three addition analytes (IL-1ra, IL-10 and IL-13) in plasma significantly inversely correlated with ventricular volume, whole brain volume or entorhinal cortex in AD. Furthermore, we observe an increase in the level of IL-10 between visit 1 and visit 2 in ADAS-cog fast decliners compare to slow decliners and, an increase level of IFN-γ was observed between visit 1 and visit 2 in ADAS-cog intermediate decliners compared to slow decliners.

Plasma cytokines are known to communicate with the brain [38] and circulating levels of peripheral cytokines have been shown to correlate and reflect central cytokine levels in the brain [38,39]. An important but unanswered question regards the source of the inflammatory signature in the periphery in AD – is it independent of, or secondary to, the inflammatory reaction in the brain? There are various routes whereby an inflammatory activity may communicate between brain and the periphery [38]. One of these routes involves diffusion of cytokines between blood and brain in regions with an impaired blood brain barrier (BBB). In some cases cytokines can be actively transported across the BBB [39]. Another route involves cytokine activation of the endothelium signalling to macrophages in brain [40]. Understanding which, if any, of these mechanisms underlies the peripheral signature of inflammatory proteins in AD is an important topic for further investigation.

The current, and these earlier studies show clearly that there is an inflammatory change in the brain in AD and an inflammatory signal in the periphery although how these are connected and the exact nature of the inflammatory profile are both far from certain. However, although it is clear from this and from other studies that there is a peripheral inflammatory response in AD, the question remains as to whether it might be sufficiently robust to act as a biomarker. One study reported 18 plasma proteins that could predict clinical AD diagnosis with high accuracy [16]. A bioinformatics-based follow-up showed that reducing the panel to 5 proteins improved accuracy to 96% [41]. However, this finding has not been widely replicated. Individual cytokines found by Ray et al, are also reported in other studies – for example, IL-6 and TNF-α associated with cognitive decline [42]. Our multiplex assay included only two (TNF-α and G-CSF) of the 18 proteins described by Ray et al but we do find G-CSF to be associated with decline on cognitive tests and to be significantly different between slow and fast declining AD patients. G-CSF plays an interesting role in the inflammatory response in AD as it suppresses the production or activity of proinflammatory cytokines [43]. A recent investigation showed decreased plasma G-CSF levels in early AD [44], in contrast to the finding of Ray et al. In the current study we find a significantly higher expression of G-CSF in fast compared to slow declining AD patients.

One limitation of the current study is that no adjustment of multiple testing was performed. However, given the modest effect sizes observed, correction for multiple testing whilst performing such large number of analyses beyond looking for associations between cytokines and AD status (such as rate of decline, measures of disease in the brain and change in time of the analytes in relation to disease progression) would require study sizes considerably larger than ours, and probably any existing biomarker cohort currently existing. We draw from this two conclusions - first that the data presented here should be considered preliminary and requiring replication and secondly, that as in genomic studies, cohorts for biomarker analyses will have to increase substantially. Nonetheless, this study is one of the first to examine large numbers of functionally related analytes in a large cohort of subjects in relation to multiple measures of disease severity. Moreover, our finding of an association between an inflammatory profile including some markers previously associated with AD, suggests that the inflammatory change in the periphery does occur in AD and is worthy of further investigation and in particular that IL-2, IL-4, IL-10, G-CSF and IFN-γ may be markers not of disease per se but of disease severity.

Supporting Information

Table S1 Association between inflammatory proteins and covariates. Most proteins showed a significant association with the covariate of collection site, with the exception of IL9, IL10, IL15 and IP-10. The number of proteins showing a significant association with the covariates of age and gender was very low (N = 2 and N = 1 respectively). *p<0.05; **p<0.001. (DOC)

Table S2 Summary of significant interaction between inflammatory proteins and diagnostic groups. The relationship between cytokines and MRI measures in diagnostic groups was assessed by linear regression adjusting for age, gender, collection site and presence of the APOε4 allelle. *p<0.05; **p<0.01. (DOC)

Acknowledgments

We would like to thank the Medical Research Council (MRC) for their intellectual input and their support for this paper.

Author Contributions

Conceived and designed the experiments: SL. Performed the experiments: RL. Analyzed the data: RL PP. Contributed reagents/materials/analysis tools: RL PP AS KL AG DK MP MT PM IK BV HS LOW SL. Wrote the paper: RL.

References

1. Bailey P (2007) Biological markers in Alzheimer's disease. Can J Neurol Sci 34 Suppl 1: S72–76.
2. Lovestone S, Guntert A, Hye A, Lynham S, Thambisetty M, et al. (2007) Proteomics of Alzheimer's disease: understanding mechanisms and seeking biomarkers. Expert Rev Proteomics 4: 227–238.
3. Noelker C, Hampel H, Dodel R (2011) Blood-based protein biomarkers for diagnosis and classification of neurodegenerative diseases: current progress and clinical potential. Mol Diagn Ther 15: 83–102.
4. Arends YM, Duyckaerts C, Rozemuller JM, Eikelenboom P, Hauw JJ (2000) Microglia, amyloid and dementia in alzheimer disease. A correlative study. Neurobiol Aging 21: 39–47.
5. Shaw LM, Korecka M, Clark CM, Lee VM, Trojanowski JQ (2007) Biomarkers of neurodegeneration for diagnosis and monitoring therapeutics. Nat Rev Drug Discov 6: 295–303.
6. Petrella JR, Coleman RE, Doraiswamy PM (2003) Neuroimaging and early diagnosis of Alzheimer disease: a look to the future. Radiology 226: 315–336.
7. Akiyama H, Barger S, Barnum S, Bradt B, Bauer J, et al. ((2000)) Inflammation and Alzheimer's disease. Neurobiol Aging 21: 383–421.
8. Mrak RE, Griffin WS (2005) Potential inflammatory biomarkers in Alzheimer's disease. J Alzheimers Dis 8: 369–375.
9. Bonifati DM, Kishore U (2007) Role of complement in neurodegeneration and neuroinflammation. Mol Immunol 44: 999–1010.
10. Eikelenboom P, Veerhuis R (1996) The role of complement and activated microglia in the pathogenesis of Alzheimer's disease. Neurobiol Aging 17: 673–680.
11. Itagaki S, McGeer PL, Akiyama H, Zhu S, Selkoe D (1989) Relationship of microglia and astrocytes to amyloid deposits of Alzheimer disease. J Neuroimmunol 24: 173–182.
12. Rozemuller JM, Eikelenboom P, Stam FC, Beyreuther K, Masters CL (1989) A4 protein in Alzheimer's disease: primary and secondary cellular events in extracellular amyloid deposition. J Neuropathol Exp Neurol 48: 674–691.
13. Eikelenboom P, Veerhuis R, Scheper W, Rozemuller AJ, van Gool WA, et al. (2006) The significance of neuroinflammation in understanding Alzheimer's disease. J Neural Transm 113: 1685–1695.
14. Vehmas AK, Kawas CH, Stewart WF, Troncoso JC (2003) Immune reactive cells in senile plaques and cognitive decline in Alzheimer's disease. Neurobiol Aging 24: 321–331.
15. Griffin WS (2006) Inflammation and neurodegenerative diseases. Am J Clin Nutr 83: 470S–474S.
16. Ray S, Britschgi M, Herbert C, Takeda-Uchimura Y, Boxer A, et al. (2007) Classification and prediction of clinical Alzheimer's diagnosis based on plasma signaling proteins. Nat Med 13: 1359–1362.
17. Soares HD, Potter WZ, Pickering E, Kuhn M, Immermann FW, et al. (2012) Plasma biomarkers associated with the apolipoprotein E genotype and Alzheimer disease. Arch Neurol 69: 1310–1317.
18. Doecke JD, Laws SM, Faux NG, Wilson W, Burnham SC, et al. (2012) Blood-based protein biomarkers for diagnosis of Alzheimer disease. Arch Neurol 69: 1318–1325.
19. Lovestone S, Francis P, Kloszewska I, Mecocci P, Simmons A, et al. (2009) AddNeuroMed–the European collaboration for the discovery of novel biomarkers for Alzheimer's disease. Ann N Y Acad Sci 1180: 36–46.
20. Simmons A, Westman E, Muehlboeck S, Mecocci P, Vellas B, et al. (2009) MRI measures of Alzheimer's disease and the AddNeuroMed study. Ann N Y Acad Sci 1180: 47–55.
21. Jack CR Jr, Bernstein MA, Fox NC, Thompson P, Alexander G, et al. (2008) The Alzheimer's Disease Neuroimaging Initiative (ADNI): MRI methods. J Magn Reson Imaging 27: 685–691.
22. Simmons A, Westman E, Muehlboeck S, Mecocci P, Vellas B, et al. (2011) The AddNeuroMed framework for multi-centre MRI assessment of Alzheimer's disease: experience from the first 24 months. Int J Geriatr Psychiatry 26: 75–82.
23. Jobst KA, Smith AD, Szatmari M, Molyneux A, Esiri ME, et al. (1992) Detection in life of confirmed Alzheimer's disease using a simple measurement of medial temporal lobe atrophy by computed tomography. Lancet 340: 1179–1183.
24. O'Brien JT (2007) Role of imaging techniques in the diagnosis of dementia. Br J Radiol 80 Spec No 2: S71–77.
25. Barber R, Gholkar A, Scheltens P, Ballard C, McKeith IG, et al. (1999) Medial temporal lobe atrophy on MRI in dementia with Lewy bodies. Neurology 52: 1153–1158.
26. Scheltens P, Fox N, Barkhof F, De Carli C (2002) Structural magnetic resonance imaging in the practical assessment of dementia: beyond exclusion. Lancet Neurol 1: 13–21.
27. Frei K, Malipiero UV, Leist TP, Zinkernagel RM, Schwab ME, et al. (1989) On the cellular source and function of interleukin 6 produced in the central nervous system in viral diseases. Eur J Immunol 19: 689–694.
28. Haga S, Ikeda K, Sato M, Ishii T (1993) Synthetic Alzheimer amyloid beta/A4 peptides enhance production of complement C3 component by cultured microglial cells. Brain Res 601: 88–94.
29. Ishizuka K, Kimura T, Igata-yi R, Katsuragi S, Takamatsu J, et al. (1997) Identification of monocyte chemoattractant protein-1 in senile plaques and reactive microglia of Alzheimer's disease. Psychiatry Clin Neurosci 51: 135–138.
30. McGeer PL, Schulzer M, McGeer EG (1996) Arthritis and anti-inflammatory agents as possible protective factors for Alzheimer's disease: a review of 17 epidemiologic studies. Neurology 47: 425–432.
31. Meda L, Baron P, Prat E, Scarpini E, Scarlato G, et al. (1999) Proinflammatory profile of cytokine production by human monocytes and murine microglia stimulated with beta-amyloid[25–35]. J Neuroimmunol 93: 45–52.
32. Yao J, Keri JE, Taffs RE, Colton CA (1992) Characterization of interleukin-1 production by microglia in culture. Brain Res 591: 88–93.
33. Suo Z, Tan J, Placzek A, Crawford F, Fang C, et al. (1998) Alzheimer's beta-amyloid peptides induce inflammatory cascade in human vascular cells: the roles of cytokines and CD40. Brain Res 807: 110–117.
34. Grammas P, Ovase R (2001) Inflammatory factors are elevated in brain microvessels in Alzheimer's disease. Neurobiol Aging 22: 837–842.
35. McGeer PL, McGeer EG (1995) The inflammatory response system of brain: implications for therapy of Alzheimer and other neurodegenerative diseases. Brain Res Brain Res Rev 21: 195–218.
36. Zhao B, Schwartz JP (1998) Involvement of cytokines in normal CNS development and neurological diseases: recent progress and perspectives. J Neurosci Res 52: 7–16.
37. Soares HD, Potter WZ, Pickering E, Kuhn M, Immermann FW, et al. (2012) Plasma Biomarkers Associated With the Apolipoprotein E Genotype and Alzheimer Disease. Arch Neurol: 1–8.
38. Konsman JP, Parnet P, Dantzer R (2002) Cytokine-induced sickness behaviour: mechanisms and implications. Trends Neurosci 25: 154–159.
39. Banks WA, Farr SA, Morley JE (2002) Entry of blood-borne cytokines into the central nervous system: effects on cognitive processes. Neuroimmunomodulation 10: 319–327.
40. Perry VH (2004) The influence of systemic inflammation on inflammation in the brain: implications for chronic neurodegenerative disease. Brain Behav Immun 18: 407–413.
41. Gomez Ravetti M, Moscato P (2008) Identification of a 5-protein biomarker molecular signature for predicting Alzheimer's disease. PLoS One 3: e3111.
42. Dziedzic T (2006) Systemic inflammatory markers and risk of dementia. Am J Alzheimers Dis Other Demen 21: 258–262.
43. Sanchez-Ramos J, Song S, Sava V, Catlow B, Lin X, et al. (2009) Granulocyte colony stimulating factor decreases brain amyloid burden and reverses cognitive impairment in Alzheimer's mice. Neuroscience 163: 55–72.
44. Laske C, Stellos K, Stransky E, Leyhe T, Gawaz M (2009) Decreased plasma levels of granulocyte-colony stimulating factor (G-CSF) in patients with early Alzheimer's disease. J Alzheimers Dis 17: 115–123.

Other titles by iMedPub:

- **_Social Medicine in the 21st Century_** by Samuel Barrack.
- **_World Health Report 2012: No Health Without Research_** by Samuel Barrack.
- **_Quality design in Anatomical Pathology_** by Anil Malleshi Betigeri.
- **_Escherichia coli infections_** by Viroj Wiwanitkit.
- **_Atlas of Biomarkers for Alzheimer's disease_** by Manuel Menendez.

www.ingramcontent.com/pod-product-compliance
Lightning Source LLC
Chambersburg PA
CBHW081103290526
45795CB00006B/1983